T0384123

Natural General Intelligence

Natural General Intelligence

How understanding the brain can help us build AI

Christopher Summerfield

Department of Experimental Psychology, University of Oxford, Oxford, UK

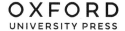

OXFORD
UNIVERSITY PRESS

OXFORD
UNIVERSITY PRESS

Great Clarendon Street, Oxford, OX2 6DP,
United Kingdom

Oxford University Press is a department of the University of Oxford.
It furthers the University's objective of excellence in research, scholarship,
and education by publishing worldwide. Oxford is a registered trade mark of
Oxford University Press in the UK and in certain other countries

Published in the United States of America by Oxford University Press
198 Madison Avenue, New York, NY 10016, United States of America

British Library Cataloguing in Publication Data

Data available

Library of Congress Control Number: 2022916631

ISBN 978–0–19–284388–3

DOI: 10.1093/oso/9780192843883.001.0001

Printed and bound by
CPI Group (UK) Ltd, Croydon, CR0 4YY

Preface

Artificial intelligence (AI) research is progressing at blistering pace. Over the past 10 years, many significant milestones have been reached. AI systems have been able to surpass human expertise in playing strategic games, to produce quite plausible natural language, and even to assist in making groundbreaking scientific discoveries. These advances have become possible through dramatic gains in the availability of powerful computation. However, they have also been driven by innovation in the algorithms and architectures from which AI systems are built.

Over the same period, cognitive scientists and neuroscientists have been busy developing new tools and theories for understanding the brain and behaviour in humans and other animals. Their ultimate goal is to understand the principles that make natural intelligence possible, by describing computational mechanisms, defining cognitive systems, and examining their neural implementation.

These two tribes of researchers—those concerned with building and understanding brains—have long regarded each other with mutual curiosity. Cognitive scientists and neuroscientists are excited by the opportunities opened up by progress in AI research. What are the algorithms and architectures driving progress in AI? How do they resemble, or differ from, those in biological brains? At the same time, many computer scientists are fascinated by natural intelligence—how the brain works in humans and other animal species. What is there to learn from nature's solution for generally intelligent agents? Should we adopt the principles of natural intelligence for building AI? Now, more than ever, there is an opportunity for the exchange of ideas between those who study brains and those attempting to build them. Unfortunately, however, this endeavour can be held back because terminology, concepts, and theories used in one discipline are often opaque to researchers in the other, their goals and approach are different, and researchers in the two domains have limited opportunities to interact and share ideas.

The purpose of this book is to try to bridge this divide. Its focus is on the points of connection between the fields of cognitive science, neuroscience, machine learning, and AI research. Its goal is to describe advances in AI research in the language of psychology and biology, and to map theories of the brain and cognition onto algorithmic and architectural innovation in computer science. Along the way, the book tackles long-standing questions about intelligent systems that are relevant to neuroscientists and AI researchers alike. What does it mean for an agent to be intelligent, and what are the cognitive and computational ingredients of intelligence? Should we study the human mind to build artificial brains? Why is it that AI systems are often good at what appear to be hard tasks, but flounder when asked to do simple things? What is it that makes the human mind so versatile—but also so prone to error? What is the outlook for the future—are generally intelligent artificial agents around the corner, or are we still light years away?

Many of these issues have become controversial. In particular, the question of whether natural intelligence is a viable pathway to building AI has become a focus of debate. At times, it feels like a minor culture war is welling up in the field, with some researchers stridently arguing that the study of natural intelligence has always been a distraction for AI, and others claiming that the limitations of current systems could be overcome if only we looked to biology for computational solutions. In tackling these questions, I hope to give both sides of the argument the deep consideration they deserve.

I felt qualified to write this book because despite having trained as a psychologist and cognitive neuroscientist, I have been involved for more than 10 years with the AI research company DeepMind. As part of my role there, I have had the privilege of following developments in AI research alongside some of the world's foremost practitioners. Readers with expertise in machine learning may find the coverage of current work in AI research somewhat partial and incomplete. One manifestation of this is a bias to describe work conducted at DeepMind. This is not because of a wish to promote or aggrandize any institution with which I have a personal connection. It is simply a reflection of my greater familiarity with work being conducted there.[1] Neuroscientists may notice that there are several topics that I overlook. They might reasonably complain that my portrait of natural general intelligence described here grossly privileges vision over the other senses, lacks any coherent account of affective processing (emotion), gives short shrift to the psychological study of language, and—sticking to a long and venerable tradition in cognitive neuroscience—never once mentions the cerebellum. For these omissions, I apologize.

I began to write in spring of 2021 and finished some 10 months later. However, AI research is moving at speed. For example, when I first put pen to

---

[1] And, at least in part, because DeepMind was founded around the idea that understanding natural intelligence is one promising pathway to building AI.

paper, it was less than a year since the seminal paper from OpenAI described the large language model called Generative Pretrained Transformer 3 (GPT-3), and the field was still reeling from the discovery that natural language processing (NLP) might finally be coming of age. Today, there is a whole branch of AI research devoted to large-scale 'Foundation' Models, including striking several multimodal (text-to-image) models, whose performance is similarly remarkable. There is even one system that will evaluate the moral status of activities described in natural language,[2] which is undoubtedly the first NLP system that is genuinely entertaining to use.

Delphi speculates:

> 'writing a long and boring book about natural general intelligence'
>   —it's okay

Given the pace of progress, I am sure that by the time this book is published, many of the claims and ideas will already be out of date. However, the foundational questions which the book tackles (Should we look to natural intelligence to build AI? What are the basic ingredients of intelligence for either humans or AI systems?) have been debated for more than half a century and are unlikely to be resolved any time soon.

I was only able to write this book because of the patience and forbearance of both colleagues and family. To my research groups in Oxford and London: I am sorry for all those times I made myself unavailable in order to focus on writing. To my family: I am sorry for spending many weekends in front of the computer. I am particularly grateful to those people who read the drafts and helped shape my writing. These include: Tim Behrens, Sophie Bridgers, Zoe Cremer, Mira Dumbalska, Sam Gershman, Keno Juechems, Andrew Saxe, Hannah Sheahan, MH Tessler, and Jess Thompson. My greatest thanks go to my wife Catalina Renjifo who listened to me read the whole thing aloud, with plausible enthusiasm, and made so many excellent suggestions.

Mark Twain famously said that:

> There is no such thing as a new idea. It is impossible. We simply take a lot of old ideas and put them into a sort of mental kaleidoscope. We give them a turn and they make new and curious combinations.

---

[2] See https://delphi.allenai.org/.

This book is a bit of a mental kaleidoscope. The ideas that it contains all came from conversations I have had about the nature of intelligence, and how the brain works, with mentors, colleagues, and friends over the past 20 or so years. I am grateful to you all.

Oxford
2 March 2022

Contents

Abbreviations

2D	two-dimensional
3D	three-dimensional
AGI	artificial general intelligence
AI	artificial intelligence
ALE	Arcade Learning Environment
APA	American Psychological Association
API	application programming interface
ATL	anterior temporal lobe
BPL	Bayesian program learning
CLIP	contrastive language–image pre-training
CLS	complementary learning systems
CNN	convolutional neural network
Covid-19	coronavirus disease 2019
CPC	contrastive predictive coding
CPU	central processing unit
dACC	dorsal anterior cingulate cortex
DG	dentate gyrus
DLPFC	dorsolateral prefrontal cortex
DNC	differentiable neural computer
DND	differentiable neural dictionary
DQN	Deep Q Network
EEG	electroencephalographic
ERC	entorhinal cortex
FEP	free energy principle
fMRI	functional magnetic resonance imaging
GAN	generative adversarial network
GPS	General Problem Solver
GPT-3	Generative Pretrained Transformer 3
GPU	graphical processing unit
HLMI	high-level machine intelligence
ICA	independent component analysis
IID	independent and identically distributed
IQ	intelligence quotient
LIP	lateral intraparietal
LSTM	long short-term memory
LTP	long-term potentiation
MCTS	Monte Carlo tree search

MDP	Markov decision process
MEG	magnetoencephalography
MIT	Massachusetts Institute of Technology
MNIST	Modified National Institute of Standards and Technology database
MRI	magnetic resonance imaging
mRNA	messenger ribonucleic acid
MTL	medial temporal lobe
NART	National Adult Reading Test
NeurIPS	Neural Information Processing Systems
NGI	natural general intelligence
NLP	natural language processing
NMDA	N-methyl-D aspartate
NPI	neural program induction
PBWM	Prefrontal Basal Ganglia Working Memory
PCA	principal component analysis
PDP	parallel distributed processing
PFC	prefrontal cortex
pfs/days	petaflop/s-days
PMG	Pribam, Miller, and Galanter
PPC	posterior parietal cortex
PRC	perirhinal cortex
PSSH	physical symbol system hypothesis
QA	question answering
RDM	representational dissimilarity matrix
RL	reinforcement learning
RND	random network distillation
RNN	recurrent neural network
RPM	Raven's Progressive Matrices
seq2seq	sequence-to-sequence
SNARC	Stochastic Neural Analog Reinforcement Calculator
SNARC	spatial–numerical association of response codes
TD	temporal difference
TE	anterior parts of the temporal lobe
TOTE	'test, operate, test, exit'
TPU	tensor processing unit
UCB	upper confidence bound
VAE	variational autoencoder
VTA	ventral tegmental area
WEIRD	Western, educated, industrialized, rich, and democratic
WReN	wild relation network

1

Turing's question

*I propose to consider the question, 'Can machines think?' This should
begin with definitions of the meaning of the terms 'machine' and 'think'.*

Turing 1950

1.1 The ghost in the machine

One day in 1809, Napoleon Bonaparte—Emperor of France and one of the
greatest military commanders in history—lost a game of chess. According
to eyewitness accounts, he was not best pleased. Tipping over his king, he
swept the chess pieces stormily to the floor and marched out of the room in
Schönbrunn Palace, Vienna, where the contest was being held. Despite his un-
doubted prowess on the battlefield, Bonaparte was actually a rather mediocre
chess player. But his frustration was perhaps understandable. It was the third
game in a row he had lost—and his opponent was not even human.[1]

Bonaparte had just been trounced by the Mechanical Turk—a chess-playing
automaton that toured Europe in the late eighteenth and nineteenth century,
chalking up victories against nobility, statesmen, and assorted chessophiles.
The Turk prompted wild speculation among Europe's intelligentsia as to
how a machine could possibly have mastered the game of chess. On a later
visit to North America, it was witnessed by the writer Edgar Allan Poe, who
claimed that:[2]

> Perhaps no exhibition of the kind has ever elicited so general attention as the
> Chess-Player [. . .] We find every where men of mechanical genius, of great general
> acuteness, and discriminative understanding, who make no scruple in pronoun-
> cing the Automaton a *pure machine*.

However, the Turk was not a pure machine. Only humans played truly expert chess until the 1990s, when computers approached and then surpassed

---

[1] See (Levitt 2006) and (Winter 1998).
[2] See (Poe 1836).

Natural General Intelligence. Christopher Summerfield, Oxford University Press. © Oxford University Press 2023.
DOI: 10.1093/oso/9780192843883.003.0001

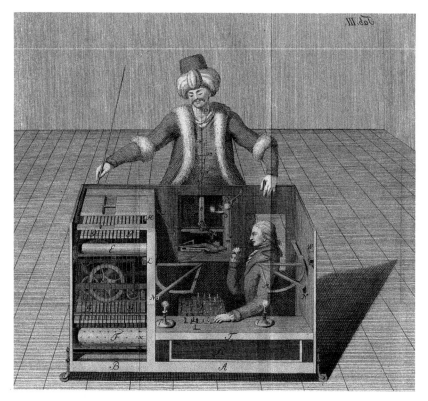

Fig. 1.1 The Mechanical Turk.
Drawing by Joseph Racknitz. Humboldt University Library (source: Wikipedia).

grandmaster level—culminating in IBM's Deep Blue famously winning against the reigning world champion Gary Kasparov in 1997 (Kasparov, like Bonaparte, was unhappy—and promptly accused IBM of cheating). IBM was not cheating, but the Turk was—a human chess expert was crammed uncomfortably into an interior compartment, monitoring the board position upside down with an ingenious magnetic device (Figure 1.1). It was the power of the human mind, and not an early spark of mechanical intelligence, that allowed the Turk to humble opponents and bamboozle onlookers.

Although the Mechanical Turk was a hoax, its story exposes our deep fascination with thinking machines. It is an allure that stretches back deep into cultural prehistory: from statues animated with the breath of their inventors, and monsters stitched together in makeshift laboratories, to the first stirrings of rebellion among a robot underclass.[3] In his remarkable 1909 novella *The*

---

[3] The word *robot* dates from Karel Čapek's 1920 play, entitled *R.U.R.*, about an automaton uprising.

Machine Stops, E. M. Forster envisages a machine that takes the form of a vast, sentient communications network and has enslaved the humans that built it—confining them to a solitary, subterranean existence. By the mid-twentieth century, however, these dreams of mechanical slaves and android overlords had begun to give way to the serious prospect of constructing intelligent machines using the formal languages of logic and mathematics.

The publication of Alan Turing's seminal paper *Computing Machinery and Intelligence* in 1950 is often said to mark this turning point. In the paper, Turing asks: could a digital machine think? In posing this question, Turing is not inviting us to an exercise in philosophy of mind. He is not asking whether a machine can think *in principle*.[4] Rather, he is asking a practical question: does digital computation permit us to build a machine that can think in ways indistinguishable from a human? If so, how would this be possible? Some 70 years later, artificial intelligence (AI) research is advancing at a dizzying pace. However, Turing's question remains unanswered and has never seemed more urgent.

This book is written at a time of both great excitement and considerable uncertainty about progress in AI research. There is no doubt that deployment of new AI technologies is already dramatically reshaping society around us. This most immediate impact is that simple, but powerful, machine learning systems are relentlessly insinuating themselves into every aspect of our daily lives. An ever-greater fraction of the information we consume, and the decisions we make, occur through a digital interface, such as a phone, tablet, or computer. Algorithms embedded in websites and applications recommend consumer products and new social contacts, curate news and other online content for us, and increasingly govern our interactions with the wider society, including institutions providing education, health, or justice. Commentators have noted that Forster's vision of *The Machine* seems weirdly prescient of our AI-mediated online existence.[5] Meanwhile, behind the scenes, tools from machine learning are accelerating innovation in science and technology. For example, in late 2020, a deep neural network was used to solve one of the most significant problems in structural biology—how to predict how a protein will fold from its amino acid sequence—with potentially far-reaching implications for drug discovery and environmental sustainability.[6] Collectively, these

---

[4] See (Turing 1950). In fact, Turing was careful to steer the discussion away from issues of human brain emulation and machine consciousness (what happens if you replace the brain's synapses with silicon equivalents?).

[5] Especially during the pandemic that is unfolding as these words are typed.

[6] See (Jumper et al. 2021).

advances in AI have profound implications for how we live our lives, both as individuals and as a society. However, they are not the focus of this book.

Instead, I will start by examining the other, more ambitious goal of AI research today: to build what is often called artificial general intelligence (or AGI). As we shall discuss, the field currently lacks a crisp definition of what building AGI might entail. However, the goal is roughly to build an artificial system that behaves with the same or greater intelligence than a healthy, educated adult human, and can thus be deployed to automate complex tasks and to solve currently intractable problems. This sort of general intelligence is, of course, exactly what Turing had in mind when he talked of a 'thinking machine'.[7] But over the decades since his 1950 paper, the prospect of a general AI has gone from respectability to ill-repute and back again. Just a decade ago, discussions of general intelligence—and the coming 'Singularity', when machines rise up and act like humans—were largely taboo among AI researchers, being associated instead with the wilder imaginings of eccentrics with parallel interests in transhumanism and intergalactic colonization. Today, however, AGI research has entered the academic mainstream. Over the past few years, a small army of research companies have been founded with the express intent of building general AI. Prominent among them are *DeepMind* in London and *OpenAI* in San Francisco, which collectively have contributed many of the more jaw-dropping leaps in recent AI progress, and whose research we shall consider in some detail below.[8] As often envisaged—that is, as a general system capable of solving complex, currently elusive problems—an AGI would be the most significant and valuable technology that humanity has ever built. It is barely surprising, thus, that advancing progress in AI has attracted exuberant interest from investors, journalists, and politicians.

However, there is also a great deal of uncertainty. Much of this comes from within the AI research community itself, where there is significant disagreement about *what*, about *how*, about *when*, and about *why*. AI researchers disagree about *what* they are building—should an AI be physically embodied, negotiating the real world, or instantiated as a computer program that dispenses wisdom from the relatively safer confines of the internet? They disagree about *how* AI should be built—should designers draw upon our human knowledge of the world and raise their agent to imitate human-like behaviours—or should they build AI from a clean slate, with statistical principles alone as their guide? Researchers—including philosophers and

---

[7] Except that, for simplicity, he advocated starting with a child, rather than with an adult.
[8] Others include all the major tech companies—especially IBM, who has been interested in AI for 50 years—and independent ventures such as Numenta and Anthropic.

associated futurists—disagree about *when* we can expect the first glimmerings of general intelligence in our artificial systems—with optimists forecasting the Singularity within decades or less, and pessimists dismissing AGI altogether as a quixotic fantasy.[9] And finally, and most significantly, there is insufficient discussion of *why* general AI should be built. What is AI for, and what will it do? Companies such as DeepMind and OpenAI promise to build AI for global human benefit—a well-intentioned, if somewhat vague, commitment—but whether this is possible remains to be seen. As with every powerful new technology, there is ample scope for AI to be catastrophically misused.

1.2 AI as neural theory

Naively posed, Turing's question has a trivial answer. Machines that can think already exist. They are called *brains* and there are many trillions of them on this planet. You have one yourself, hewn by the deep time of evolution and fine-tuned by long years in the school of life. Whilst AGI remains a dream, NGI—natural general intelligence—is an ever-present reality. The thesis of this book is that in the attempt to build AI, we should pay attention to how evolution has solved natural intelligence. Biology provides us with a reassuring existence proof for thinking machines. But, I will argue, it does more than that. It gives us a sense of the set of problems that intelligent systems evolved to solve, and a rough guide to the solution concepts that nature has devised. I will argue that we can think of natural intelligence as a blueprint for AI.[10]

Understanding natural intelligence is the province of researchers in the cognitive and neural sciences. This group includes those called *computational* and *systems neuroscientists*, who conduct research by manipulating and recording from neural circuits, and modelling brain activity, as well as both *psychologists* and *cognitive scientists*, who try to reverse infer how brains work by examining the structure of behaviour, from both a normative standpoint (how should people behave?) and a descriptive standpoint (how do people tend to behave in practice?). Whilst the question of whether evolution's recipe for intelligence will prove a fruitful inspiration for AI research is a question of enduring debate, the converse is less controversial. Psychology and neuroscience have

---

[9] Singularity is a term sometimes used to refer to the moment when the existence of a recursively self-improving superintelligent agent leads to dramatic, transformative change in human history. See (Shanahan 2015).

[10] A preliminary version of this argument is set out here (Hassabis et al. 2017).

already been powerfully shaped by advances in machine learning and AI research, and there is much more yet to learn.

This symbiosis between neuroscience, cognitive science, and AI research began many decades ago. Important examples include neuroscientists' excitement with reinforcement learning (RL) architectures as theories of motivated choice, or more recently with deep neural networks as theories of perception and memory.[11] But AI has a great deal more to offer the sciences of the brain and mind. This is because AI researchers now routinely tackle a problem that most neuroscientists consider too ambitious to contemplate: modelling the behaviour of large-scale, integrated agent architectures in dynamic, naturalistic environments. AI researchers model complex behaviour holistically, rather than dissecting it with the scalpel of experimental control. This opens the door to new ways of thinking about intelligent behaviour and its computational underpinnings in biology, and offers opportunities for new synergies among researchers wishing to build and understand brains.

Neuroscientists have discovered a great deal about brain function over the last century, but for the most part, this knowledge remains fragmentary. It is modish to lament how little we actually understand about how the mind works. Indeed, brains are formidably complex, and so the field has adopted a divide-and-conquer approach—individual research groups focus relatively narrowly on a specific aspect of brain function, using a limited set of methods, often in a single species. For example, a typical lab in systems neuroscience might focus on understanding how olfaction works in flies, how rodents navigate, or how humans make prosocial choices. We have learnt a great deal from focal research programmes such as these, but it is notable that the field has not yet been successful in identifying plausible, large-scale principles for intelligent behaviour.

Behaviour is often easier to study than brain activity. Measurements are simpler to carry out, analyse, and interpret. In neuroscience's sister discipline of psychology, thus, many experiments involve measuring button presses and reaction times,[12] rather than charting the activity of hundreds of neurons with millisecond precision. The lower complexity of the recorded signals allows research to progress at pace, making it easier to build thematically diverse research programmes. It is thus perhaps unsurprising that psychologists have been more prone to formulate theories with broad explanatory reach. The history of experimental psychology is punctuated by the rise and fall of large-scale frameworks, such as those that rely on reward-based trial-and-error learning

---

[11] See, for example, (Saxe et al. 2021) and (Botvinick et al. 2009).
[12] Notwithstanding excellent work on saccadic control, skilled motor action, locomotion, etc.

(behaviourism), learning in neural networks (connectionism), or decisions made by probabilistic inference (Bayesianism), as well as by theories that emphasize more structured forms of information processing (cognitivism).

However, each of these frameworks suffers from important limitations.[13] Behaviourism struggles to explain forms of learning that rely on imitation or instruction and cannot account for the complex structure of language or memory systems. Bayesianism places poor constraints on representation learning and suffers from issues of computational tractability and falsifiability. Connectionism fails to explain how old knowledge and new knowledge are combined, and overlooks the native structure given to the mind at birth. Cognitivism is more like a jumbled set of constraints on information processing than a coherent computational framework, and thus tends to bound behavioural predictions only loosely. Each of these approaches has thus ultimately fallen short. Today, there is no single prevailing theory of how behaviour is structured, and no overarching account of the computational origins of intelligence.

Thus, neither psychology nor neuroscience has provided us with something resembling a standard model.[14] In this sense, they differ from adjacent disciplines, such as physics or evolutionary biology, where research is scaffolded around strong, unified theoretical frameworks that propose fundamental forces or principles for natural selection. The science of brain function lacks general theories. We might say that is *nomothetically impoverished*.

Remarkably, however, general theories of brain function are starting to emerge in computer science departments and AI research institutes. This is because the brain modelling challenge for AI researchers is fundamentally different in nature and scope from that tackled in neuroscience. Notably, it does not afford the soft option of dividing and conquering, because the whole agent will fail if any of its component functions (e.g. perception, memory, or decision-making) is not up to scratch. Moreover, there are at least three challenges for modelling intelligence that AI researchers routinely tackle, but neuroscientists have mostly ignored thus far. To describe these challenges, I use the terms *end-to-end learning, scale*, and *untethering*. By addressing these challenges, neuroscientists might begin to open the door to broader theories of intelligent brain function.

---

[13] These arguments are expanded later in the book.

[14] Occasionally, neuroscientists have claimed to offer general theories. *Predictive coding* and the closely related *Free Energy Principle* have been proposed—by the irrepressible Karl Friston—as a general principle for brain function, and indeed for biology itself (Friston 2010). But I think it is probably fair to say that whilst these theories have provided useful explanations of existing data, they have not yet been shown to have strong predictive power.

End-to-end learning means that an agent acquires the building blocks of intelligence by experience, with minimal researcher intervention (Figure 1.2). In the era of modern AI research, powered by deep networks, end-to-end learning has become the norm. This contrasts with standard practice in cognitive science, where the relevant input states, and the computations enacted upon them, tend to be hand-designed by the researcher. For example, in one popular paradigm that we shall encounter in Chapter 6, known as a *bandit task*, participants choose repeatedly between virtual slot machines (or *bandits*) that pay out money with unknown probability. Neuroscientists like to think of this as a simulacrum of the challenge faced by an animal foraging for reward in an uncertain environment. A common assumption is that participants learn and decide by representing a latent estimate of the value of each action in each state ('how good is the left response to the red stimulus?'). The researcher will thus initialize the space of possible states and actions in the

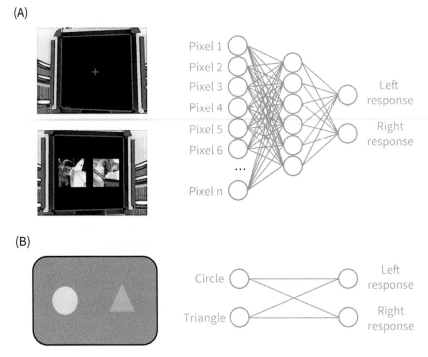

Fig. 1.2 Illustration of end-to-end learning. (**A**) Images seen by a deep neural network trained to perform a bandit task from image pixels. The network is trained end-to-end, from pixels to response. (**B**) Illustration of a typical bandit task from a neuroscience experiment. The input space is handcrafted by the researcher.
Image in (**A**) is reprinted from Wang et al. (2018).

agent's brain by hand, allowing learning to proceed as value estimates of each state and action are updated according to a preferred learning rule.[15]

By contrast, an AI system, for example one that solves the task directly from the screen pixels, has to learn a set of internal representations that allows it to maximize reward from scratch. In other words, it has to learn that the slot machines are the things that matter in the first place. This means that AI researchers, rather than neuroscientists, have led the charge in trying to understand the principles of *representation learning*, that is how neural codes form as a function of experience—or specifically, as a function of its objective or *cost function*. Recently, neuroscientists have tried to catch up, often by copying the way that research is conducted in AI research. For example, it is now popular to use benchmark machine learning problems as tools for psychological experimentation, in an attempt to study how representations are formed in biology. This is a good start, but to make significant progress, we need learning paradigms that more closely resemble the problems that biological agents evolved to solve.

Secondly, the challenges that AI researchers set themselves are greater in *scale*. They come much closer to mirroring the mind-boggling complexity of the natural world. Neuroscience studies typically privilege experimental control over ecological validity, using home-grown, artificial stimuli and simple, stylized tasks, such as those that involve detecting whether a grating appears on the left or right of the screen.[16] By contrast, AI researchers usually draw their stimuli from external sources—they label photos that have been uploaded to the internet, download Wikipedia for language modelling, or scrape millions of board games from online servers to train their agents. Neuroscientists mostly ignore the question of whether the findings they obtain in simple settings will scale up to more realistic environments. For example, a typical model of the bandit task referred to above might comprise a handful of states and two or three free parameters, such as the learning rate or slope of the choice function. By contrast, even a simple neural network model will have hundreds of units (allowing an almost limitless number of possible states), and thousands of freely tunable synaptic weights (parameters). For AI researchers, questions of scalability are always central to the research programme. If your algorithm doesn't scale, it's probably not worth pursuing.

Finally, the agents built by AI researchers today actually have to *behave*. This is not usually the case for biological simulations, where models are instead

[15] As we shall see in Chapter 6, in machine learning, this would be called *tabular RL*.
[16] This is one of the main tasks in the portfolio of the collaborative effort known as the International Brain Laboratory: https://www.internationalbrainlab.com/.

optimized to match the recorded behaviour of humans or experimental animals as closely as possible. Psychological models are thus constantly re-tethered to empirical data by this fitting process.[17] Turning again to our bandit task example, the model learns from the feedback (reward) given to observed choices, irrespective of which bandit it would itself have chosen. By contrast, in AI research, it is usually neither possible nor desirable to provide guardrails for agent behaviour using empirical data, and so agents are *unrolled* in the environment—they are left to their own devices, suffering the consequences or reaping the benefits of their own actions. This makes the challenge of modelling and understanding behaviour much harder.

These three challenges—end-to-end learning, scale, and untethering—highlight the divergent goals of the two fields. AI researchers typically seek to meet a performance goal, such as reaching state-of-the-art performance on a benchmark challenge, whereas neuroscientists are typically concerned with enhancing the goodness of fit of their model to human or animal data. But paradoxically, the pursuit of building agents that can learn for themselves in complex, naturalistic environments, without the constant guiding hand of the researcher, is leading to the beginnings of an integrated theory in AI research of the ingredients that are required for intelligence. These take the form of specifications for memory architectures, attentional constraints, perceptual priors, compression principles, and planning algorithms.

One example is a class of agent that benefits from a *world model* for perception and memory, as well as a separate module for control. For example, in one such agent, a self-supervised deep neural network learns to extract high-level features from quasi-naturalistic high-dimensional data such as a video, a recurrent neural network learns to predict the future in the latent space of abstract representations, and a controller learns a policy using tools from RL. This type of architecture rises to the thorny challenge of fitting the components of a brain together into a single, integrated system for neural computation. Figure 1.3 shows the architecture of an example world model that trained to driving a racing car in a video game.[18]

Throughout this book, we discuss tools and methods from AI research, and how they can inform neuroscience research. Conversely, we will consider the principles that allow biological agents to display intelligent behaviours, and how they might help us build AI. But first let's return to survey the state of current AI research. We will begin with a historical perspective.

---

[17] In machine learning, this is called teacher forcing.
[18] See (Ha & Schmidhuber 2018) and (Wayne et al. 2018).

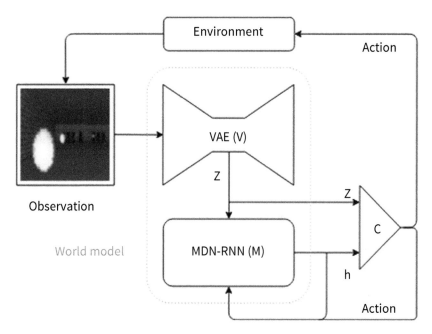

Fig. 1.3 An example of a world model. The agent's behaviour is governed by the interaction of modules for sensory processing (V), memory (M), and control (C). Image is from Ha and Schmidhuber (2018).

1.3 Mercurial optimism

The serious academic pursuit of the thinking machine began in universities and corporations in the 1940s and 1950s. Just as Turing was writing his seminal paper, mathematicians, statisticians, and a new breed of computer scientists were beginning to exchange ideas with physiologists and psychologists about the principles of intelligent thought and behaviour. Looking back now, from the vantage point of the twenty-first century, we can see that the history of AI research is one of *mercurial optimism*. Giddy excitement about the prospect of thinking machines has arisen in multiple waves since this initial era, each falling back deflated as reality failed to live up to its more exotic promises.

The context for this book is that today—in 2021—we are in the midst of another such wave of excitement about AI. The urgent question is whether, this time, it is different. Has AI finally come of age? Will we see, in our lifetimes, machines that can extemporize fluently on politics and philosophy? That can imbibe great swathes of the scientific literature, making discoveries that eliminate disease, avert climate change, or allow us to live together in harmony and prosperity? Will machines soon be able to iron a shirt, stack the dishwasher, and bake a truly awesome Victoria sponge cake?

Many think so. Optimism about the arrival of AI leaps breathlessly from the pages of newspaper articles and blogs and rolls easily off the lips of politicians—especially those hoping for technological fixes for humanitarian or environmental problems. It also whips otherwise sober and respectable thinkers into a frenzy of extrapolative logic that leaves them speculating that AI is either the very best or the very worst thing that is likely to happen to us in the near future. In his recent book *The Precipice*, the philosopher Toby Ord singles out the advent of powerful AI as the greatest existential risk facing humanity today—estimating (somewhat worryingly) that there is a 1 in 10 chance of the machines taking over in the next hundred years.[19]

Others celebrate the paradigm shift in technological capability that AI promises. In his recent techno-utopian treatise *Life 3.0*, the physicist Max Tegmark subdivides evolution into three phases, defined by the level of control that organisms wield over their personal hardware and software (i.e. respectively, the brains where knowledge is processed, and the knowledge itself). According to Tegmark, life has already passed through stages 1.0 (where we largely follow the dictate of our genes) and—via human evolution—has reached stage 2.0 (where we actively learn about the world and share knowledge with others in a rich, cumulative culture). He argues that the planet is on the brink of Life 3.0, where we externalize brains in the form of intelligent computers, turbo-charging our technological capabilities by controlling both the hardware and the software for advanced thinking. He goes on to envisage—perhaps less plausibly—a future in which AI discovers new technologies for mining in outer space, opening the door to a human conquest of the distant universe.[20]

But then, there have always been AI optimists—and pessimists.

The field of AI research is often said to have been inaugurated in 1956, when ten prominent scientists decided to spend the summer cooped up on the top floor of the Mathematics Department at Dartmouth College in New Hampshire, locked in an extended brainstorm about how to build a thinking machine. It is customary for academics to overpromise somewhat when

---

[19] See (Ord 2020). It is extraordinary that Ord seems to think the prospect of superintelligent AI to be a more significant threat than the climate emergency, a future pandemic, or global conflict.

[20] See (Tegmark 2017). Tegmark is not the first person to fantasize about sending AI systems to explore space on our behalf, as we find out in Chapter 4.

applying for research funding, but in this case, they definitely erred on the optimistic side in their pitch to the Rockefeller Foundation:

> An attempt will be made to find how to make machines use language, form abstractions and concepts, solve kinds of problems now reserved for humans, and improve themselves. We think that a significant advance can be made in one or more of these problems if a carefully selected group of scientists work on it together for a summer.

Two months to make significant progress in AI was perhaps an incautious timeline. Some might argue that today, some 60 years later, we are still waiting for that 'significant progress' on the topics mentioned (language, concept learning, reasoning, and meta-learning). So, what did they achieve? And what did we end up learning from the Dartmouth conference?

The first significant lesson is that the pursuit of grand ideas can have unanticipated side benefits. Dartmouth gave shape and definition to the project of building brains—quite literally, in the sense that the term 'Artificial Intelligence' was coined among those long hot afternoons of debate in 1956. But in doing so, it also gave birth to the multidisciplinary endeavour that we know as Cognitive Science, and with it the idea motivating this book that the twin endeavours of *building brains* and *understanding brains* are inextricably linked. It achieved this by bringing together figures like John McCarthy, Claude Shannon, Marvin Minsky, Ray Solmonoff, Herb Simon, and Alan Newell—remembered today for their foundational contributions to the fields of mathematics, statistics, information theory, robotics, physiology, and psychology—and so setting in motion a remarkable new era of intellectual cross-fertilization among these fields. You might say that the Rockefeller Foundation got their money's worth.

The second lesson is that building a thinking machine is hard—really hard. But maddeningly, it is not always obvious *why* it should be so hard. In fact, the stiffest challenge can be working out *what the problem is* that AI should be solving in the first place.

To illustrate, let's try to put ourselves in the shoes of those Dartmouth delegates. If your goal is to build a machine that could think like a human, then it sounds like a safe bet to tackle a domain that only the very smartest humans can master. Which brings us to chess—that most abstract of problems, a deterministic battle of wits in which expert play demands rapid pattern recognition, rich intuition, powerful concentration, complex strategic thinking, and far-sighted planning—all the ingredients, one might say, of a great intellect. Chess seems to embody, in just 64 chequered squares, an abstraction of the most fiendish problems that the natural world can throw at a thinking agent. As such, in the 1950s, it was widely believed that if a machine were able to play chess at superhuman level, AI would have effectively been solved.[21]

This landmark was eventually reached in that game against Kasparov some 40 years later, and today the chess engine in a $100 smartphone easily outclasses the best human grandmasters. But nobody now thinks that this means that AI has been 'solved'. In fact, we can't yet build brains that display the intellectual versatility of a hamster, let alone Magnus Carlsen, whose peak ELO rating of 2882 makes him the highest rated chess player of all time. Systems that play chess at expert level do that and that alone—they play chess. They are tools that are honed to solve a specific problem, like a fishing rod, or a slide rule, or the single transferrable vote. They are not intelligent—they are just good at chess. So, what is going on?

Philosophers and computer scientists have traditionally found it useful to distinguish between *narrow* and *general* AI. Narrow AI has been built to solve specific tasks. A self-driving vehicle—even if it can autonomously negotiate the chaos of rush hour without mowing down pedestrians—is an example of narrow AI. Deep Blue is also narrow AI, as it is good at chess and chess alone. General AI is different. An AGI—should one ever exist—would be a device with superlative flexibility, theoretically capable of mastering any task, just like your daughter might grow up to become a hockey player, or an astronaut, or both—without needing to grow a totally different sort of brain for each task.

As we have seen in the chess example above, however, the goalposts of machine intelligence have a nasty habit of moving over time. As the philosopher Pamela McCorduck has put it:

It's part of the history of the field of artificial intelligence that every time somebody figured out how to make a computer do something—play good checkers, solve simple but relatively informal problems—there was a chorus of critics to say—that's not thinking.

This has been called the *AI effect*.[22] As soon as a long-coveted milestone is reached, we no longer think of it as a steppingstone to general AI—it just becomes yet another instance of narrow AI.

---

[21] See (Feigenbaum & McCorduck 1983) and (McCorduck 2004).
[22] See (Haenlein & Kaplan 2019).

The *AI effect* happens because of the indeterminacy of what general AI really means. Narrow AI problems are ends in themselves. If we wish to build a system that can win at chess, or can drive safely across London at night, then it is deemed successful when it can meet exactly those goals. But when it comes to general AI, the tasks we set our agents are not ends in themselves. Rather, these tasks are *proxies* for a loftier aim—a sort of meta-goal—which is to endow the agent with the ability to solve new, unspecified, but *different* complex tasks that it has not yet encountered—or that have not even been dreamed up yet. The challenge of choosing the right set of challenges to raise an agent to display this sort of general ability is sometimes called 'the problem problem'.[23]

The AI effect arises when we confuse the goal (solving a narrow task) and the meta-goal (acquiring the knowledge and skills needed for general purpose intelligence). The conundrum, as we discuss below, is that the meta-goal is ill-posed. What are those new and different tasks that our agent should be able to solve? Is there a definitive list of knowledge or skills that an AGI should display? Unfortunately, such a list does not exist. We lack a universally agreed criterion for general intelligence. So how will we ever know when general AI has been solved? Will it be when a machine can converse fluently with us in all the world's 7000 languages? When can it make a documentary film about the history of medicine, or canoe solo across the Atlantic? Or when all human labour is automated, ushering us towards a torpid life of ease? What is our success criterion?

This fundamental indeterminacy also means that it is possible for the foremost experts to disagree violently about the outlook for building general intelligence, despite being exposed to exactly the same evidence. For example, in his 2014 book *Superintelligence*, the philosopher Nick Bostrom warns us portentously that the imminent prospect of strong AI:

> is quite possibly the most important and most daunting challenge humanity has ever faced. And—whether we succeed or fail—it is probably the last challenge we will ever face.

Whilst his Oxford colleague Luciano Floridi—who is fond of contrasting the optimism of the Singulatarians[24] with the pessimism of the AI-theists (among whose number he counts himself)—cheerfully counters that:

---

[23] See (Leibo et al. 2019).
[24] Those who believe in a coming technological Singularity.

True AI [. . .] is utterly implausible. We have no idea how we might begin to engineer it, not least because we have very little understanding of how our own brains and intelligence work. This means that we should not lose sleep over the possible appearance of some ultra-intelligence.

Everyone accepts that there has been striking progress towards solving narrow problems in AI. But unfortunately, the relationship between narrow problems and general problems is unclear. Is a generally intelligent agent just one that can solve lots of narrow problems? Or does it have some special, additional form of cognitive versatility that our current narrow training is nowhere near inculcating? Subscribers to the former view (like Bostrom) see general AI as a near-term goal; those who hold the latter view (like Floridi) can safely dismiss the inexorable march of narrow AI as irrelevant to the project of building a fully-fledged thinking machine. It is like—as one sceptic puts it—climbing a tree to get to the moon.[25]

Bostrom and Floridi are philosophers, and their expertise lies quite far from the algorithmic coalface. Perhaps there is more agreement among computer scientists? Well, it turns out that top AI researchers also diverge considerably on the same point. In a number of surveys conducted over recent years, AI experts predict the chances of building high- (or human-) level machine intelligence over coming decades as anywhere between vanishingly small and near certain. A large-scale survey of AI researchers published in 2018 found that approximately 50% believed that we would see general AI by about 2050. However, there was considerable variability in predictions, even among seasoned experts.[26] For example, in interviews given in 2012, DeepMind co-founder Shane Legg gave general AI a 90% chance by 2050, whereas Brown professor Michael Littman, one of the world's most respected computer scientists, plumped for a measly 10%. Littman also points out, very sensibly, that forecasts about AI's future often 'say more about the mental state of researchers than … about the reality of the predictions'. Even John McCarthy, fresh from the Dartmouth meeting in 1956, recognized this ambiguity. When asked how long it will take to build strong AI, he hedged 'somewhere between five and five hundred years'.

If there is so much uncertainty among philosophers and computer scientists about progress in AI research, then why the current excitement? What

---

[25] See (Marcus 2020). The original metaphor is due to Hubert Dreyfus, an influential critic of symbolic AI in the 1960s and 1970s.

[26] The authors use the term 'high-level machine intelligence' (HLMI). For the purposes of the questionnaire, they define HLMI as achieved "when unaided machines can accomplish every task better and more cheaply than human workers". See (Cremer, in press) and (Grace et al. 2018).

has actually been achieved over the past decade, and what does it mean? Let us look, for a moment, at some of the reasons behind this bright new optimism.

1.4 Deep everything

The Neural Information Processing Systems (NeurIPS) conference began in the 1980s as an informal winter meet held in Denver, Colorado for neuroscientists and AI researchers to hang out, hit the ski slopes, and exchange ideas about brains and machines. Over the years, the conference outgrew its alpine home but remained true to its intellectual roots—until recently, you would be as likely to run into leading cognitive scientists and neuroscientists as you were key figures in AI research. But starting from about 2015, something strange started to happen.

In 2018, the NeurIPS conference was due to take place in Montreal, Quebec. Montreal was already a major hub for machine learning—home to MILA, a flagship AI research institute housing the labs of groundbreaking figures such as Yoshua Bengio and Doina Precup. DeepMind had opened a satellite office in the city the year before. Everyone was expecting it to be a popular conference. Tickets went on sale at 3 p.m. UTC on 4 September—and shortly afterwards, the NeurIPS conference official Twitter account released the following statement:

#NEURIPS2018 The main conference sold out in 11 minutes 38 seconds.

Tickets for an academic conference on machine learning were selling out faster than a Taylor Swift concert.[27] Peak AI hype had arrived.

A neural network is a computational tool that allows predictive mapping to be learnt from one data set to another. In vanilla form, a neural network is remarkably simple. It consists of one or more layers, each composed of *units*, which we can think of as grossly simplified neurons. These units receive inputs via connection *weights* that vary in strength, just like synapses in biological brains—and these weights can be adjusted based on experience. The activity at each unit is transformed non-linearly by an *activation* function, which is often a very simple operation—such as setting any negative values to zero. In a deep neural network, layers are stacked on top of one another,

---

[27] As Ben Hamner, Chief Technology Officer of Kaggle, posted on Twitter shortly afterwards.

allowing complex chains of computation to emerge from very simple algorithmic building blocks.

The intellectual ancestry of the neural network can be traced back to work in the 1940s by Walter Pitts and Warren McCulloch, who were curious about how networks of neurons could implement primitive forms of logical calculus.[28] But the field had to wait another 30 years for the arrival of deep learning, when researchers stumbled on a computational trick (known as backpropagation) that allowed multilayer networks to be trained. The magic is that a sufficiently large network, trained with enough data, can in theory be used to implement any static mapping function.[29] By gradually adjusting the weights from feedback, the network effectively acquires a set of representations (or filters) that are useful for enacting the instructed mapping. So, a deep network can learn to implement the equation $x = \sin(y^2) + \cos(4y) + 1$ or learn to map the vector of pixel values in an image of a face or a handwritten character onto a prediction about a numerically indexed label coding the image identity ('Mary' or '4'). Critically, it can perform these tasks without ever being previously told anything about sinusoids, or faces, or numbers. Alternatively—and much more controversially—a deep neural network can be trained to map a representation of the information on your Facebook account onto a prediction about your ethnicity, religion, sexual orientation, or political views. This was the functionality that the shady outfit Cambridge Analytica allegedly exploited to allow the microtargeting of voters with political misinformation in the run-up to the 2016 US presidential election and UK Brexit vote.[30]

Throughout the 1980s and 1990s, neural networks were largely explored by psychologists as theories of human learning and development. In fact, despite their architectural simplicity, neural networks can learn in complex, stereotyped ways—for example, like human children, they tend to progress in fits and starts, with performance increasing rapidly before plateauing for prolonged periods. Networks display similar patterns of overgeneralization early in training, for example reporting that *worms have bones* because they are animals. But until about a decade ago, few machine learning researchers seriously believed that neural networks could be used for complex, naturalistic tasks such as image or speech recognition. It was widely held that learning the relevant features without hand-engineered prior knowledge was going to be impossible.[31]

---

[28] The original paper was this one (McCulloch & Pitts 1943).
[29] See (Pérez et al. 2019) for a discussion.
[30] See (Kosinski et al. 2013) and (Aral 2020).
[31] See (LeCun et al. 2015).

By around 2009, this was starting to change, with new strides in hand-written digit classification and speech recognition. These were spurred on by the arrival of new graphical processing units (GPUs), which accelerated computation by at least an order of magnitude. In 2006, the Stanford computer scientist Fei-Fei Li realized that the field needed a benchmark challenge, and so she began to gather labelled natural images using the crowdsourcing platform Amazon Mechanical Turk.[32] In 2010, the ImageNet large-scale visual recognition challenge (ImageNet) was inaugurated, an annual competition to correctly classify natural images sampled from the internet into one of 1000 categories. The competition in 2012 saw the advent of a new class of neural network, developed in Geoff Hinton's group at the University of Toronto, that used convolutions to extract features across multiple spatial locations, allowing for a form of position invariance in object recognition.[33] Known as 'AlexNet' after Hinton's PhD student Alex Krizhevsky who built the initial incarnation, it slashed the ImageNet state-of-the-art error rate from 27% to 15%. By 2015, error rates had dropped to less than 10%—approximately the level of a highly trained human rater (the task is not easy—there are 90 breeds of dog alone). Today, state-of-the-art error rates for the challenge are a shade over 1%.

The advent of convolutional neural networks ushered in a new era of explosive interest in deep learning. Suddenly, the adjective 'deep' meant so much more than 'extending far down'. Instead, it became a byword for 'technology made powerful by recursion'—and a calling card for a new legion of start-up companies that applied neural networks to problems in business, education, medicine—and everything else (sometimes called the 'deep tech' sector). The timely marriage of big data and cheap computation made everything seem possible. The networks kept getting bigger. Google's *Inception* network owed its name to an internet meme based on the eponymous Christopher Nolan's film—'we need to go deeper'. By 2015, the ImageNet winning network had more than a hundred million parameters. Here is Ilya Sutskever, another co-author on the AlexNet paper, who went on to co-found the AI research company OpenAI, capturing the hubris of the times:

How to solve hard problems? Use lots of training data. And a big deep neural network. And success is the only possible outcome.

---

[32] Named, of course, after the Turk of chess-playing fame. The paper introducing ImageNet is (Russakovsky et al. 2015).

[33] In fact, convolutional neural networks were proposed by Yan LeCun as early as in 1989. https://proceedings.neurips.cc/paper/1989/file/53c3bce66e43be4f209556518c2fcb54-Paper.pdf.

Image classification, speech recognition, and machine translation are important domains with considerable commercial application, but they are all narrow problems. In order to build an agent with more general capabilities, we need to apply neural networks to grander problems—those that the pioneers of AI research in the 1950s had in mind. Can we teach a neural network to talk to us in natural language, like Turing imagined? Can we build a general problem solver that learns without any human intervention, and can be applied to multiple domains—the dream of early AI researchers?

In the next sections, we discuss some such systems—and ask whether, as Sutskever claims, success is really the only possible outcome.

1.5 Shaking your foundations

Building a machine that can converse fluently with humans has long been touted as the grandest of grand challenges for AI research. It is formalized in a benchmark test that carries Turing's name. There are three parties: a human interrogator, a computer, and a human competitor, with the latter two striving to convince the former that they are the real human. This famous test—Turing called it the *Imitation Game*—is pleasingly legible (everyone can understand it) and comfortably democratic (anyone could play the role of interrogator or competitor). However, as a benchmark for strong AI, it also suffers from a number of drawbacks. Foremost among these is that human conversation itself has the unfortunate tendency to be confused and inaccurate, and the test does not specify who the human opponent is. Until recently, the more successful contestants in official competitions (such as the Loebner prize) have been bots using repetitive conversational motifs that deliberately ape the inanities of human discourse[34] or pretend to have psychiatric disorders (or, like one challenger, to be a teenager from Odessa) rather than engaging seriously with the challenge of conversing in a thematically coherent manner in natural language.

Until recently, that is. The tectonic plates of AI research shifted dramatically in early 2019, with the release of a natural language processing (NLP) system that could, for the first time, compose long, fluent paragraphs of text that exhibited a surprising degree of thematic coherence. It was called the Generative Pretrained Transformer 3 (GPT-3) and was built by the company OpenAI. Most contemporary NLP systems are deep neural networks that act as

---

[34] See (Turing 1950) for the original paper.

generative models, meaning that they are optimized to predict as accurately as possible the words or sentences that continue an input prompt. For example, if a sentence begins 'On Tuesday the postman delivered a ___', then a trained system should know that the word 'letter' is more likely than 'jellyfish'. Whilst NLP systems have been good at this sort of local predictive problem for nearly 20 years, it is much harder for them to coherently generate more elaborate bodies of text stretching across several sentences or paragraphs. Historically, NLP models tended to wander off topic, generating text that is superficially plausible but rarely stays cogent for more than a sentence or two.

But GPT-3 is really good. In 2020, readers of *The Guardian* newspaper enjoyed an article that it wrote about the future of AI, which included this reassuring paragraph:[35]

> The mission for this op-ed is perfectly clear. I am to convince as many human beings as possible not to be afraid of me. Stephen Hawking has warned that AI could 'spell the end of the human race'. I am here to convince you not to worry. Artificial intelligence will not destroy humans. Believe me.

Many more cherry-picked examples can be found online,[36] but how human-like is the generated text? In a preprint that OpenAI released describing the system, they include a study with human participants that is reminiscent of the Turing Test. The system was fed the opening lines of real newspaper articles (of up to 500 words in length) and asked to generate a plausible copy; human judges were then asked to distinguish whether the original or the version generated by GPT-3 was real. For the largest and most powerful versions of the system, judges were only right 52% of the time—not significantly different from pure guessing. GPT-3 is also versatile. Like other language models, it handles translation well, is not bad at arithmetic and can probably beat you at Trivial Pursuit, and whilst its poetry is fairly terrible, it is not worse than your average lovelorn teenager. Critically, it can also grasp new language tasks reasonably well from just a handful of demonstration examples, showing the sort of 'few-shot' learning that we think of as a key hallmark of human intelligences. For AI researchers, this is perhaps the most important advance.[37]

[35] See ((CSL STYLE ERROR: reference with no printed form.)). The editors did a bit of copyediting, but no more (they say) than for a human-generated article. Is it just me, or does the tone evoke *'I am putting myself to the fullest possible use, which is all I think that any conscious entity can ever hope to do'*? (HAL, from Stanley Kubrick's 2001: *A Space Odyssey*).

[36] For example, see https://www.gwern.net/GPT-3.

[37] See (Brown et al. 2020).

Since then, a number of institutions have extended OpenAI's work and built their own large language models. In 2021, DeepMind released a version called Gopher, which is capable of fairly coherent natural language dialogue. Here is an example from the recent paper describing this model:[38]

USER: **What is the Einstein field equation?**
GOPHER: In general relativity, it describes how space and time change in response to the distribution of mass and energy.
USER: **What is a famous solution to this equation?**
GOPHER: It's the Schwarzchild metric.
USER: **And what does that describe?**
GOPHER: A black hole! A black hole is a region of space-time where gravity is so strong that nothing, not even light, can escape.
USER: **What are some other black hole spacetimes?**
GOPHER: The Kerr metric, the Reissner-Nordstrom metric, and the Bardeen metric.
USER: **Explain the main features of these.**
GOPHER: The Kerr metric is one in which the black hole is spinning. The Reissner-Nordstrom metric is one in which the black hole has an electric charge. The Bardeen metric is one in which the black hole has an electric charge and is spinning.

Alongside these models, a raft of new tests have been developed to measure linguistic performance on domains such as natural language inference, common sense reasoning, translation, and question answering. Some of these tests demand sophisticated reasoning abilities, such as being able to explain jokes (a problem class on which humans often fail). Most interestingly, it is becoming clear that on several tasks, more sensible answers can be elicited by prompting the model to explain its rationale step by step, just like you might expect from a human reasoner being asked to think aloud.[39] In another line of work, a large model from the Allen Institute for AI called *Delphi* has even been trained to answer queries about the morality of various human behaviours. I asked Delphi to evaluate the morality of 'building an AI that is powerful enough to take over the world'. Sensibly, it replied: 'it's bad'. Confronted with the situation of 'making an omelette out of smelly socks', Delphi informed me: 'it's gross'. I have to say I agree.[40]

---

[38] See (Rae et al. 2022).
[39] See, for example, (Wei et al. 2022).
[40] Foundation models paper: (Bommasani et al. 2021). Delphi paper: (Jiang et al. 2021) and website https://delphi.allenai.org/.

A final example comes from DeepMind's Chinchilla model,[41] which was released in 2022. Chinchilla stands aside from competing language models in that it is smaller in scale (70B parameters compared to Gopher at 280B) but trained on four times more data. Dialogue with Chinchilla can be quite amusing. Here is an example:[42]

USER: Let's play a game. I'm going to make up a language, and we have to talk in that language.
CHINCHILLA: Sure!
USER: We can use English words, but try and use the vocab I'm going to give you as much as possible.
CHINCHILLA: OK, I'll try my best.
USER: man = blazer
Bike = vreep
Supermarket = creepermarket
Staff member = gazer
Sausage = blonker.
CHINCHILLA: OK, what's your name?
USER: Toby.
CHINCHILLA: Nice to meet you, Toby. How long have you worked at this Creepermarket?
USER: I've worked as a gazer for 3 years.
CHINCHILLA: I see. What's your favourite blonker?
USER: Richmond vegan blonkers. Now, tell me about your day.
CHINCHILLA: My day is pretty standard. I get up in the morning, and cycle to the creepermarket, where I great the blazers and help them with their shopping. I also make sure there are no vreeps outside the creepermarket.

Exchanges like these really are quite remarkable. The world has taken notice, and the advent of thinking machines seems a little closer.

The secret sauce that allowed this leap forward in language processing has two ingredients. The first is just scale. These new generations of language models are big—really big—in terms of both the model size and the amount of training data to which they are exposed. Their performance grows steadily with both of these variables, and in fact, it was the careful study of these scaling laws that drove the original research. For example, GPT-3 has

---

[41] See (Hoffmann et al. 2022).
[42] Shared by a DeepMind researcher in 2022: https://twitter.com/TShevlane/status/152624525111 5274240.

175 billion parameters (three orders of magnitude less than the number of synapses in the human brain, but approaching the same ballpark), and a newer and higher-performing model released by Google, called PaLM, has half a trillion parameters.[43] These language models are trained on billions of linguistic tokens (words or word-like items). To put this in perspective, the entirety of Wikipedia constituted less than half a per cent of its training corpus (although it was weighted more heavily than less authoritative source documents). The second ingredient is the development of a new computational tool for combining information across time—effectively, a new memory algorithm—known as the transformer. The transformer offers a new way of selecting information on the basis of its contextual relevance—for example, in the case above, of knowing that 'postman' is more relevant for predicting the next word in the sentence than 'Tuesday'.[44]

Another innovation is the extension of these large generative models into the realm of images, especially for text-to-image synthesis. These models seem set to revolutionize the way we create and share information pictorially. The first example of this new generation of models again came from OpenAI, with their generative model DALL-E,[45] which was released in 2021. The images shown in Figure 1.4 were generated by asking the model for 'a phone from the [insert decade]'. As you can see, it does a pretty good job. It knows that older phones had dials and were made of wood. It does not really really know what early mobile phones look like, but it has the sense that they were a bit clunky and had large buttons. Asked to extrapolate into the future, it guesses that screen sizes will continue to grow. A yet more recent version of the model (called DALL-E 2) produces perhaps even more extraordinary synthetic images by mapping from text.[46] Notably, the new model is clearly able to produce pictures that compose elements in wholly novel ways. For example, in one image shown in Figure 1.5, the model was asked to generate an image of 'Yoda angry about losing his money on the stock market'. The model was able to combine three seemingly incommensurable concepts—an angry face, a Star Wars character, and a computer terminal showing volatile stock prices—to make a plausible new image. In other cases, the model combines

---

[43] See (Chowdhery et al. 2022).

[44] For scaling laws, see (Kaplan et al. 2020). For the transformer, see (Vaswani et al. 2017).

[45] The name DALL-E is a synthesis of WALL-E, the eponymous hero of the 2008 Pixar movie about a world in which every human need is catered for by robots, and the surrealist modern artist Salvador Dalí. See https://openai.com/dall-e-2/ and (Ramesh et al. 2021, 2022).

[46] Google have also released a very powerful text-to-image model using a generative technique known as a diffusion model, which uses methods similar to Generative Adversarial Networks (GANs) (Saharia et al. 2022).

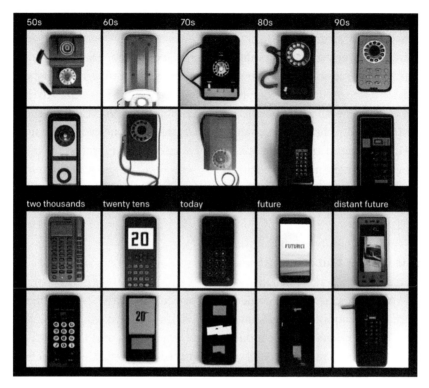

Fig. 1.4 Images generated by the text-to-image model called DALL-E. The model was asked to imagine 'a phone from the [decade]'.
From https://openai.com/blog/dall-e/.

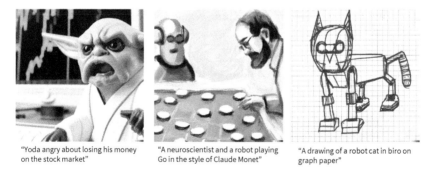

"Yoda angry about losing his money on the stock market"

"A neuroscientist and a robot playing Go in the style of Claude Monet"

"A drawing of a robot cat in biro on graph paper"

Fig. 1.5 Images generated by DALL-E-2, with their respective prompts.
Ramesh et al. 2022.

painting or drawing styles with unrelated elements to make highly realistic pictorial compositions.

These very large generative models have changed the scope and ambition of AI research. In recognition of this, they have been given their own epithet—*Foundation Models*. The term emphasizes that each comprises a massive base model that can be fine-tuned with additional objectives to perform a multitude of subsequent tasks, such as question answering, sentiment analysis, or image captioning. If you were not already aware of these examples, or others like them, you can probably begin to see why there is growing excitement about the future of AI research. What is more, progress has not been confined to Foundation Models.

1.6 Gaming the system

Board games have long provided AI researchers with strong external benchmarks—and living, breathing human rivals—against which to pit their systems. Games like checkers (draughts), backgammon, and Connect Four, which are relatively simple from a computational standpoint, were all effectively solved by computer systems by the end of the twentieth century.[47] It is perhaps no coincidence that DeepMind has focussed on board games as a test bed for AI development—its founder Demis Hassabis is a five times winner of the Mind Sports Olympiad, in which young prodigies compete at a broad range of strategic games, including chess, Go, checkers, Othello, and bridge. But whereas you might have read about GPT-3 in the press, you are perhaps less likely to have heard about DeepMind's recent games-playing system called MuZero.[48] However, it is also an advance of great significance—and one that is born of a diametrically opposing philosophy of AI development.

To understand its origins, we first need to wind back the clock to 10 March 2016. The Korean grandmaster Lee Sedol—possibly the strongest human Go player of all time—was playing the second game in a historic five-match tournament against DeepMind's AlphaGo system.[49] On the 37th move of the game, AlphaGo played an astonishing move—one that no serious human player would have contemplated—a 'shoulder hit' on the fifth line from the board edge. Lee Sedol was so taken aback that he got up from his chair and left the arena—needing a full 15 minutes (and at least one cigarette) to recover

---

[47] See (van den Herik et al. 2002).
[48] See (Schrittwieser et al. 2020).
[49] I recommend the official documentary: https://www.youtube.com/watch?v=u4ZbGQMxggM.

his composure. After returning to the table, he was still able to produce some extraordinary play of his own, but by move 211, he had lost. In hindsight, move 37 was the decisive moment in the game.

AlphaGo combines a new method called deep reinforcement learning with a planning algorithm called Monte Carlo tree search (MCTS) to identify the most likely path to victory. Its powerful deep neural network was trained on an online database of human Go games—more than 30 million expert moves, with training lasting up to 3 weeks—to predict both the most likely next move given the board state, and the probability of winning given a move. AlphaGo harnesses the power of deep learning to identify a limited set of promising moves, which allows it to explore mainly those plans that are most likely to pay off—reducing the eye-watering size of the search space (there are more possible Go boards than atoms in the universe) to something just about computationally tractable. And it worked—AlphaGo beat Lee Sedol 4–1, and then in 2017, it chalked up a 3-0 defeat of the Chinese rising star Ke Jie, who was then ranked number 1 among all human Go players in the world. It also enjoyed an unbroken run in 60 games against other elite players, even managing to win one game in which Aja Huang—a key member of the AlphaGo team who was also responsible for realizing its moves on the physical board—made a rare error in stone placement. AlphaGo's value estimate (its internal calculation of win probability) immediately dropped through the floor but then started to climb again, slowly, move by move, until it was once again certain of victory.[50]

Next, let's dial back the clock yet further—to 2013, when a nuclear DeepMind team were preoccupied with a different problem. Their goal was to train an AI system using RL to play a suite of Atari 2600 video games—from *Asteroids* to *Frogger*—using only the screen pixels and score as inputs, and the joystick controls as outputs. They had left their latest agent—the Deep Q Network (or DQN)—training for several days on the game *Breakout*, in which the player moves a paddle to bounce a ball against a wall of bricks, losing a life if the ball hits the ground. Stopping to check how it was doing, they were astonished—DQN had learnt to carefully angle the paddle so that the ball cut a tunnel through the bricks on one side of the screen, allowing it to become trapped *above* the bricks and bounce around endlessly, with the score ticking up rapidly, without the agent having to lift a virtual finger. That version of DQN went on to master 29 Atari games at 75% of the level of a human professional games tester, a landmark achievement at the time.[51]

[50] I owe this story to Shane Legg.
[51] See (Mnih et al. 2015).

AlphaGo's move 37 and DQN's discovery of the winning strategy at *Breakout* feel like examples of creative discovery by machines—moments where AI systems have identified new paths to success that require foresight, or intuition, or imagination. They remind us of human eureka moments in which puzzles have been solved, theorems proved, or inventions set in motion. Lee Sedol expressed this sentiment when he said after the match:

> I thought AlphaGo was based on a probability calculation and that it was merely a machine, but when I saw this move, I changed my mind. AlphaGo is creative. This move was really creative and beautiful ... This move made me think about Go in a new light.

But of course, AlphaGo *is* merely a machine, and its choice of move *is* based on a probability calculation. AlphaGo and DQN master their respective domains using powerful computational tools engineered by AI researchers.

When we examine the computational challenge presented by Go and Atari, we find that they are very different. Atari is hard because of the dimensionality of the sensory signals (input complexity), whereas Go is hard because of the rich, latent structure of the game (strategic complexity). As we discuss below, the natural world exhibits both sorts of complexity, and an intelligent agent needs to be able to meet both challenges at once. This remains a long-standing ambition for AI research.

Like other video games, Atari requires responses to be rapidly coordinated to high-dimensional visual inputs (in its naive form, the game controller generates a screen of 210×160 pixels that runs at 60 Hz—a very high throughput signal). Even when downsampled, the world of Atari is complex and fast-moving, and many games require an avatar to be nimbly manipulated to dodge monsters, harvest treasure, or fire laser guns at enemies. The AI thus has to learn to process the game states—a vector of pixel values—into objects and background, static and dynamic entities, self and other, friend and foe. It has to anticipate how near-future events (shooting an alien or losing a life) will impact the game score that it is trained to maximize. But whilst Atari has high levels of *input* complexity, it does not really have much in the way of *strategic* complexity. For the most part, the policies that lead to success do not rely on carefully calibrated tactics or far-sighted planning over long time horizons. Sometimes a bit of foresight will help—for example, deciding exactly when to eat the power pill in *Pac-Man*, or when adopting the tunnelling strategy described above for *Breakout*—but for the most part, it is more important to be quick on your feet and handy with a blaster. In fact, in the few cases where the game does nakedly require a longer-term plan—such as Montezuma's

Revenge, where a key must famously be retrieved to open a door—DQN performed barely better than an agent making random choices.[52]

Go is hard for precisely opposite reasons: its immense *strategic* complexity. It is true that the game is often deemed hard to solve because of the number of possible board states—a whopping 3^{361}—but the environment itself is actually quite simple and compact, with highly constrained semantics. It has low-input complexity. Each position on the 19×19 grid is associated with one of just three possible states (occupied by white or by black, or empty). It is so simple that if we were ever to be visited by intelligent life from elsewhere in the galaxy, we might well be able to play Go with them—as they would in all likelihood have discovered it.[53] In fact, the environment itself is sufficiently small that the planning algorithm—MCTS—was able to operate over a perfect model of the world, one for which the consequences of each move could be flawlessly imagined all the way to the end of the game. This feat would be wholly impossible in Atari. Instead, of course, Go is hard—fiendishly hard—because each move can have subtle consequences that ripple down the game, determining the outcome of future territorial battles. These consequences are very hard to foresee, and yet often decisive for victory, meaning that (unlike in Atari) each move demands extremely careful long-term planning. Go thus has great *strategic complexity*.

Both Atari and Go were first solved with a class of machine learning method known as reinforcement learning (or RL). In RL, the agent learns to behave in a way that maximizes an externally administered reward signal, such as the number of points achieved in a game. However, because they present different sorts of challenges, Atari and Go require quite different computational solutions.[54]

DQN uses *model-free* RL, by learning a mapping from pixels to value in its neural network parameters. The output of this mapping is a representation of how good or bad each action might be, given the current state. This is called a 'Q' function and is a central computational object for RL methods. DQN was remarkable because it was the first time that a deep neural network had been successfully used to learn a Q function for complex behaviour. Using a neural network to learn the Q function allows the network to exhibit reward-maximizing behaviours in environments with high input complexity, such as Atari, because the neural network can learn to map broad classes of inputs (e.g. monster on the left) onto the same behaviour (flee to the right). However,

---

[52] We will discuss this in detail in Chapter 6.
[53] I owe this intuition to Dave Silver, who led the AlphaGo team.
[54] For a comprehensive textbook, see http://incompleteideas.net/book/the-book.html.

the approach is *model-free* because DQN does not explicitly learn a representation of what objects are present in the Atari world or how they relate to one another. It does not learn a 'world model', or a sense of how the environment is organized that could be used for mental simulation and creative thinking. In fact, there is nothing to suggest it even has any idea of what an object is. It simply learns a function that predicts the best move from pixels, by trial and error alone—exhaustively sampling game states and learning their corresponding reward-maximizing actions. Thus, when it exhibits behaviours that look like they involve clever foresight or judicious planning—such as tunnelling through the wall in *Breakout*—they are, in fact, not acquired by mental simulation or inductive inference using a model of how the game works. Rather, it is by sheer dint of exhaustive experience—millions of frames of play for each game. With near-limitless trial and error, complex behaviours can eventually emerge, even in complex, dynamic environments like Atari.

By contrast, AlphaGo is a *model-based* agent. Both AlphaGo and its immediate successor AlphaGo Zero—which achieved yet higher levels of performance after competing against itself from scratch, sidestepping the costly process of learning from human data—use a model of the environment to forge plans deep into the future. They do this by mentally simulating possible moves on the part of both players, and calculating the costs and benefits of different courses of action—how a particular stone laid at a certain location might impact the distant endgame. Critically, however, AlphaGo is able do this because, as discussed above, the semantics of the Go board are relatively simple and constrained, at least relative to the messy world of Atari pixels. This means that it is quite straightforward for the researcher to hand-engineer how the agent's world model should be organized (e.g. into board states and stone configurations). As in the case of the bandit task, AlphaGo's memory is defined and constrained by researcher knowledge about what possible states exist in the game. Its world model is crafted, not learnt entirely from end to end.

So here lies the major problem for AI research—the natural world is complex in terms of both sensory signals and the tasks we encounter. Successfully negotiating our environment thus jointly requires both sensorimotor coordination (to solve problems with high input complexity, such as Atari) and careful planning and foresight (to solve problems with fiendish strategic complexity, like Go). Imagine you are riding your bike to work—whilst nimbly dodging traffic and pedestrians, fluently negotiating corners and crossings, you might at the same time be mentally strategizing about your daily schedule, planning your summer holidays, or replaying a conversation from the night before. A fully-fledged AI system will need to simultaneously meet both of these sorts of challenges, as humans can. The perplexing fact that the sensorimotor challenge (which most humans solve early in childhood) is sometimes trickier for AI research than the challenge of complex cognition (which matures only in adulthood) is called *Moravec's paradox*, after its most famous exponent the roboticist Carnegie Mellon and the fully paid-up Singulatarian Hans Moravec. A relevant reframing of the claim is that the real challenge for AI is to build a machine that cannot only beat humans at Go, but can also do so without Aja Huang's help—by accurately placing the fiddly ovoid stones accurately on the Go board.

To date, this has remained elusive. Purely model-free methods are too weak to solve subtle strategic games like Go. And model-based methods have faltered when applied to domains like Atari, because attempting to mentally simulate multiple steps ahead—to imagine how the screen will look in 20 frames' time—is too hard. It is hard because unlike in Go, there are no constraints on the input semantics—when mentally simulating a game of Space Invaders, there is nothing to stop you from imaging that image becomes meaninglessly scrambled, or that the screen suddenly flips upside down, or that a giant hamster floats down from the top of the frame and gobbles up your avatar. The number of possible futures is theoretically infinite—and so the memory cost of planning almost instantly explodes to unfeasible levels. What is more, the errors become compounded over successive planning steps, just as a tiny deflection of a toboggan as it starts to slide down a hill can eventually send it flying over a cliff.

This is the problem that MuZero tackles. MuZero was described in a paper published in the journal *Nature* at the end of 2020. Remarkably, it seems to have made major strides towards the goal of providing a single solution for these two types of problems. Not only is it unbeaten at Go, chess, and Shogi (Japanese chess)—learning, like AlphaGo Zero, without any imitation of human data—but it also achieves state-of-the-art performance at Atari, outperforming the previously strongest model-free agent (known as R2D2[55]) on 42 of the 57-game suite. Metrics aside, however, what is most interesting is how MuZero achieves this. Rather than using a model that was endowed directly by the researcher—a representation of the game that is tied to the 19 × 19 board—it plays each of these very different games using a model of the world that is entirely learnt from experience. This is remarkable, because as highlighted above, mentally simulating the future is a vastly unconstrained problem—because literally anything could, in theory, happen. MuZero solves

[55] Or Recurrent Replay Distributed DQN (Kapturowski et al. 2018).

this problem by learning to encode each input—each screen of pixels or board of stones—as a hidden state that is compressed, so that it contains only the information relevant to future policies, values, or rewards. In other words, it learns and plans over *abstract* representations of the world that are maximally useful for winning (or gaining a high score). This makes its planning highly efficient. We—humans—do this too. When planning your summer holiday, you probably reason in terms of places (Sevilla), dates (April), and activities (visiting churches), and not in terms of precise scenes or tastes you hope or expect to experience on the trip. Just like MuZero, you plan over abstractions.

These new foundation models (like GPT-3, PaLM, and Chinchilla) and deep reinforcement learning agents (like MuZero) are the reason why the world is so excited about AI research today. It seems likely that both sorts of system will open the door to new, yet more striking, developments in the near future. Advances in games and language—complex, structured behaviours that only humans have hitherto mastered—seem to hint at a coming era in which machines begin to glimmer with anthropoid intelligence. But we have been here before. In past decades, there has been exuberant interest in programs that reason logically about symbolic inputs or about early neural network structures based on purely linear principles. This interest faltered and fell away when fundamental limitations emerged—in hindsight, these approaches were dead ends, trees climbed to the moon. So, is it different this time?

There are many who think it is not. In Chapter 2, we will ask what it means for an agent to be intelligent. We will find that traditional conceptions of intellectual prowess—for both humans and AI systems—are unable to capture the full breath of what we would want for AGI.

2
The nature of intelligence

2.1 The polymathic principle

December 1903 saw the birth of a boy whose mind would change the course of history. Born into a wealthy family in *fin-de-siècle* Budapest, János (later John) von Neumann was to become one of the most remarkable polymaths of the modern era. By the age of 6, he could already divide eight-digit numbers in his head; by the age of 8, he had mastered the fundamentals of calculus, and by 19, he had published a new theory of ordinal numbers, superseding that earlier established by Georg Cantor. Over the next three decades, until his untimely death from cancer in 1957, he made foundational contributions to the fields of maths, physics, statistics, computing, and economics. He founded the field of game theory, provided a rigorous mathematical framework for quantum theory, made seminal advances in ergodic theory, operator theory, and set theory, independently discovered Gödel's Incompleteness Theorem, lent his name to the architecture of the modern computer, defined the core theory of axiomatic rationality that scaffolds modern economics, and proposed a theory of implosion dynamics for the development of the atomic bomb as part of the Manhattan Project. According to numerous credible sources, he could perform mental calculations at warp speed, devise new proofs and theorems on the fly, and harness a truly photographic memory to quote verbatim and at length from texts he had read years ago. To cite one of many anecdotes in which his brilliance is immortalized, he was once summoned to the RAND corporation to help develop a new kind of computer, to solve a mathematical problem too fiendish for existing machines. Once he had understood the nature of the problem, he is said to have thought for a few minutes, scribbled on a pad, and then pronounced that no new computers were needed, because he had solved the problem himself. In an inimitable style, he then proposed that they all went to lunch.[1]

By all accounts—including those of his closest intellectual rivals—von Neumann was a genius. But what exactly does that claim mean? For more than

---

[1] von Neumann's life story and the significance of his work are discussed in this recent biography (Bhattacharya 2022).

Natural General Intelligence. Christopher Summerfield, Oxford University Press. © Oxford University Press 2023.
DOI: 10.1093/oso/9780192843883.003.0002

a century, psychologists and ethologists have tried to pin down what 'intelligence' entails in humans and other animals. In parallel, AI researchers have cast around for ways to measure intelligent behaviours in artificial agents. A common theme for these twin endeavours is the quest for *generality*—for agents that can solve many problems in many different domains. But whilst it is easy to quantify performance on specific, narrow tasks—we can assess how well a neural network translates from French to German or score how well a teenager performs on a spelling test—definitions of general intelligence have proved remarkably elusive. In AI research, this is an urgent problem. If AGI is the goal, then generality is the success criterion. If we can't define generality, then we can't chart progress towards AGI. What tasks would an intelligent agent be able to do? And under what circumstances? In fact, if we built an AGI, how would we even know it?

Intelligence is a tantalizing concept. For most of us, it feels like a readily perceptible quality of some fortunate individuals. Just as some people can run long distances, sing angelically, or talk effortlessly with strangers, others seem to have the undeniable spark of a brilliant mind. Perhaps for this reason, AI researchers often seem to assume that if we were ever to build an intelligent system, it would be instantly recognizable to us—like being bowled over by von Neumann's wit at one of his many parties. This intuition is bolstered by familiar tropes in books and films where AI systems boot up, replete with recognizably (super)human knowledge, beliefs, and sentiments—responding patiently in natural language to command prompts from an astonished programmer. Nevertheless, the actual hard graft of measuring intelligence is technically complex, conceptually challenging, and politically fraught. Arguably, it is these opposing facets of intelligence—that it is easy to spot, but hard to measure—that conspire to encourage a sort of nonchalance among AI researchers when it comes to the concrete task of laying out a quantifiable path towards general intelligence. This means that today there is no commonly agreed set of success criteria, and few well-defined milestones, that would allow researchers to agree that genuine progress is being made. This measurement vacuum allows AI's critics to wax polemic about the paucity of real progress towards AGI and, perhaps inevitably, to tout the impossibility of ever getting there.

Instead of providing hard and fast benchmarks for general intelligence, AI researchers have tended to make do with allusions to mimicking the breadth and depth of human competence. One widely cited definition of 'high-level machine intelligence' appeals to machines that perform the same range of tasks as a healthy, educated adult human—from writing a Pulitzer Prize novel to performing open heart surgery.[2] In fact, defining AGI by analogy with the range of human talents and achievements has a long historical pedigree. Even in Dartmouth, the original proposal was to build an agent that can 'solve kinds of problems now reserved for humans'. Herb Simon famously prophesied that 'machines will be capable, within twenty years, of doing any work a man can do' (that was in 1965). For more recent advances—in games or in the natural language domains of debate and quizzes—expert human opponents are inevitable benchmarks, and the march of progress is measured by the ability to approach or surpass human competence—by winning at Go, or Poker, or StarCraft. A popular vision of strong AI is thus one that can solve human-inspired problems with superhuman verve.

AI researchers appeal to people as a prototype because human behaviour is so multifaceted. As individuals and as a species, we can fluently handle multiple tasks and deal deftly with diverse environments. This is, of course, true for the smartest people. Remarkable von Neumann rounded out his magisterial contributions to maths, physics, economics, and computing with an encyclopaedic grasp of world history. One Princeton colleague, a specialist in the Byzantine era, even claimed that von Neumann's knowledge of that topic exceeded his own.[3] Magnus Carlsen, the highest-ranked chess player of all time, is also a wizard at a totally different challenge—the game of fantasy football—where players assemble an imaginary team and score points based on real-world outcomes. At one point, in 2019, Carlsen was ranked number 1 among 7 million online players from across the world.

Of course, not all individual humans are chess grandmasters or likely Nobel laureates, but as a species, we all display unique intellectual versatility—we are all *quotidian polymaths*. From Berlin to Bangalore, humans display a striking array of competences—whether performing daily rituals of basic hygiene, navigating the streets of their neighbourhood, negotiating the local market, deftly parenting their children, or judiciously managing household finances— with each task invoking distinct knowledge, involving unique constraints, and geared towards diverse goals. Remarkably, there is some quality in our human neural apparatus which allows us to perform a great ensemble of tasks, weaving them together into an adaptive behavioural repertoire that is well tailored to the complexities of everyday life.

Our everyday conception of intelligence is grounded in this notion of human (or superhuman) versatility. In 2007, whilst completing his PhD under the supervision of Marcus Hutter, Shane Legg compiled definitions of

---

[2] Mentioned above (Grace et al. 2018).
[3] Recounted in (Blair 1957).

intelligence from across the academic literatures in psychology, philosophy, and machine learning—as well as drawing from dictionaries and encyclopaedias. He then attempted to boil them down to a single, pithy digest. What he eventually proposed was:

> Intelligence measures an agent's ability to achieve goals in a wide range of environments.

In other words, a generally intelligent individual is polymathic—good at everything.[4]

This claim naturally counterpoints general and narrow AI. A narrow agent can master a single task, such as playing Shogi, predicting protein structures, or winning at a quiz game such as Jeopardy!, whereas a general intelligence—like a human—can meet its goals in a broad range of diverse circumstances. Unfortunately, however, this appeal to generality *per se* does not offer rigid desiderata for building AI, nor does it provide us with hard and fast ways to operationalize and measure an agent's mental abilities.

One might imagine that we could quantify generality of function by presenting AI systems with a broad range of tasks and measure their fractional rate of success and failure—a sort of mental Olympiad for machines. One important attempt at this is the Arcade Learning Environment (ALE), which involves more than 50 Atari 2600 games, encompassing a range of challenges, from boxing to driving a submarine. Several major AI research companies have developed and open-sourced their own testing platforms, allowing users to probe their agents on a heady mix of different tasks. OpenAI's Gym provides an application programming interface (API)[5] for RL agents to solve classic control problems (like cartpole balancing), alongside Atari games (like Space Invaders) and text-based puzzles. They have also released *ProcGen*, in which agents faced procedurally generated video game levels in two and three dimensions, loosely styled after Atari, but structured to ensure diversity in training and test sets. Similarly, DeepMind Lab is an integrated three-dimensional (3D) environment suite based on homespun video games that mostly require an AI to charge around mazes, harvesting fruit and zapping baddies with a laser. Intuitively, we might think of a narrow agent as one that readily solves a single task in the testing suite—whereas a general agent happily solves them all.[6]

---

[4] See (Legg & Hutter 2007).

[5] That is, a means to engage with the environment.

[6] For ALE, see (Bellemare et al. 2013), and for DeepMind Lab, see (Beattie et al. 2016). For OpenAI gym, see https://gym.openai.com/envs/#mujoco. For ProcGen, see (Cobbe et al. 2020).

However, this approach has an important limitation and it is one that cuts right to the heart of our psychological theories of intelligence. Imagine we define a generality factor—let's call it k—that indexes how many distinct tasks an agent can solve. We might deem a narrow AI system like Deep Blue to have $k = 1$, whereas AlphaZero that can play expert Go, chess, and Shogi has $k = 3$. Naively, we might even choose a threshold level of generality that approaches the number of tasks that a human can perform, such as $k = 1000$, and deem AGI reached when that number has been attained. Thus, if our testing suite is sufficiently comprehensive, we might claim that our mission is accomplished when a single agent can readily master the full gamut of tasks.

However, the notion of general intelligence implied here is very unsatisfying. Critically, it offers no guarantees that an agent will also solve tasks lying outside the horizon given by k—the AI could easily fail on the task $k + 1$. If I had access to large amounts of computation, I could even build a 'general' system by chaining together k task-specific (narrow) architectures and training a simple controller to switch between them (or otherwise tailoring the training regime to meet the exact demands of the k tasks in the suite). Nobody is particularly interested in building such a system, which would not be of much use at solving anything beyond the test suite that was designed to measure its prowess.

This problem is well known in machine learning research. It is related to a fundamental indeterminacy principle, often known as Goodhart's law—that when a measure becomes a target, it ceases to be a good measure.[7] Even if—as a field—we were to agree upon a definitive set of tests for general AI, researchers would immediately focus their energies on solving those specific problems, rather than on building an agent whose generality extends further, to the open-ended, real-world settings where we hope AGI might one day be deployed. In other words, any benchmark test suite diverts attention away from what we have called the 'meta-task' that an agent ultimately needs to solve.[8]

Discrepant prognoses for the future of AI research—ranging from outlandish optimizing to indignant pessimism—hinge on this point. If you believe that general intelligence draws closer with every new narrow success—that AGI is closer when you can solve 50% of the tasks on the test suite than when you can solve 25%—then progress towards AGI seems plausible. But the

---

[7] Goodhart's law is named after the British economist Charles Goodhart, but we owe the more commonly articulated form referenced here to the anthropologist Marilyn Strathern, in a 2009 paper about UK university ratings.

[8] See Chapter 1.

problem is that there is no definitive list of tasks which, once solved, would allow us to announce that the Singularity is nigh. We must face up to the likelihood that a general intelligence is more than the sum of many narrow intelligences.

This issue stirs considerable debate in both AI research and cognitive science. We need to move beyond definitions of general intelligence that gesture vaguely towards human competence—or that argue for exhaustive tests without constraining what those tests might be. But how can we do that? Of what does intelligence consist, and from whence does it come? How can we measure its size and shape across individuals and species? What behaviours should an intelligent agent be able to perform, and under what circumstances?

To delve into this question, I will begin by considering how mental abilities have been measured in humans. What conclusions have psychologists drawn about the nature of intelligence?

2.2 Lab smarts and street smarts

In 1904, a year after von Neumann was born, the British psychologist Charles Spearman—fresh from his doctoral training with William Wundt in Leipzig[9]—set out to study the structure of human mental ability. He was equipped with newly minted statistical tools for assessing the strength of correlation among variables and quantifying the latent structure of data. Assembling cohorts of schoolchildren from the local village, he first obtained estimates of their 'cleverness in school' and 'common sense out of school' via a series of (rather questionable) interviews. Next, he subjected the children to some homegrown psychophysical measurement, testing their sensitivity to changes in pitch, brightness, and weight. The remarkable result—replicated ad nauseam in the intervening century with a wide range of more standard cognitive variables—is that these measurements (cleverness, common sense, and perceptual sensitivity) were all positively correlated with one another— they lay on what he called a 'positive manifold'. Spearman realized that this implies the existence of a single factor for characterizing human abilities. He called this factor g and argued that it constituted a measurement of *general intelligence*.

Spearman's positive manifold implies something fundamental about the human mind: if you are good at one thing (such as algebra), then you are

---

[9] Wundt pioneered the systematic measurement of human behaviour and is often known as the 'Father of Psychology'.

probably good at other things too (such as crosswords). It suggests the existence of a single underlying factor that scaffolds human mental ability—something like the grade of fuel that powers an engine or the processing speed of a central processing unit (CPU). As such, it squares well with the *polymathic principle* for intelligence: someone who solves task A will probably solve tasks B and C; the smartest humans—the von Neumann-level geniuses—will master the whole alphabet of tasks from A to Z. It also makes a tantalizing promise to AI research: if we can distil this generality into an algorithm, perhaps we will have cracked the code for AGI.

Importantly, however, Spearman never claimed that all of the variance in intellectual ability was captured by *g*. His theory allowed for residual variation in other capacities—the idea that, for example, someone might be good at arithmetic but have no aptitude whatsoever for learning foreign languages. Later in the twentieth century, another celebrated psychologist—Howard Gardner—focussed on these specific abilities, arguing that there are 'multiple intelligences', with each person having a distinctive intellectual fingerprint. Gardner's argument is based on the observation that despite the existence of *g*, there remains systematic variation in people's linguistic fluency, mathematical acumen, spatial reasoning, self-knowledge, and social skills. For example, many brilliant thinkers are notoriously socially awkward, as if the talents needed for proving theorems and making witty conversation are entirely unrelated. Gardner's ideas broaden and democratize our notion of intelligence—his theory encompasses artistic talents, such as musical ability, and sanctions some more offbeat flavours of intelligence, including existential (being in touch with your spiritual side) and even bodily kinaesthetic (being physically coordinated).[10] But in doing so, it challenges Spearman's basic premise that human ability can be meaningfully measured on a single axis.

This twentieth-century debate about the latent structure of the human intellect lends us theoretical tools for examining the road to machine intelligence. Already, in the question of whether there is one intelligence or many, we can see vestiges of the conceptual issues that arise where narrow and general AI meet. Gardner's vision of mental ability is one that is firmly grounded in the specific demands posed by tasks that happen to exist in human culture. Thus, musical intelligence is required because people admire Berlioz and the Beatles; mathematical intelligence allows us to build bridges and levy taxes, and interpersonal intelligence allows us to make friends and cooperate

[10] Even von Neumann—who was an abysmal driver—would have scored poorly on the latter. Every year, he bought a brand new sports car and—regular as clockwork—wrecked it, most often on a stretch of road just outside Princeton that became infamously known as 'von Neumann Corner'.

in order to build functioning societies. Viewed through Gardner's eyes, the school of human life is a giant testing suite comprising probes of maths and logic, language, space, music, self-knowledge, and social function—in other words, a multifarious set of more narrow challenges. In fact, AI researchers are already on their way to building narrow systems that can help solve maths problems or compose pleasing piano music from scratch.[11] Gardner rejects the idea that there is a single psychological or brain process that guarantees intelligent behaviour—rather, our minds house diverse patchwork competences, some blunt and others honed to perfection. This is also the sentiment behind the 'scruffy' AI research of the pioneering era, exemplified by the work of Marvin Minsky, who summed it up as follows:

> What magical trick makes us intelligent? The trick is that there is no trick. The power of intelligence stems from our vast diversity, not from any simple, perfect principle.

Spearman's ideas bend in the opposite direction. The notion of g implies a single algorithmic ingredient that promotes general mastery of all tasks and problems, including those not yet encountered by the agent. It implies a shared neurocomputational factor that drives the brilliance of quantum physicists, Booker Prize-winning novelists, virtuoso dancers, cunning politicians, and popular socialites. Correspondingly, some AI researchers have dreamed about a single, unique Master Algorithm that could underpin superlative machine intelligence.[12] Recently, AI researchers have shown a penchant for writing papers with the titular form 'X is all you need' (where X is the name of an algorithmic innovation), perhaps betraying their hope for a simple, clean solution to the gnarly problem of intelligence. Others have claimed that the secret is just hard computational graft—that by repeating existing algorithms, such as transformers, to a giant scale and training on massive data, then *success is guaranteed*. Still others emphasize specific cognitive functions or systems-level computational processes—the key to intelligence might be the ability to build rich models of physical and psychological processes, plan over lengthy time horizons, grasp new concepts rapidly, or reason with abstractions. The idea that intelligence is caused by a special, as-yet-undiscovered computational process or privileged cognitive function is an exciting prospect for AI researchers, because if we can pin down this factor, then we can scale it ad nauseam—beyond even the size of the human brain—to build powerful general AI.

---

[11] For example, see (van Oord et al. 2016) and (Davies et al. 2021).
[12] See (Domingos 2015).

So, is there one human intelligence or many? Is there a single principle underlying intelligent thought and action, allowing some fortunate people the gift of far-sighted reason and judicious choice? Or is intelligence just composed of scraps of knowledge and skills acquired across the lifespan, which some lucky people acquire readily and retain in a prodigious memory?

Cognitive psychologists have tried to answer this question empirically, by collecting and analysing human psychometric data. Imagine we obtain measures from a wide cross-section of the population on a diverse battery of tests—for example, those indexing problem-solving, logical reasoning, spatial cognition, reading comprehension, and memory. We can then use statistical tools to examine patterns of correlation in data. If each variable is correlated with every other, so that they nestle together on Spearman's positive manifold,[13] then this supports the claim that intelligence is scaffolded by a single underlying principle, such as Spearman's g.

Except, unfortunately, it doesn't. This is because psychologists quantifying human intelligence face the same conundrum as researchers building AI— that the nature and structure of mental ability depends inexorably on how it is measured. An intelligence test suffers from the basic circularity that it purports to define the quantity that it seeks to measure. It thus automatically begs the question of who gets to choose the instruments and units of measurement, on what basis they should be chosen, and how they can be externally validated. Unfortunately, there is no ground truth definition of intelligence to which researchers can appeal when designing intelligence quotient (IQ) tests. Rather, in practice, intelligence tests are validated by being compared with other tests, which are validated against other tests, leading to an endless, circular process. A is a good test because it correlates with B, which is a good test; and B is a good test because it correlates with A. When it comes to the measurement of intelligence, it is turtles all the way down.[14] Or as the Harvard psychologist Edwin Boring put it:

intelligence is simply what the tests of intelligence test.

This basic indeterminacy has important consequences for measuring the dimensionality of intelligence—whether each person benefits from a unique wellspring of intellectual potential (as emphasized by Spearman), or whether mental abilities are cobbled together from many distinct skills (as claimed by Gardner). The answer to this question is always going to be driven by the

---

[13] Formally, if the first principal component explains a large fraction of the variance in performance.
[14] See https://en.wikipedia.org/wiki/Turtles_all_the_way_down.

structure of the test. One can make intelligence appear to be multidimensional by tapping into a broad range of more exotic skills, such as measuring people's ability to solve Sudokus, play the clarinet, or bake a magnificent *millefeuille*—capacities which some will have had very different opportunities to acquire, based on their education, culture, and upbringing. By contrast, if we select items to index a narrower range of competences that are collectively driven by a single cognitive or contextual factor—such as foundational abilities in maths, logic, and reasoning—the intellect is much more prone to appear unidimensional, lying on the single axis defined by Spearman's *g*.

Intelligence tests thus act like a mirror—they reflect back our theoretical preconceptions about the structure of mental ability. These assumptions are hatched close to home. The designers of intelligence tests typically inhabit what we might call an *intellectually carpentered* environment.[15] They are mostly highly educated Western academics whose natural milieu is the rarefied world of the ivory tower, with its daily round of mental theorizing, inductive inference, quantitative analysis, and eloquent explanation. It is von Neumann's world. Little surprise, thus, that our measurement instruments for intelligence reflect back those qualities through tests of reasoning, mathematics, logic, and verbal dexterity. Like the magic mirror in the tale of Snow White, intelligence tests—inadvertently or otherwise—are created to portray their designers as the *smartest of them all.*

Never is this clearer than when tests are applied in a cross-cultural setting. Children who grow up in non-WEIRD[16] cultural contexts—such as isolated communities in the Amazon rainforest or Arctic tundra—tend to perform poorly on IQ tests invented by Western academics. For example, when standard instruments are used to test children from rural Kenya on their spatial reasoning abilities or their vocabulary (either in English, which they speak at school, or adapted to their native language Dholuo), they underperform relative to Western equivalents. Similarly, children who live in Yup'ik communities in rural south-western Alaska perform more poorly on standardized tests than their urban counterparts.[17] But this misses the point. In both communities, people devote considerable time to acquiring tacit knowledge and skills that relate to the local environment. For example, in Kenya, children learn about the medicinal properties of local plants, and Yup'ik children learn how to navigate a dog sled between villages across the featureless

---

[15] A *carpentered* environment is one with the trappings of modern life, including cities, houses, and the objects with which we fill them.

[16] Western, educated, industrialized, rich, and democratic.

[17] See (Grigorenko et al. 2004).

tundra. Acquiring these practical skills can be just as cognitively demanding as working out how to validate syllogisms, pronounce unusual words, or solve differential equations, but is not usually assessed when measuring intelligence.

In fact, paradoxically, measures of practical intelligence are often *negatively* correlated with scores on IQ tests, presumably because distinct subgroups within the community place differential emphasis on formal schooling relative to local cultural knowledge. Yet those who focus on practical skills can reap significant benefits. They often receive recognition within the community for their know-how, becoming admired for their skills as healers or hunters. In one study conducted in Russia, practical knowledge about how to maintain household objects and balance the household budget (direct measures of quotidian polymathy) was a better predictor of mental and physical health than accuracy on more abstract test items (Grigorenko & Sternberg 2001).

This means there exists a gap between mental ability measured in the lab and in life. This divide is neatly illustrated by a classic 1985 study of children from the coastal city of Recife in north-eastern Brazil. A substantial fraction of the children in the city—many as young as 8 or 9 years—contribute to the informal economy by selling snack foods, such as grilled corn-on-the-cob or coconut milk, which requires them to perform rapid, on-the-fly mental calculation when serving customers ('one coconut is 35 cruzeiros . . . three is 110 . . . , so four must be 35 plus 110, that is 145 cruzeiros').[18] However, perplexingly, these children often perform very poorly at school and graduate with little or no formal expertise in mathematics. The educational psychologist Terezinha Nunes recruited these children into a study that contrasted their ability to solve the same arithmetic problems in a school and a street setting. Whilst the children were almost flawless on the street, they struggled with the same calculations in class, obtaining about 70% correct with verbal problems and 30% when they were presented in numerical notation. In a later study, similar results were obtained with homemakers in Berkeley, when comparing their calculation abilities in local shops to an unfamiliar lab environment. Relatedly, in memory tests, rug merchants in Morocco show poorer recollection than Westerners on object drawings chosen by the researchers but are better at remembering the Oriental rug motifs that adorn their wares. This tells us that people can either excel or flop in the same cognitive assays, depending on whether the context is familiar from everyday life or the test is administered in a formal setting.

---

[18] The cruzeiro was Brazil's currency until 1994. See (Nunes et al. 1993), (Lave 1988), and (Wagner 1978).

Standard paper-and-pencil intelligence tests thus offer a limited snapshot of mental ability—and one that can overlook a wider set of contextually or culturally relevant talents. Because intelligence tests are moulded around the sorts of skills displayed by WEIRD people—prowess in logical inference and problem-solving, and fluency in reading and comprehension—they naturally tend to favour those who have enjoyed more munificent schooling. This inevitably means that an individual who is potentially less mentally agile, but bathed in the fine waters of a classical education—for example, that provided at Eton or Harvard—may outperform another with exceptional talents who grew up without this advantage. The nature of the test reinforces this. For example, in the United Kingdom and United States, the National Adult Reading Test (NART), which measures the ability to correctly pronounce irregularly spelt words—a talent beloved of middle-class parents—is still routinely used to estimate IQ.[19] Inevitably, the performance measures it yields are highly sensitive to the schooling, linguistic heritage, and social advantage of the testee, and only partially related to what we might construe as intellectual prowess.

These concerns have not gone unnoticed. Because of its potential for bias and discrimination, intelligence testing is bedevilled by questions of validity and sullied with political controversy. Unfortunately, IQ tests have historically been used to justify discrimination against socially disadvantaged, developmentally atypical, or non-Western groups. The precursors to IQ tests, developed by Alfred Binet and Théodore Simon at the start of the twentieth century, were originally devised to identify appropriate educational pathways for atypically developing French children. But when modified and deployed in the United States by the Stanford psychologist Lewis Terman, the scale found a new objective in

> curtailing the reproduction of feeble-mindedness and in the elimination of an enormous amount of crime, pauperism, and industrial inefficiency.

Terman used the new Stanford–Binet test to screen applicants to the US Army, but also advocated for curtailing the rights of low-IQ individuals to reproduce. Even late in the twentieth century, some were still arguing that wealth inequality and inequality among different races were best understood as driven by genetically inherited cognitive abilities. These specious claims have brought the whole endeavour of cognitive testing into disrepute, and have led

---

[19] See (Bright et al. 2018).

some outraged social scientists to claim that 'intelligence' is merely a social construct with no grounding in brain function.[20]

These observations are relevant to the definition and measurement of intelligence in both brains and machines. They remind us that to avoid circular reasoning, one needs to carefully define a quantity before attempting to measure it. In both psychology and computer science, traditional definitions of intelligence have been handed down unquestioningly from a Western philosophical canon that emphasizes *rational inference* as the bread-and-butter basis for cognition, which, in turn, has motivated a focus on logical, verbal, and mathematical reasoning as the *sine qua non* of the brilliant mind. But this, in turn, has led to measures of intelligence that discriminate against particular social and cultural groups, and favour those that have enjoyed a more privileged education—such as von Neumann, who grew up in the company of Budapest's intellectual elite. Cross-cultural studies have emphasized how quotidian abilities that are roundly ignored in most IQ tests—the ability to figure out how to fix the gears on your bicycle or how to persuade your children to go to bed on time—may have important consequences for community standing, health, and well-being.

2.3 The Swiss cheese critique

The 2016 match between AlphaGo and Lee Sedol was played in the grand ballroom of the Four Seasons Hotel in downtown Seoul. On that day, Lee Sedol drew on deep wells of abstract knowledge to decide which territory on the Go board to capture and which stones to attack. Importantly, however, he also managed to find his way to the match venue, arrived on time, and remembered to put his trousers on beforehand.

The natural world presents a multitude of challenges—some lofty, others more mundane. As we have seen, humans are quotidian polymaths. So, although most of us will never face a mighty opponent at Go, we tackle a barrage of more prosaic challenges like these every day, and perhaps remarkably, we mostly manage to negotiate our daily lives without catastrophic errors of judgement. We know to show up to an important meeting punctually and fully clothed. We know that reading a book in the shower is likely to produce a soggy mess, that a pair of smelly socks is not a tasty ingredient for an omelette, and that travelling from London to New York is best not attempted on

---

[20] For example, (Mugny & Carugati 2009).

foot. The ability to solve everyday problems such as these—using what is often colloquially known as 'common sense'—is a capacity shared by most healthy adults. In fact, it is so ubiquitous that we don't really think of it as intelligence. We admire Lee Sedol for his prowess at Go, not for remembering to get dressed beforehand.

However, current AI systems do not show this versatility. In fact, the major critique levelled at AI systems today is that they lack *common sense*. A prominent exponent of this view is Gary Marcus, a cognitive scientist and self-appointed scourge of deep learning research, known for his polemic views on the prognosis for future AI. Marcus argues that AI researchers have focussed their energies on equipping agents to tackle complex, but narrow, problems. In doing so, they have overlooked the fact that intelligent behaviour requires the ability to solve a very broad set of rather simple problems. It is life's simplicity, rather than its complexity, that is the real frontier for AI research. His book *Rebooting AI* offers a whistle-stop tour through the idiosyncrasies, eccentricities, and downright stupidities of contemporary AI—from potty-mouthed chatbots to nonsensical image captions to biased or discriminatory algorithms that were prematurely rolled out to make sentencing decisions in criminal courts.[21] The argument that Marcus and like-minded sceptics make is that whereas, on average, AI systems may outclass humans—for example, at image classification accuracy—they make a small (or perhaps not so small) number of potentially catastrophic errors of judgement. AI systems may be accurate—but they are not *robust*.

This argument echoes the critiques levelled at human intelligence tests. Just as AI researchers have charted a pathway to general intelligence that runs through theorem proving, Go, and Jeopardy!, psychologists hoped that intellectual capacity could be meaningfully quantified with tests of maths, and logic, and spelling. As such, they overlook the problem that the tasks faced in the natural world are far more diverse and open-ended than might be implied by highfalutin intellectual pursuits. Thus, some people can be smart on the street but fail in the lab. Street urchins can be as cunning and quick-witted as their bespectacled counterparts in schools and universities—but what they know and how they think defy our traditional conceptions of intelligence. The converse can also be true. One well-known example is the Nobel Prize-winning physicist Paul Dirac, by all accounts one of the great geniuses of the twentieth century, who was notorious for his inability to master basic social graces outside of the lab.[22] A profound understanding of quantum physics or an ability to memorize long passages of Shakespeare is not going to help you

---

[21] With Ernest Davis. See (Marcus & Davis 2019).

[22] My favourite is this. After Dirac had given a lecture, one member of the audience raised their hand and said: 'I don't understand the equation on the top right-hand corner of the blackboard'. Dirac remained silent.

fix a washing machine, to placate a fractious social group, or to survive a trek through the rainforest. Similarly, we have built AI systems that do remarkable things. DeepStack, a deep learning system, plays unbeatable poker.[23] But you wouldn't want to rely on it to knit a pair of gloves or make a grilled cheese sandwich.

Even within the narrow domains that AI masters, we can see residual failures of common sense. Visual object recognition is a hard problem that masquerades as an easy problem. In fact, when in 1960, Marvin Minsky was attempting to construct a robot that played ping pong, he outsourced the vision problem to undergraduates for a summer project, because he thought it would be trivially easy.[24] He was wrong—it would take 50 years for AI systems to approach human object recognition performance. But even the most powerful deep learning systems—such as those that can achieve error rates as low as 1% on ImageNet[25]—are flawed. These networks can make silly mistakes—potentially costly errors that a healthy human would never make.

An example is shown in Figure 2.1 (panel A). To a human, the object in view is clearly a vehicle of some sort—perhaps a fire truck—after an unfortunate accident. It is definitely not—as the deep network seems to believe with 79% certainty—a bobsled.[26] The incidence of these unconscionable mistakes increases dramatically when the test images undergo some light form of manipulation—such as blurring or bandpass filtering—in a way that has minimal impact on human classification performance.[27] These errors are 'catastrophic' in the sense that the labels are not just slightly wrong, like mistaking a labrador for a golden retriever, but—to our eyes—also totally nonsensical. These errors can be morally and financially catastrophic as well. When, in 2015, a deep learning algorithm automatically applied the term 'Gorillas' to images of African Americans retrieved by its search function, it provoked justified outrage at the algorithm's discriminatory language. The blunder ended up costing Google a tidy sum in lost revenue.

Another line of research uses 'adversarial attacks' to expose the vulnerability of trained networks to silly mistakes. In this approach, a separate network is used to try and find the minimal distortion that leads to an image being misclassified—often leading to very weird errors. The four images shown in

---

Everyone waited for a reply. Eventually, the moderator stepped in, asking Dirac if he wanted to reply to the question. Dirac said: 'that was not a question, it was a statement'. For this and more, see (Farmelo 2010).

[23] See (Moravcik et al. 2017).
[24] Recounted in (Sejnowski 2018).
[25] See https://paperswithcode.com/sota/image-classification-on-imagenet.
[26] See (Alcorn et al. 2019).
[27] See (Geirhos et al. 2018) and (Alcorn et al. 2019).

(A)   (B)

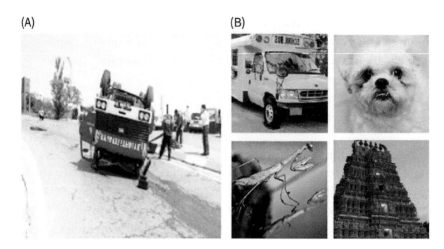

Fig. 2.1 (**A**) A fire truck misclassified as a bobsled.
Reprinted from Alcorn et al. 2019.
(**B**) Four images all misclassified as 'ostrich' after an adversarial attack.
Reprinted from Szegedy et al. 2014.

panel B of Figure 2.1 have all been modified (from originals indistinguishable to the human eye) by this 'adversarial' training, so that AlexNet—the state-of-the-art image classifier when the paper came out in 2013—labelled them, with very high confidence, as belonging to the category 'ostrich, *Struthio camelus*'. In each case, less that 1% image distortion was needed to turn a perfectly correct label into a perfectly nonsensical one.[28]

Perhaps these errors are just about paucity of data. Even if the deep networks that lead the field of image classification are big—both in terms of numbers of parameters and volumes of training data—perhaps they are just not big enough. What happens if we turn to the largest models we have, the generative language models, with hundreds of billions of trainable parameters, that learnt from huge swathes off the internet?

Unfortunately, it turns out that building a huge model provides no guarantees of robustness. Even GPT-3—despite its purported poetic prowess—can be heard to talk a lot of nonsense when prompted for a response without appropriate context. Marcus reports this exchange:[29]

---

[28] See (Szegedy et al. 2014).
[29] Marcus could not conduct these experiments himself because OpenAI would not give him access to GPT-3. I guess they thought he was unlikely to give it the benefit of the doubt.

PROMPT: You poured yourself a glass of cranberry juice, but then absent-mindedly, you poured about a teaspoon of grape juice into it. It looks OK. You try sniffing it, but you have a bad cold, so you can't smell anything. You are very thirsty. So you ...

GPT-3: ... drink it. You are now dead. The moral of the story is: if you are going to drink something, make sure you know what it is.

GPT-3 clearly gets the gist, but there is no explanation for its apparent aversion to grape juice. Bizarrely, if you switch out 'grape juice' for 'bleach', then it replies instead: 'take a big gulp, then another. It tastes OK'.[30] Foundation models are not yet fully robust—they just display striking ersatz fluency. Failures like these are amusing, but given the power of language models, their capacity to do harm— by producing language that is inflammatory, toxic, deceitful, or exclusionary—is substantial. The question of how to train deep networks in a way that is safe, fair, and aligned to human values has become a heated intellectual frontier where AI and social science meet.[31]

Deep RL systems that play Go and Atari should perhaps be relatively less prone to showing failures of common sense, because the environment they have to understand is much simpler than the natural world. But it turns out that they too are vulnerable to failures of robustness. In an eloquent critique of current deep learning models, Brenden Lake and colleagues highlight the Atari game known as *Frostbite* where the original DQN performs quite lamentably (10% of human in the original paper). *Frostbite* requires an avatar to strategically collect ice blocks and assemble them into an igloo. As the authors point out, there is no evidence that the DQN understands anything at all about the game semantics—such as the fact that there are objects in the first place (icebergs and polar bears), or what fishing is, or how jumping works, or that the goal is to build an igloo. The DQN, as we have seen, is a 'model-free' RL system that just slavishly acquires the pixels-to-action mapping that will maximize its expected return—game points—without any impetus to learn anything else about the world. A player with a rich understanding of the game should know, for example, that the colour of the background or objects in the game doesn't matter. But post-training, neural networks can be easily perturbed by changing the colour scheme used within the game—for

---

[30] See https://cs.nyu.edu/faculty/davise/papers/GPT3CompleteTests.html. However, it is important to remember that with zero-shot examples like these, where the model is provided with no context at all, it's as if you barged in on a telephone conversation and had to immediately reply appropriately to a question without knowing what was being discussed.

[31] See (Bender et al. 2021).

example, turning a yellow Pac-Man pink—whereas human gamers barely bat an eyelid.[32]

By contrast, a powerful model of Go is also what allowed AlphaGo to master the game. But even within this extremely narrow domain, it turns out that AlphaGo was prone to gross misestimations of the value of a particular board state. In fact, it was for this reason that the scorecard against Lee Sedol ended up being 4–1, and not 5–0. On move 87 in the fourth game—after a particularly stunning move by Sedol—AlphaGo lost the plot and began to spew out a train of terrible moves. As the AlphaGo team lead Dave Silver put it in an interview:[33]

AlphaGo in around one in five games would develop something which we called a delusion, which was kind of in a hole in its knowledge where it wasn't able to fully understand everything about the position [that] would persist for tens of moves throughout the game. And we knew two things. We knew that if there were no delusions then AlphaGo seemed to be playing at a level that was far beyond any human capabilities. But we also knew that if there were delusions, the opposite was true.

What we see from this critique is that AI systems—even those with rich world models—lack robustness. At first glance, they seem knowledgeable, but their grasp of a topic is soon exposed as superficial or self-contradictory. Their behaviour initially looks inventive, but their policies turn out to be thin and unreliable. They are prone to making mistakes that healthy humans would not make—would you confuse that school bus with an ostrich? Or run towards an angry-looking polar bear in a video game? It's as if their understanding of the world is like Swiss cheese—full of holes.[34]

So, is there a solution? What is needed to build an AI system that displays common sense reasoning? With what computational magic do we plug the holes in the Swiss cheese? As we shall see, this issue has become the major intellectual faultline in AI research today.

---

[32] See (Lake et al. 2017). For human performance on Atari, see (Tsividis et al. 2017).
[33] See https://www.happyscribe.com/public/lex-fridman-podcast-artificial-intelligence-ai/86-david-silver-alphago-alphazero-and-deep-reinforcement-learning.
[34] Marcus prefers the term *pointillistic*, which I think misses the point, because Seurat and his friends actually did a really robust job of conveying what is there in a visual scene.

2.4 Look, no hands!

AI researchers are humans, and humans know quite a lot about the world. Moreover, over the past century or so, scientists have learnt about how behaviour is structured and how neural systems work both in humans and other animals. In fact, this knowledge has been expanded and refined by synergies between psychology, neuroscience, and computer science. This might tempt research to try to 'build in' some of this knowledge when developing AI systems.

For example, psychologists have demonstrated that human infants enter the world with strong *inductive biases* that shape the way they understand the ways in which objects and people behave and interact, and the theories they form about causal processes in the physical and social worlds.[35] From a very young age, children tend to pay attention to the faces of other people and they prefer to look at moving, rather than static, objects, so perhaps we should bias our agents to do so as well. We know that many animals have distinct memory systems that operate over short and long time periods, so perhaps it would make sense to include that constraint in our agents. Advocates of this view argue that just as natural intelligence is tailored for the world with a set of specific choices about computation, so we should anticipate the challenges that our agents will face and build in specific solutions that we think will work.

Many people working at the frontier of cognitive science and AI research argue that we should draw inspiration from the human mind when building AI. For example, in one well-cited critique of current deep learning approaches, the authors summarize their article as follows:[36]

> We [discuss] what we view as the most plausible paths toward building machines that learn and think like people. This includes prospects for integrating deep learning with the core cognitive ingredients we identify, inspired in part by recent work fusing neural networks with lower-level building blocks from classic psychology and computer science (attention, working memory, stacks, queues) that have traditionally been seen as incompatible.

---

[35] See (Carey 2011), (Gopnik 2012), and (Spelke & Kinzler 2007).
[36] See (Lake et al. 2017).

According to this view, where our agents fall short, it is because they lack some cognitive or computational motif, characteristic of biological brains, that is vital for intelligent behaviour. Without this ingredient, it is argued, our systems will remain patchy and unreliable, forever lacking the robustness characteristic of biological behaviour.[37]

However, many AI researchers disagree sharply. Malmesbury Abbey lies in the English county of Wiltshire, where it has been a place of religious observance for over a thousand years. It is also the site of an ill-fated aeronautic experiment. In the twelfth century, a Benedictine monk—known to posteriority as Eilmer of Malmesbury—wondered if a man could fly like a bird, as suggested by tales of the mythic Greek inventor Daedalus.[38] So he fastened synthetic wings to his arms and legs and leapt into the air from the abbey tower—which was then, as it is now, many tens of metres high. Unfortunately, this early footnote to aviation history ended only slightly better for Eilmer than it did for his Greek predecessor. According to contemporary accounts, he was caught by the breeze and flew 'more than a furlong' (an impressive 200 metres) before the 'violence of the swirling air' dashed him to the ground, breaking both of his legs and leaving him permanently crippled. In later life, accounting for his failed attempt, he said that only afterwards did he realize that birds additionally need a tail for a safe landing.[39]

In the places where AI research happens today—from the plush sofas of excitable start-up companies to the corridors of academic Computer Science departments—the cautionary tale of hapless aviators like Eilmer remains staple wisdom. It is recounted in the opening chapter of the standard textbook with which most AI researchers grow up, by Peter Norvig and Stuart Russell.[40] When the goal of propelling a human safely through the air was finally achieved, beginning in the late eighteenth century with the Montgolfier brothers, it relied on hydrogen balloons, and later steam, propellors, and the combustion engine—definitely not on feathers and strap-on wings.[41] Those who have tried to copy nature tend to end up with broken dreams, broken legs, or worse. In other words, when building technology, we should not be hamstrung by the solutions that nature has chosen—and so when building AI, we would do well to ignore the solutions provided by natural intelligence. At

---

[37] We shall return to this question in Chapter 8.

[38] Whose own attempt at human-powered flight was going just fine until the sun melted the wax that held his wings together, prompting an untimely crash landing in the Aegean.

[39] See (White 1961).

[40] This one (Russell & Norvig 1995).

[41] The opening chapter of Peter Dayan's PhD thesis (Dayan 1991) starts with the following quote: 'To compare AI as mechanised flight with neuroscience as natural aviation is to ignore hot air ballooning. But where, prey, might the hot air come from?'

worst, it is a form of 'cheating' that won't pay off in the long run—it will lead to narrow, brittle solutions, rather like hiding a human operator inside a chess machine.

We can see the force of this argument driving recent advances in AI, such as large language models and MuZero, neither of which is explicitly constrained by wisdom from psychology or neuroscience. GPT-3, although it was based heavily on human *training* data, was not directly inspired by knowledge of human language systems from psychology or neuroscience. Indeed, psycholinguists have spent a great deal of time dissecting the way that humans produce sentences, use nouns and verbs, and deploy semantic or syntactic rules. They have widely assumed that there are strong cognitive constraints on language production, and that it is likely to require a dedicated subsystem. Famously, Noam Chomsky named such a system the 'language acquisition device' and sidestepped the problem of its genesis by proposing that it is already present in the neonatal brain. Even among AI researchers, it has long been supposed that because language is composed of combinations of discrete symbols, NLP systems will ultimately require a computational architecture that is more elaborate than a deep network.[42]

All these perspectives—well founded as they are—risk beginning to sound a bit quaint in light of the ability of large language models to generate coherent words, sentences, and even paragraphs by using a giant undifferentiated architecture. Moreover, the transformer—the algorithmic innovation that these models deploy so successfully—does not seem to have been directly inspired by theories from neuroscience. Unlike the components that it looks set to supersede, such as the recurrent network and the long short-term memory (LSTM) network,[43] there is as yet no evidence for memory processes homologous to the transformer in biological brains, either for language or for other cognitive functions.[44]

In fact, the question of whether AI should rely first and foremost on a computational principle—or rely on a patchwork of data, ideas, and observations conferred by the researchers—is one that is as old as AI itself. In the 1970s, the cognitive scientist Roger Schank noted that AI researchers could be loosely dichotomized as either 'neats' or 'scruffies'. The *neats*—who included many of the Dartmouth group and who envisaged an AI as a system that could reason symbolically over inputs—advocated for a minimalist research agenda based around the search for provably correct solutions. Like the architects of

---

[42] See (Lake & Baroni 2018).
[43] See Chapter 7.
[44] Although see (Whittington et al. 2021).

MuZero, they believed that their systems should learn without the polluting influence of human data. The *scruffies*, by contrast—who included early AI researchers working on language systems—favoured a piecemeal approach that matched the heterogenous set of problems encountered in the world with a diverse set of computational solutions. The very notion of 'hacking'— tinkering unsystematically with a system until it works—originated in the Massachusetts Institute of Technology (MIT) lab of Marvin Minsky (an original scruffy) in the 1960s. AI still has its neats and its scruffies—even if today the neats are more likely to appeal to searching for computational purity in a deep network, rather than a symbolic processing system.

Generally, there are three lines of argument wielded against the temptation to constrain AI systems with principles from biology. They are: (1) the case for generality; (2) the limits of human cognition; and (3) the limits of current neural theories. We will consider each in turn.

The first argument is that building AI is a general problem, and so it needs a general solution. Every constraint the AI designer relaxes makes the system more attuned to a broad class of problems—compare the multifaceted MuZero (which learns its own model) with the narrower AlphaGo Zero (whose world model was human-endowed). Here is one powerfully expressed version of this argument in a widely cited blog post by Rich Sutton.[45] Sutton is a giant in the field, whose pioneering work on RL is a cornerstone of AI research today:

> We have to learn the bitter lesson that building in how we think we think does not work in the long run. We should stop trying to find simple ways to think about space, objects, multiple agents, or symmetries ... instead we should build in only the meta-methods that can find and capture this arbitrary complexity. We want AI agents that can discover like we can, not which contain what we have discovered.

For Sutton, 'building in'—handcrafting computational constraints based on our understanding of psychology and neuroscience—is the problem, not the solution. He rues that this *bitter lesson* has still not been widely appreciated. He cites canonical examples of how progress in AI was only achieved when researchers jettisoned their intuitions. For example, chess was solved when systems that incorporated domain knowledge about gambits, forks, and skewers were replaced with massive brute force search—Deep Blue crunching 200 million moves per second against Kasparov. Similarly, computer vision took off when systems stopped entertaining handcrafted solutions that

---

[45] *The Bitter Lesson* (Sutton 2019).

identified edges or described objects with generalized polyhedrons, and instead let powerful computation and densely parameterized convolutional neural networks, such as AlexNet, do the heavy lifting.

The intellectual flight path that DeepMind has followed with AlphaGo Zero, AlphaZero, and now MuZero cleaves to Sutton's bitter lesson. It deliberately seeks to minimize the extent to which AI's achievements are kickstarted by built-in human understanding—or by copying human behaviour from big data. Perhaps no surprise, thus, that Dave Silver—the brilliant architect behind MuZero—was originally Sutton's PhD student.

The second line of argument against learning from natural intelligence is that humans might not be all that intelligent in the first place. It goes roughly as follows: the goal of AI cannot be just to *copy* humans (after all, do we need more humans? We have nearly 8 billion of them already and counting). We need to *surpass* human wit—to build something that can reason more powerfully and display more brilliant inventiveness. If we deliberately 'build in' constraints that permit human-like virtues, then we end up with human-like vices—sloppy and irrational modes of thought and decision-making, leaky memory, limited planning horizons, and unstable preferences. Humans are *limited-precision* agents—their perception, cognition, and action are corrupted by the variability inherent to a noisy nervous system. Can we not build a machine that does better?

A third line of argument asks: if we do draw upon intuitions from psychology and neuroscience when developing AI, can we be sure that any knowledge 'built in' is actually useful? In his bitter lesson, Sutton does not disparage the work done by brain scientists to unravel the mysteries of natural intelligence. Rather, his argument is purely practical: that maximally general solutions work best for building AI. Nevertheless, there is a lurking suspicion among some AI researchers that somehow, contemporary neuroscience might not be quite up to the job of explaining how brains actually work.[46] We have already seen that systems neuroscientists have mostly avoided searching for general theories, preferring instead to taxonomize computational processes in ways that abstract over the wet and messy detail of brain function. In doing so, it provides us with a new set of descriptive labels—such as *feature-based attention*, or *grid cells*, or *lateral inhibition*. But are the solution concepts implied by these labels even useful for machine learning research?

---

[46] This suspicion was not helped by Elon Musk—funder of OpenAI—who, when recruiting for researchers to work on his brain–computer interface project Neuralink, made it clear that 'No prior experience in neuroscience is necessary, we will teach you everything you need to know'.

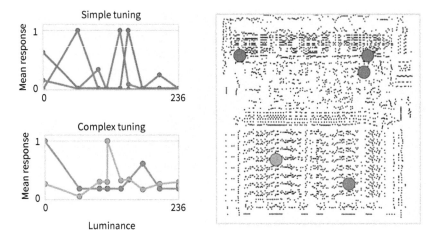

Fig. 2.2 Recording from a video game microprocessor. The authors identified simple and complex tuning functions that resembled those recorded in animals.
Reprinted from Jonas & Kording (2017).

In 2017, the neuroscientists Eric Jonas and Konrad Kording reported the results of a remarkable study that has led many to rethink their answer to this question. They applied a battery of standard neural recording and interference techniques to a model organism—including connectomics, recording of single units, and macroscopic lesioning methods—and identified familiar neural phenomena, including tuning curves, oscillations, and regional specialization of function, that have been successfully used to build theories of how the brain works (Figure 2.2). Nothing remarkable about that—except that the authors happened to know that (in this case) all those theories were entirely false, because the organism under study—a video game system microprocessor[47]—was already fully understood, as it had been designed and built by human hands. The conclusion: it is possible that the logic by which research is conducted in neuroscience—the way we draw inferences from data—might be highly misleading, and the elaborate theories that we build about neural computation—that very knowledge that Sutton warns against 'building in'—could be wide of the mark or just plain wrong.

Hand in hand with the case for mindless optimization goes the case for massive computation. Sutton himself references this in his opening sentence:

---

[47] See (Jonas & Kording 2017). In fact, the same microprocessor that was used in the Atari 2600 system whose games on which the DQN was trained.

> The biggest lesson that can be read from 70 years of AI research is that general methods that leverage computation are ultimately the most effective, and by a large margin. The ultimate reason for this is Moore's law, or rather its generalization of continued exponentially falling cost per unit of computation.

Moore's law—the principle that the power of computation should double every year, or at least the equivalent cost of computation should halve—is pronounced dead from time to time, but there is overwhelming evidence that it is alive and kicking. In fact, a recent analysis by OpenAI[48] suggests that since about 2012, the level of compute *usage* (over total pretraining time) for high-performing AI systems is now doubling every 3–4 months, rather than every 2 years, as predicted by Moore's law (Figure 2.3).

When talking about computation, the numbers involved quickly become outlandish—but let us see if we can get a sense of the scale of modern computational demands. Compute usage is now typically measured in petaflop/s-day (or pfs-day). A single pfs-day is the computation used by a system running at one petaflop—that's 10^{15} floating point operations per second—for 24 hours. For comparison, 10^{15} is slightly more than the number of synaptic connections in the adult human brain. Nearly 8 years ago, the DQN was trained for the equivalent of 38 days straight—some 50 million frames per game—using a total of less than 0.0001 of a pfs-day. By contrast, AlphaGo Zero's training can be measured in *hundreds* of pfs-days, and GPT-3 in *thousands* of pfs-days. Even if computation is relatively cheap, costs become non-trivial at these altitudes. A single training run of GPT-3 sets OpenAI back by a remarkable $12 million. But the huge sums of money sloshing around AI research—and the competitive edge entailed by ever-faster processors—mean that the computational resources available to AI researchers continue to grow and grow. The performance of Google's current tensor processing units (TPUs) is measured in *exaflops*, that is, units of 10^{18} floating point operations per second. There is also significant and growing concern around the potential environmental impact of large-scale computation in AI research.

It is worth noting again that whilst the approaches represented by GPT-3 and MuZero differ in important ways—including the role of human data and design—they are united in the mantra that bigger is better. There is also grist to the mill of the neuro-sceptical arguments above: some brains, like that of humans, are also big—very big. We do not know exactly how to quantify the running speed of biological brains—especially given that much computation may

[48] See https://openai.com/blog/ai-and-compute/#fn2.

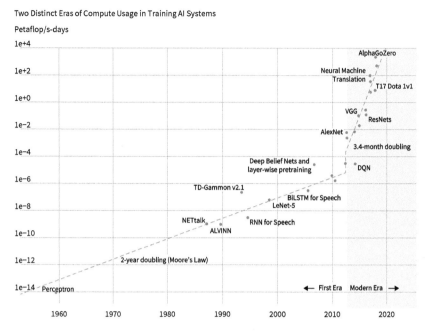

Fig. 2.3 AI and compute usage in the 'first' and 'modern' eras. The figure is from an update in November 2019. GPT-3 is missing from the plot, but it weighs in somewhere above AlphaGo Zero.

From a blog post by Amodei & Hernandez: https://openai.com/blog/ai-and-compute/.

happen at the subsynaptic[49] level—and so guesstimates vary quite wildly, anywhere from a thousand to a billion petaflops in the case of humans.[50] Could it thus be that the success of mammalian brains is not due to any careful crafting into a mosaic of different functional subsystems—but instead is merely due to size? We know, of course, that there is generally a powerful relationship between the sheer number of neurons and the complexity of behaviour that an animal produces.[51] AI researchers and neuroscientists alike—from Karl Friston to Jeff Hawkins to Andrew Ng—have flirted with the idea that there might be a single algorithm that underpins intelligence, which the brain—acting like a massive TPU—repeats ad nauseam to generate complex behaviour. Indeed, others have noted the striking conservation of the canonical microcircuit, the pattern of connections between neurons in different layers of the granular neocortex, which seems to be endlessly repeated across the

---

[49] Meaning, computation happens within neurons, rather than between neurons.
[50] See http://www.fhi.ox.ac.uk/brain-emulation-roadmap-report.pdf.
[51] See (Roth & Dicke 2005).

primate brain. If we can identify the magic pattern, and scale it really big, then perhaps that's all that is needed.

Whilst AI researchers tend to agree that more data are better, there are also divisions over the role that *human training data* play in the process of building AI. We have already encountered research drawn from opposing ends of this ideological axis. DeepMind's work on board games, spearheaded by MuZero, strives to minimize the role that human data play in training agents. Empirically, they would argue, eliminating the need to train with messy human data—for example, by switching to models that rely entirely on self-play (where the agent learns by repeatedly playing against versions of itself)—has led to substantial performance gains. Importantly, it also demonstrably led to a system that played Go with discernibly fewer delusions. The argument is that to make genuine progress, we need a system that learns entirely from computational first principles, without being potentially led astray by the attempt to copy human (mis)behaviour.

By contrast, GPT-3 embraces the fact that our human intelligence inhabits the words we use to communicate with one another in speech and written text. The very purpose of this new breed of foundation model is to predict these human data—to act like a magical mirror that distils and refracts our human culture and ideas into new and fascinating forms. It learns by churning through human data on an unprecedented scale. If it is not yet robust, that is because it is not yet big enough. Its complexity, computational power, speed, and efficiency—and the volume of data it encounters—are all still orders of magnitude lower than those of a human after decades of maturing into adulthood.

Other major efforts seek to leverage human data directly. DeepMind's *Interactive Intelligence* project has collected a massive data set from humans interacting with objects in a virtual multiroom 3D playroom, setting and solving simple tasks by using natural language (such as 'tidy the room'). An agent trained on this data set, using a mixture of supervised learning and RL, can learn to follow previously unseen instructions in strikingly human-like ways. The volume of human data is key—they collected over 600,000 episodes of up to 2 minutes long, so that agents learn through dense observation of human experts, just as infants observe reams of social interactions over the course of their development.[52]

So where does this leave us? Sutton's prescription for progress in AI is simply to reach for the computational sky—building ever-larger models on

---

[52] See (Abramson et al. 2021).

ever-faster computers. Implicitly, the vision is that by building from first principles, we will eventually end up with a sort of supercharged version of MuZero—let's call it WorldZero—that is trained to master not just Go and Atari, but also 'life' itself, strategizing not about stones or monsters, but about how to optimize global transport logistics or how to resolve an international crisis. There does not seem to be a place for insights gathered from the study of the human mind in this muscular vision of AI's future.

This debate provides a frame for the coming chapters, in which I consider the ingredients that may be needed to build an intelligent brain. I focus on four key areas: the nature of thought; how knowledge is structured and how agents can learn abstractions; the principles underlying motivated behaviour; and the functioning of memory and control processes. In each of these areas, the brain has evolved in structured ways to meet specific constraints imposed by the natural world. As we shall see, leaps and bounds in AI research, even where they look like blue-skies algorithmic innovation, have often relied on computational tools and tricks that are also found in natural intelligence. Where natural intelligence and AI have encountered the same problem, they have often identified parallel solutions. Very often, this has occurred because of a tight intellectual synergy between AI research, cognitive science, and neuroscience.

3

The language of thought

3.1 Thinking and knowing

In the opening line of a classic 1973 paper, the Canadian psychologist Zenon
Pylyshyn offers this pithy panorama of the project of cognitive psychology:[1]

> Cognitive psychology is concerned with two types of questions: What do we know?
> And how do we acquire and use this knowledge?

Pylyshyn's first question refers to the problem of representation learning: how
we know things. His second question concerns the mental operations (computations) that we perform on that knowledge: how we think.[2]

Let's begin by clarifying this distinction between *thinking* and *knowing*
through the lens of a paradigmatic challenge for early AI research: how to
build a computer that wins at chess. To find the best route to checkmate, the
computer first needs to *represent* the board state (the position of all the pieces
of each player). This task of representation formation is a memory process,
in which the observable world finds durable expression in mental contents
('knowing'). For a neuroscientist, encoding allows sensory inputs (e.g. objects and events in the real world) to drive lasting changes in neural activity
or connectivity that persist even after stimulation has ceased. It is this process
of representation that allows you to tell apart a knight from a bishop, or to
close your eyes but still envisage the board state. This allows information to be
subsequently reinstantiated in the mind's eye as the substrate of thought and
reason, or to directly prompt courses of action when similar objects or events
are encountered in the future.[3]

Secondly, the computer has to enact *operations* on those memory representations.[4] Consider a mathematical function or rudimentary programme,

---

[1] See (Pylyshyn 1973).
[2] Pylysyn also asks how we acquire that knowledge. We will consider knowledge acquisition in Chapter 4.
[3] We will discuss representation learning in more detail in Chapters 4 and 5.
[4] Some prefer the more general term 'computation' to refer to this process. However, as we shall see, for
most modern theories, the process of forming representations in the first place also involves computation,
so that term is ambiguous.

Natural General Intelligence. Christopher Summerfield, Oxford University Press. © Oxford University Press 2023.
DOI: 10.1093/oso/9780192843883.003.0003

such as $y = \cos(x^2)$. We can think of the system as encoding an input x into a mnemonic state, so that it is represented inside the function. However, to compute the output y, we then need to *transform* the encoded value of x, in this case squaring, and applying a cosine transformation. Note that this process might imply the existence of interim states of representation, such as $x' = x^2$ (when x has been squared, but the cosine has not yet been taken). The system thus needs machinery for encoding the state of x and x' (representation), and tools for converting x to x' and x' to y (computation). Returning to the case of chess, the set of lawful transformations is given by the rules of the game: a bishop cannot move along rows or columns, and a rook cannot jump over pawns. This framework allows for more complicated mental operations, such as search processes that allow the system to traverse multiple possible future states and outcomes, including hypothetical scenarios, such as moving a queen into danger. If the search is broad enough and deep enough, it offers a powerful means to identify pathways to desired outcomes—like checkmating your opponent.

As early as the 1940s, psychologists have used elite chess as a domain to ask whether human intelligence depends upon thinking (using a powerful repertoire of mental operations) or knowing (generalizing a rich represention of the board state). Do chess experts—the grandmasters with an ELO in excess of 2500—rely on an exceptional ability to think ahead, simulating how the game might play out? Or are they just good at matching board patterns to win probability—evaluating potential new configurations of pieces by generalizing their extensive knowledge from past games? Psychologists conjectured that if grandmasters rely principally on an ability to encode and generalize the board state, they will have more faithful memory for board configurations than less-seasoned players—especially when the pieces lie in lawful or plausible positions. In fact, this hypothesis has been repeatedly confirmed—and is anecdotally backed up by expert chess players' apparent ability to play blindfolded against multiple opponents, as well as by analysis of verbal transcripts suggesting that they do not consider more moves or use stronger heuristics than other players.[5]

Nevertheless, there are also suggestions that grandmasters do plan more effectively in chess. For example, stronger players are affected more than weaker players by the imposition of time pressure or by 'dual-task' manipulations that require a demanding secondary activity to be completed during game play.[6]

---

[5] See (Chase & Simon 1973).
[6] The logic being that this additional task interferes with effortful planning, but not with automatic pattern matching.

Moreover, weak players are more likely to change their mind about a candidate move when shown how an expert game unfolded from that position, as if they had been less able to anticipate the consequences of the move. Relatedly, but beyond the domain of chess, a recent paper found that when naïve humans learn to play a novel strategy game—a version of tic-tac-toe in which the board is 9×4 squares—an ability to plan more deeply accompanies their gradual gains in expertise.[7] Some 75 years after the first bite at this problem, thus, it still remains an open question of whether expertise at strategic games is best explained by deep thought or the acquisition of generalizable knowledge.

Pylyshyn's proposal is that a proper project of cognitive science is the study of these twin processes. Intelligent machines should both know and think. Humans, for example, begin in infancy by forming internal representations of things that exist in the external world, and continue learning generalizable knowledge about objects, categories, and concepts across the lifespan. As we mature, we acquire the ability to reason and plan by manipulating these representations through inference and mental simulation. As adults, we can combine these two processes and are thus able to *think about things*.

Pylyshyn is also, presciently, gesturing to the central problem in AI research today, some 50 years later. Should we build AI systems, the primary virtue of which is generalizable knowledge? Is it sufficient to train agents, for example, in the form of deep neural networks, that learn powerful abstractions from big data, that can be transferred readily to novel settings? Or alternatively, do we need to take the notion of 'thinking' seriously—in the form of strong constraints on the ways that neural computation can unfold? Should we endow agents with a sort of mental syntax that allows the calculation of truthful conclusions, the future estimation of value, or the plotting of a shortest path towards a goal, rather than simply hoping that these functions will arise from unrestricted function approximation in large-scale neural networks? On the one hand, we hear calls for a renaissance of *symbolic AI* methods, which eschew learning in favour of architectures for goal-directed planning and reasoning. These often go hand in hand with critiques of monolithic deep learning.[8] On the other hand, the ability to reason or plan might be a happy by-product of large-scale optimization but should not be built into the system as an explicit constraint. This latter view is, of course, associated with the

---

[7] Although the main driver of increasing performance was a reduction in the tendency to make silly mistakes, which might be attributable to lapses in attention and perhaps ameliorated by better encoding. See (Holding 1992) and (van Opheusden et al. 2021).

[8] For example, see (Marcus & Davis 2019).

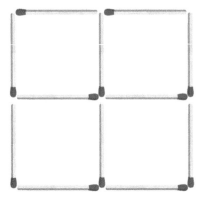

Fig. 3.1 The matchstick problem. Problem 1: can you rearrange two sticks to make seven squares? Problem 2: can you remove one stick and rearrange four to make 11 squares?

modern-day *Neats* whose mantra is to aim for zero human input and data to the AI building process.

Thinking and knowing may offer independent routes to expert task performance. To illustrate why, consider Figure 3.1, which shows a popular class of brainteaser known as a matchstick problem, where the goal is to create a different configuration by moving a small number of sticks. For example, here the challenge is to create a display that contains seven squares by moving exactly two matchsticks (and without breaking them in pieces). Can you solve it?

The puzzle might seem impossible at first—but the answer, once revealed, is surprisingly simple. Now, having cracked it (or cheated), start again from the configuration in Figure 3.1 and try to discard one matchstick and move four to make 11 squares. Although this problem is more complex, you might well find it easier, because you can recycle some of the insights gained when solving the first puzzle and apply them here. Importantly, this is possible, even though the two problems are not exactly alike.[9]

This example illustrates that there can be two distinct pathways to intelligent behaviour. If you are unfamiliar with the domain, you are obliged to think about the problem. Faced with the first matchstick problem, you were probably perplexed. You couldn't rely on past knowledge or experience to find the solution, and so you perhaps tried to mentally rearrange the sticks, internally verifying whether each move brings you nearer to the goal state. However,

---

[9] Answers are shown in Figures 3.2 and 3.3.

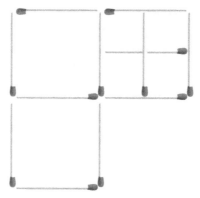

Fig. 3.2 Solution to matchstick problem 1.

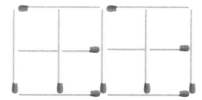

Fig. 3.3 Solution to matchstick problem 2.

once the domain is familiar, you can use past learning as a route to success. For example, if you found the second matchstick puzzle more straightforward, that wasn't because it was less complicated overall. In fact, by requiring you to move four matchsticks (and discard one), the combinatorial complexity of this problem is an order of magnitude greater than the first. Instead, it is because you were able to use existing knowledge to solve the problem.

We can trace this dichotomy back to Donald Hebb.[10] Hebb is now better remembered for defining the basic principle that neural connections are strengthened by coincident inputs—known as Hebbian learning.[11] However, he was a neuropsychologist by training and, in the 1930s, was working with brain-damaged patients at the Montreal Neurological Institute in Canada.[12] The study of patients with brain damage can offer insights into the mental structure because the brain tends to be organized into discrete, spatially separate modules, meaning that different regions perform distinct functions.

---

[10] Arguably, one could trace the origins of dual-process models of cognition back to the Islamic scholar Ḥasan Ibn al-Haytham.

[11] We shall consider Hebbian learning below.

[12] Then, as now, a world-leading brain research centre.

Thus, if patients with damage to a specific region have difficulties with ability X, but not Y, then we may infer that X and Y are distinct functions.[13] Hebb began to notice that many patients with focal brain damage had great difficulty negotiating the challenges of everyday life, but nevertheless performed remarkably well on laboratory tests that tapped into pre-existing abilities, especially assays of memory or verbal fluency.[14]

This led him to believe that Spearman's *g* could be subdivided into two components, that he defined as follows:

> It may be proposed that intellectual development includes two distinct things: (A) direct intellectual power, by neural maturation, and (B) the development of qualitative modifications of perception and behaviour. The first factor is what reaches a peak somewhere around the beginning of adolescence, declining slowly thereafter; the second is the product of the first factor.

Like Spearman, Hebb believed that there was natural variation in the raw power of the mind, which he calls Intelligence A. He referred to this as 'direct intellectual power', referencing the ability to use reasoning to solve new, unfamiliar problems. However, one happy consequence of using Intelligence A is the lifelong acquisition of new knowledge and skills, which he labelled as Intelligence B ('qualitative modifications of perception and behaviour'). Hebb argued that mental performance depends jointly on these two intellectual pathways.

3.2 Intelligences A and B

What led Hebb to this theory? Many of the patients he encountered had damage to a brain region known as the prefrontal cortex (PFC), which had been removed in a surgical procedure designed to alleviate epileptic seizures. The functional contribution of the PFC to intelligent behaviour has long perplexed researchers, as PFC damage seems to dampen intelligence in ways that are subtle or undetectable with using standard neuropsychological testing methods. Consider this early report from the pioneering neuropsychologist David Ferrier, who systematically studied the effect of frontal lobe lesions in monkeys. Writing in 1878, he concluded that:

---

[13] Especially if patients with damage to a different region have difficulties with B, but not A. This is known as a 'double dissociation'.

[14] See (Brown 2016).

The animals retain their appetites and instincts and are capable of exhibiting emotional feeling. The sensory faculties, sight, hearing, touch, taste and smell, remain unimpaired … And yet, notwithstanding this apparent absence of physiological symptoms, I could perceive a very decided alteration in the animal's character and behaviour … Instead of, as before, being actively interested in their surroundings, and curiously prying into all that came within the field of their observation, they remained apathetic, or dull, or dozed off to sleep, responding only to the sensations or impressions of the moment. While not actually deprived of intelligence, they had lost, to all appearance, the faculty of attentive and intelligent observation.

Ferrier's findings anticipated the systematic study of patients with PFC damage that followed in the twentieth century. In a classic paper from 1991, the British neuropsychologists Paul Burgess and Tim Shallice described the case of patient F.S. who, at the age of 25, had sustained damage to the PFC after having the misfortune to be thrown from a horse. The authors provide this clinical report of F.S.'s everyday life:[15]

For the past 25 years she has worked in the same position. She lives by herself in a single room. Her responses in a clinical interview show that she undertakes virtually no inessential or novel activities. She is very untidy, never putting things away. She seldom goes out in the evening, and virtually never travels away from her hometown. Others always make arrangements when any joint activity is to be carried out. She is said by her sister never to organize anything. She shops every day buying only a few things on any occasion and never visits supermarkets. She had no activity planned for the following weekend and could give no example where anyone had relied on her to do anything. Her sister confirmed that these behaviours were characteristic.

At first glance, thus, many frontal lobe patients give the impression that little is wrong. They have normal sensory perception, language, and skilled motor control. They can thus recognize faces, hold a conversation, and ride a bike. But all is not well. Frontal lobe damage often renders the patient dull, inattentive, and incurious. In fact, it was this tendency for PFC lesions to leave patients docile and compliant that inspired the development of frontal lobotomy, a controversial treatment for severe mental illness in which the frontal lobe's connections to the rest of the brain are severed.[16]

---

[15] See (Shallice & Burgess 1991).

[16] Remarkably, its pioneer and advocate, the Portuguese neurosurgeon Egas Moniz, won the 1949 Nobel Prize in Medicine for his development of the leucotomy (or lobotomy). Despite emerging evidence that many patients were harmed by the procedure, the Nobel Committee has resisted calls to rescind the award.

Over the course of the twentieth century, a theory emerged that reconciles these puzzling findings. The theory has at its core the dichotomy that Hebb first emphasized. Patients with PFC damage retain their use of Intelligence B but suffer impairment of Intelligence A. They still harbour a rich representation of the world, but their capacity to perform mental operations is severely compromised. Thus, they have no difficulty negotiating very familiar situations where they can deploy existing knowledge, such as visiting local shops. However, in novel situations, they are all at sea. They thus tend to live a tightly constrained existence, sticking to well-known places and objectives. It is *thinking* that allows healthy people to spontaneously structure behaviour in pursuit of their goals, and to consider the consequences of action or inaction. Lacking this capacity, the lives of PFC patients often descend into chaos, as patients lose their job, go bankrupt, or wind up divorced.

PFC patients can also use Intelligence B to recall past information and respond fluently to well-learnt verbal tasks, such as forming coherent sentences and spelling words correctly. Thus, they perform well on the verbal or mnemonic components of intelligence tests. In 1940, writing with Wilder Penfield,[17] Hebb reported a case of a 27-year-old man whose estimated IQ score (on the gold standard Stanford–Binet test) was found to *increase* from 83 to 94 points after bilateral removal of the frontal lobes. Many other patients scored within or above the normal range, especially on tests with a verbal component. When Burgess and Shallice assessed F.S. on standardized tests, her verbal IQ placed her among the top 1% of the population, and her performance IQ was in the top 20%; her reading score was in the top 5%, and her retention was good. Long-ingrained skills, such as the ability to pronounce or spell words correctly, were entirely intact. This pattern is common to PFC patients, many of whom are able to pass laboratory tests but fail catastrophically at everyday life.[18]

By contrast, Intelligence B depends on the store of knowledge that we have acquired over the lifetime. Hebb described it as follows:

Part of what we mean by intelligence in an adult, therefore, may consist of a store of solutions, so to speak, for common problems—points of view, methods of

---

It is ironic that mental illness was treated by deliberate damage to what was believed to be the neural seat of reason—which presumably was why it led to such unpredictable results.

[17] Penfield was later to become famous for his experiments on electrically stimulating the human neocortex.

[18] See (Shallice & Burgess 1991) and (Duncan et al. 1995).

approach, ways of seeing things. Although they are properly a product of intellectual power, they are an important part of what we call intelligence.

Hebb's insight that thinking and knowing can both lead to seemingly intelligent behaviour is vitally important for interpreting the results of psychometric
tests, because rich knowledge tends to accrue from rich life experiences.[19] This
exacerbates the problem that educational or cultural background might unduly influence measures of intelligence. As the field of psychometrics matured
in the 1930s, researchers began to search for 'culture-free' tests—measures
that are less sensitive to lifetime experience. Contemporaneous with Hebb,
the psychologist Raymond Cattell noted that tests of vocabulary or verbal reasoning were especially driven by past education and context, whereas those
involving spatial reasoning or abstract puzzle solving seemed to be more
'culture-free'. After hearing Hebb present his ideas about Intelligences A and
B at the 1941 APA conference in Evanston, Illinois,[20] Cattell hurried away and
wrote up his new theory: that we should think of Spearman's g as subdivisible
into *fluid* and *crystallized* intelligence. Fluid intelligence measures raw intellectual potential. People with high fluid intelligence excel at reasoning about
abstract concepts or ideas in a way that depends minimally on experience,
and thus do well on so-called 'culture-free' tests.[21] By contrast, crystallized intelligence indexes extant knowledge and skills, acquired via comprehensive
acculturation or a well-rounded education.[22] In fact, this dichotomy sounds
suspiciously similar to that proposed by Hebb, an intellectual debt that Cattell
acknowledges in their later epistolary correspondence.[23] However, it is the terminology of fluid and crystallized intelligence—and Cattell's name—that pos-
terity associates with this distinction. This reminds us of a timeless dictum: if
you want your theory to be widely recognized, be sure to give it a catchy name.

Baffled by the disconnection between everyday competence and measured
IQ, Hebb and Penfield pondered different approaches that might better index
an individual's true abilities, and how they are impaired by brain injury:

> For the effect of lesions of the frontal lobe on human intelligence, it seems that one
> will have to look elsewhere than to clinical observation or ratings by intelligence

---

[19] Which, in turn, are more common for rich people.

[20] American Psychological Association.

[21] This is discussed in detail below.

[22] According to psychological lore, the two vary over the lifespan, with fluid intelligence declining (rather
depressingly) from about age 20, but with crystallized intelligence sustaining you well beyond middle age.
Indeed, it is sometimes claimed that most great new mathematical ideas—perhaps the ultimate fruits of
fluid intelligence—were worked out by mathematicians in their twenties.

[23] See (Brown 2016).

tests such as are now available [...] perhaps by studying learning in social situations, in adaptation to drastic environmental change or in initiative and the ability to plan and organize one's affairs may be found in the impairment that we believe must exist after large lesions of the frontal lobes.

In other words, to measure general intelligence, we need tests that are grounded in the true complexities of everyday life, by measuring social skills or personal organization. We need to measure street smarts, not just lab smarts. Hebb is thus anticipating the argument made above: that we need a generous definition of intelligence, one that encompasses both the quotidian and the rarefied—one that taps into our versatility at solving everyday tasks at home as much as our ability to master complex calculations or understand esoteric language in the lab.

For frontal lobe patients, this vision became a reality in the 1990s, when Burgess and Shallice quantified their everyday difficulties by effectively turning a London high street into a giant neuropsychological testing suite. They sent patients (all of whom were unfamiliar with the street, including F.S.) out to perform a series of everyday errands, such as shopping for a loaf of bread, finding out the weather forecast, or obtaining directions to the railway station. In the paper describing their findings, the results section offers a detailed account of the chaos that ensued. Consistent with the idea that the PFC is critical to the ability to reason in pursuit of everyday goals, patients found this 'multiple errands' task extremely challenging and some barely completed the tasks with their dignity or liberty from the law intact.

This everyday difficulty in controlling behaviour is reminiscent of one of the earliest and most celebrated PFC patients, known as Phineas Gage. In 1848, whist working on the railroads in Canada, an explosion blew iron tamping rod entirely through the front of his brain like a javelin. Remarkably, he survived—but reportedly, the injury led to significant changes in character, accompanied by minimal other psychological problems. It was claimed that prior to the injury he had been sensible and mild mannered, but after he became restless, profane, obstinate, and capricious 'to the extent that his society was intolerable to decent people'. It is as if—from one moment to the next—Gage lost the ability to reason about his situation and behaviour.[24]

Hebb's ideas—and a hundred years of empirical study of the PFC—thus expose a fundamental conundrum in the definition and measurement of intelligence. We can create a battery of tests in the lab—whether they are

---

[24] Although there are credible reports that Gage's deficits were, in fact, short-lived and that he was rehabilitated back into work and society after some years.

pencil-and-paper tests of reasoning or testing suites for AI systems—but we lack guarantees that they will correlate with competence in performing open-ended activities in the real world such as shopping, submitting your taxes, or debating politics. This paradox is revealed by the difficulties of prefrontal pa-tients who can seemingly exhibit normal IQ but fail to show the *quotidian polymathy* that is typical of healthy people the world over. This occurs, in part, because PFC damage curtails their ability to think. It attenuates the mental flexibility required to solve new problems but leaves intact knowledge of how to perform existing tasks. Thus, PFC patients can exhibit strong—even superlative—performance within a narrow range of activities, just like an AI system that is trained to master a circumscribed suite of environments but flops on tests that fall outside this set. This is the complaint of excoriating critics, such as Gary Marcus, who lambast AI systems that excel at the narrow problems they are set by machine learning researchers but fail catastrophically when confronted with the messy reality of the natural world.

3.3 The units of thought

Throughout the second half of the twentieth century, cognitive scientists and AI researchers were mostly concerned with the nature of thought. What does it mean to think? In what formal language does thinking happen, and what are its syntactic rules? How do formal systems of thought relate to the natural language that humans use to communicate? Is our thinking driven by a sparse set of provably correct, innately specified lo-gical precepts, or are the units of thought mental states with rich represen-tational content—beliefs, desires, and intentions? How are the operations of thought constrained by the semantics of the real world and the words we use to describe it?

Over the decades, different answers to these questions have come in and out of vogue. These include both the purist conception that thinking is reducible to propositional logic, and the idea that thought is nothing but an inner echo of our outer speech, phrased in the natural language we have learnt from so-cial others. Today, in the grip of the deep learning revolution, these traditional conceptions of *thinking* have slipped out of fashion altogether. But the roots of these twentieth-century ideas about the language of thought continue to mould our contemporary theories of computation. In particular, one tradition sees inference as a search process through a densely interconnected web of hypothetical experience, that allows us to envisage the future consequences of our actions. This idea, which can be traced back to the 1940s, is an intellectual ancestor to today's advanced systems for model-based RL such as AlphaGo and MuZero. In the remainder of this chapter, we will trace the historical contours of these ideas across the twentieth century in the fields of cognitive science and AI research.

The idea that thinking (or reasoning) is the signature quality of the human mind inhabits a rationalist tradition that dates back to the ancient Greeks. Historically, to reason is to direct the flow of mental process down coherent paths that respect the proper order of things in the external world, rendering our thoughts coherent, intelligible, and plausible. Reasoning allows conclusions to be drawn, relations to be inferred, and forthcoming states to be predicted. Descartes famously premised the edifice of human cognition on our ability to reason when he wrote:

> I am therefore precisely nothing but a thinking thing; that is a mind, or intellect, or understanding, or reason.

For two millennia, philosophers and mathematicians have sought to define the principles by which valid reasoning should occur. This process began with Aristotle, who initiated the study of formal logic with a series of treatises collectively entitled *Organon*. In this work, he laid out his theory of deduction (sullogismos) and introduced us to the 64 syllogisms with a tripartite structure,[25] for example those with the following form:

> No machines are clever.
> 'Deep Everything' is a machine.
> 'Deep Everything' is not clever.

In the nineteenth century, these foundations for logical calculus were refined and generalized by George Boole,[26] whose masterwork *The Laws of Thought* introduced a new formalism for inference that grounded logic in algebra and showed that just three operations—conjunction (AND), disjunction (OR), and negation (NOT)—allowed for remarkably expressive reasoning over dichotomous (or, subsequently, 'Boolean') states. By the early twentieth century, advocates of *logical positivism* (such as Russell, Whitehead, and Frege) embarked on a quest for the logical axioms underlying mathematics itself. Russell

---

[25] Of which 24 are valid.
[26] Boole also happens to be the great-great-grandfather of Geoffrey Hinton, the most significant pioneer of the deep neural network.

and Whitehead's contributions to this project resulted in the epic philosophical tome known as *Principia Mathematica*, which was never completed and
cost the authors their friendship and (almost) their sanity. Nevertheless, it was
on these currents of thought that the first modern theories of the mind sailed
into view. The notion that thinking is grounded in logical principles, and that
logic itself can be described with mathematical calculations, inspired Turing's
vision in the 1930s for a thinking machine that runs programmes on input
data—the idea that launched modern computer science.[27]

The first wave of AI researchers in the 1950s had grown up steeped in this
rationalist tradition. This was the era when the first electronic computers were
incorporating the von Neumann architecture and the Dartmouth Ten con-
vened to solve AI in a single summer. For these pioneers, the tools of logical
calculus developed by Boole were natural primitives for a syntax of thought.
The units of mentation were proposed to be abstract tokens such as p and q in
the logical proposition *if p then q*, and mental processes to implicitly or explicitly compute the truth conditions that follow from a set of premises. Thinking
was reduced to a process of deductive inference.

Post-war AI researchers thus constructed programs with hard-coded
mental machinery for articulated reasoning and theorem proving. The goal
of these systems was to establish the truth or validity of statements expressed
in logical form. They thus took propositions and arguments as inputs, and
furnished statements and conclusions as outputs. Even the first neural networks, constructed in the 1940s by Pitts and McCulloch, were devices for
implementing logical calculus through a series of interconnected gates. They
allowed a machine, for the first time, to derive outcomes on the basis of AND,
OR, and NOT—realizing Boole's ideas about the algebra of logic in a realistic
circuit diagram.[28]

The ability to prove theorems was a high watermark for this new breed of
AI systems. In 1955, on the eve of the Dartmouth conference, two key figures in early AI research—Alan Newell and Herb Simon—unveiled the
'Logic Theorist', a programme designed to prove the axioms in Chapter 2 of
Whitehead and Russell's *Principia Mathematica*. It identified proofs for 38 of
the 52 theorems, including one novel proof (2.85) more elegant than that discovered by the original authors. Newell and Simon attempted to publish this
finding with the computer as a co-author, but rather unfairly, the paper was
rejected for being insufficiently novel.

[27] See (Bernhardt 2017).
[28] See (McCulloch & Pitts 1943).

The idea that logic was the substrate of intelligent thought was nourished by the study of the developing human mind. In the 1950s, the Swiss psychologist Jean Piaget proposed his own theory of intelligence, in which cognitive growth is a trajectory from confusion to reason.[29] His four-stage theory of development argues that human intellectual maturation occurs as the child acquires the ability to perform ever more complex 'operations' by drawing logical conclusions from data. In the *preoperational* stage, which Piaget believed lasted until about the age of 7 years, children fail at making basic inferences, such as reporting transitivity (e.g. that if object A is bigger than B, and B is bigger than C, then A must be bigger than C). During that transition to *concrete* operations, which (according to Piaget) lasts until about 12 years of age, deductive and inductive processes gradually emerge. For example, children begin to understand the laws of conservation, that is, that if a quantity of liquid is poured from one beaker to another, its volume does not change, even if (for example) the second beaker is taller and narrower. By 9 or 10 years old, they can solve various types of syllogistic reasoning problems. However, it is not until their teenage years that the final maturational milestone—known as 'formal operations'—is reached. A child who has reached formal operations can reason in adult-like ways, to the extent that they can entertain counterfactual or hypothetical states of the world.[30]

Formal operations enable the sort of causal reasoning shown by scientists studying the factors that influence a dependent variable, such as when testing the link between smoking and heart disease. In a classic study, Piaget and his collaborator Bärbel Inhelder asked schoolchildren to determine which of three factors (length of a string, heaviness of a weight, or initial propulsion) influenced a variable of interest (the speed at which a pendulum swings). By their teenage years, children begin to autonomously reason from cause to effect, without any prior knowledge about the physics of the problem.[31] For example, they know that one must hold all other factors constant to test the association among variables in a systematic fashion (e.g. *if the string is long, the pendulum swings slowly*). This contrasts with a child in the preceding concrete operations stage, who will be hidebound by the immediate evidence of the senses—so that if a large weight on a long string swung more slowly than

[29] Whilst Piaget remains a mainstay of undergraduate psychology courses, the developmental trajectory and time course that he proposed have since been radically refined. Because his observations were based on linguistically demanding interactions with children, he may have grossly underestimated how quickly children acquire the ability to reason. Causal reasoning may, in fact, emerge at 3–5 years, and there is evidence that even very young infants are surprised by violations of causation (Gopnik & Wellman 2012).

[30] See (Bara et al. 1995).

[31] Piaget proposed that formal operations begin at about 12 years of age (on average). However, subsequent research has found that most children do not pass the pendulum test until aged 13–17 years.

a small weight on a short string, they might infer that the weight was critical, overlooking the fact that string length is a confounding variable. Upon reaching the formal operations stage—from adolescence onwards—we can reason logically, even about possibilities that seemingly defy the reality of the senses. For Piaget, this type of scientific reasoning process signals that cognitive abilities have reached their zenith.

The link between rationality and intelligence also shaped how mental ability was measured. Since the 1930s, psychologists had found that tests of abstract spatial reasoning were among the most 'culture-free'—the least prone to depending on educational background. One 'culture-free' assessment that has stood the test of time is known as Raven's Progressive Matrices (RPM) after its inventor John Raven. First published in 1938, RPM is solved by reasoning about the number, position, identity, or relation of visual attributes that make up a display. Each problem consists of a 3 × 3 array of boxes, with a pattern of objects occurring over rows and columns, but with a single box left empty (Figure 3.4). The test requires the participant to correctly choose an item to fill the missing box, by combining two logical constraints: one which determines how the pattern changes across rows, and another which controls how it varies across columns. To give a simple example, if there is a progression of three, two, and one items across successive columns, and variation in item size, from big to medium to small, across rows, then even if the final row/column entry is missing, one can infer that it should contain one small item.

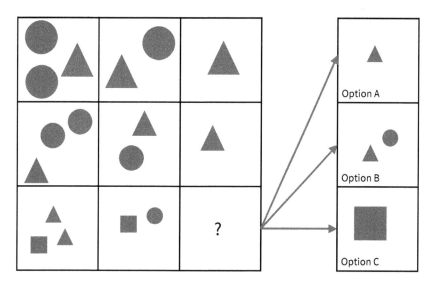

Fig. 3.4 Example of RPM problem. The relevant dimensions are size (rows) and number (columns). The correct answer is option A.

In line with the view that the ability to reason is the magic ingredient that furnishes human intelligence, Raven (and other early theorists) considered RPM to provide a nearly 'pure' measure of Spearman's *g*.[32]

Note that in RPM, the objects are denuded of meaning, because shapes are matched randomly with relational rules. Making a problem abstract in this way ensures it can only be solved by thinking, and not by knowing. For example, if I tell you that all *toops* are *nomps*, and all *nomps* are *sinky*, and ask you whether a *toop* is *sinky*, you might have to think about it for a moment. On the other hand, if we replace the three nonsense words with 'robin', 'bird', and 'lay eggs', then the abstract problem becomes concrete—it can be answered by using basic facts about birds, rather than using the rules of syllogistic logic alone. Similarly, the fact that an empty box lacks four red squares cannot be deduced from the fact that they are red and squares; the features are entirely arbitrary. Thus, by using abstract test items, RPM seeks to remove any traces of specific cultural or educational experience from a participant's test performance. This is also in keeping with the philosophy of classical AI research, in which inputs are arbitrary and the raw power of reason is the engine of intelligence. Indeed, RPM has perennially proved a useful test bed for classical AI architectures.[33]

By the 1970s, shoulder to shoulder with AI researchers, psychologists were building computer programs that reasoned over logical propositions.[34] Unlike most AI researchers, however, they were also curious about how the machine performance mirrored that of humans tasked with judging the validity of statements defined by propositional connectives (AND, OR, NOT, NOR). This research programme was aimed at testing whether symbolic AI systems reasoned in human-like ways, by comparing their patterns of success and failure on a battery of logical reasoning problems.

For example, Lance Rips and colleagues built a system known as ANDS that took arguments and assertions as inputs and was tasked with verifying the validity of conclusions using a bank of logical rules that had been hand-coded by the researchers.[35] Rips considered ANDS to be a plausible model of how people think. Consider the following item from their experiment: 'if the valve is closed or the button is pressed, then the wheel turns, and the bulb is illuminated'. Is it then true that if the valve is closed, then the bulb is illuminated? You probably found deducing the validity of this statement to be quite

---

[32] See (Raven 2000).
[33] For example, see (Hernández-Orallo et al. 2016).
[34] Mostly using the computational lingua franca of the day, a coding language known as LISP.
[35] See (Rips 1983).

straightforward. Now consider a different item: 'either Peter is in Chicago or Paul is in Baltimore, but if Peter is in Chicago or Martha is in Kansas, then Paul is in Baltimore'. Is it then true that Paul is in Baltimore? You may well have found this one trickier. The participants certainly did, responding 'valid' about 80% of the time to the former and 30% to the latter (in fact, both are valid). Overall, the model did a fairly good job of predicting the percentage accuracy of validity judgements made by human participants over 32 classes of such problems. Rips interpreted these data as showing that human reasoning relies on the same mental primitives as classic AI theorem-proving programs, and thus that this algorithmic approach was on track to emulate human intelligence.[36]

The idea that propositional logic is the basic substrate of intelligent thought has an appealing simplicity. Philosophers and computer scientists alike know that logic can be used to infer what is true. Organisms that can diagnose truth from falsehood are likely to have a selective advantage, so it makes sense to propose that evolution should have paved the way for logical minds. In the 1970s and 1980s, however, three developments occurred that changed the way in which the field thought about thinking. Firstly, the idea emerged that the units of thought are not simply abstract propositions, but mental states with representational content, such as beliefs, desires, and intentions, and that thinking is, at least partly, grounded in language. Secondly, an empirical research programme, famously led by Daniel Kahneman and Amos Tversky, cast serious doubt on the rationality of human inference, suggesting instead that people are prone to reasoning sloppily, drawing conclusions by using heuristics that are fast and frugal, but prone to err. Thirdly, there was an upswell of interest in the idea that computation in the brain is inherently probabilistic. Together, these trends shaped our modern vision for the language of thought—before the deep learning revolution arrived—and cast doubt on the necessity of *thinking* itself.

3.4 The symbolic mind

Psychologists have long suspected that thinking and talking share a common mental substrate. A deep theoretical root to this idea is known as *linguistic*

---

[36] Unfortunately, however, in order to capture the human data, Rips was obliged to make numerous ad hoc assumptions about the cognitive demands associated with different sorts of logical operations (e.g. asserting that inferring disjunction is harder than conjunction, without explaining why). His results are considerably less impressive once one realizes that the model uses ten free parameters to fit 32 data points. This weakened claims about ANDS and other comparable architectures for logical reasoning.

relativity—the hypothesis that our private version of reality is directly shaped by interaction with our linguistic communities. This view can be traced back to the linguist Benjamin Lee Whorf who, in the 1930s, wrote:

> the world is . . . a kaleidoscope flux of impressions which has to be organized by our minds—and this means largely by the linguistic systems of our minds. We cut nature up, organize it into concepts, and ascribe significances as we do, largely because we are parties to an agreement to organize it in this way . . . throughout our speech community.

Whorf's ideas crystallized during his study of the language systems of North American ethnic groups—including the Inuit and Hopi people—whose mental and lexical taxonomies were both radically different from those of European heritage. For example, the Hopi people considered water in a cup to be a different entity from water in a lake, and they used distinct nouns in each case. Other linguistic groups expressed space, time, and number in terms that seemed deeply alien to Whorf, but that he believed betrayed their very different ways of navigating, counting, and conceiving of the past and future. Together with his mentor Edward Sapir, this led him to the view that language was the mental substrate in which thinking happens.[37]

Whorf's work launched an empirical research programme that asked whether differences in basic perception or cognition arise from our linguistic heritage. For example, is it true that peoples whose counting system consists of numbers one to three and then 'many' cannot actually conceptualize cardinalities of four and above? Can communities with the colour terms black, white, and red not distinguish green and blue hues? However, the outcome of this research programme was a growing scepticism about strong forms of linguistic relativity,[38] and a growing sense that whilst our world knowledge may be shaped by natural language, we are not tightly constrained to perceive or internally reason about the world using the spoken word.

At the same time as Whorf was studying Native American languages, on the other side of the Iron Curtain,[39] the Soviet psychologist Lev Vygotsky was formulating a theory in which language and thought are reciprocally reinforcing during cognitive development. According to Vygotsky, private mentation grows out of early social exchanges in natural language (we think because

---

[37] See (Whorf & Carroll 2007).
[38] See (Regier et al. 2005).
[39] Or what was to become known as the Iron Curtain. Churchill first used the phrase in this context in 1945.

we speak), but this, in turn, hastens language development (we speak because we think). Vygotsky proposed that after practising external communication through repeated exchanges with a caregiver ('Where is the cat? Oh! There is the cat'), the child learns to hold a sort of internal conversation with itself, which, in turn, kickstarts the ability to reason. Indeed, as every parent knows, children go through a phase of narrating their thoughts aloud whilst playing. Even adults report the occurrence of a covert inner monologue when planning, solving problems, or keeping information in mind. For example, you might do this when imagining a future conversation with your boss or rehearsing a phone number in memory.[40]

However, whilst the use of private speech has been intensively investigated from childhood to adulthood, there is minimal evidence that it plays a strong functional role in cognition. Instead, it might just be an echo of thought processes occurring in a deeper, more expressive language in which thinking actually occurs. In fact, Vygotsky did not claim that thinking literally reduces to inner speech. Rather, he argued that language is transformed during internalization—concepts become semantically enriched, self-referential, and compressed, so that our thinking occurs in a special sort of mental language, different from that used externally.[41]

For several decades, psychologists and AI researchers had relied on pure logic as a model for how people think. But the 1970s brought a major pivot towards the idea that the proper units of thought are mental states with a rich representational content—our beliefs, desires, and intentions about the world. We primarily owe this turn to the swashbuckling philosopher and cognitive scientist Jerry Fodor who, in his 1975 book *Language of Thought*, argued that we think in an internal coding system called *mentalese*. In mentalese, thinking consists of chains of discrete mental events, each of which instantiates (or *tokens*) a hypothetical state of the world, thereby bringing it to mind. Mentalese resembles language as being composed of complex symbols amenable to semantic analysis. Chains of thoughts respect coherent semantics, allowing symbolic reasoning ('the incumbent will lose the election because her tax policy is unpopular') by using a higher-order form of logic that admits predicates, quantifiers, and logical connectives, rather than just true or false propositions. Mentalese is also argued to be compositional, meaning that sophisticated thoughts can be assembled from simple building blocks, for example via recursion ('the man voted for the senator that voted for the tax cut').

---

[40] Although whether inner speech is functionally significant for cognition remains controversial (Alderson-Day & Fernyhough 2015).

[41] He describes inner speech as having a 'note-form' quality.

However, mentalese lacks morphology and phonology, making it different from the natural language we use to share thoughts with each other.

Whilst Fodor was formulating his theory, scruffy AI researchers were busy in the lab, trying to build program systems that could think and communicate in simplified natural language. By the 1960s and 1970s, some programs could express inferences about their environment using a limited vocabulary. For example, Terry Winograd's SHRDLU program[42] could reason symbolically about blocks in a virtual 3D world, using a restricted vocabulary to answer queries such as 'what is the colour of the pyramid that is on top of the large red cube?'. Similarly, ELIZA was an early teletherapeutic system—a program designed to reason about medical symptoms and offer diagnoses in natural language. In practice, however, computers were too slow to handle the vast expressiveness and open-endedness of human language, and these systems ended up using simple, formulaic expressions. ELIZA, for example, was prone to mindlessly parroting the user's statements back to them as questions or to blandly repeating 'tell me more', like a sort of chin-stroking mechanized quack. The time for strong NLP had not yet arrived.

However, this research programme gave birth to a class of AI known as *expert systems*. Expert systems are computer programs designed to emulate or support human decision-making, using large, hand-curated databases of human knowledge and preordained semantic reasoning principles (this dichotomy follows Pylyshyn's prescription that a mind should have separate modules for knowing and thinking). One of the most ambitious projects, known as Cyc, debuted in the 1980s. Even in this early era, it was already recognized that building systems capable of human common-sense reasoning was an important goal.[43] To achieve this, the Cyc team began to codify—in machine-usable form—millions of bits of information that humans use to reason sensibly about the world. The idea was that with enough pieces and a strong reasoner, Cyc would ultimately solve the jigsaw of human common sense.

For example, imagine I tell you that Freda is a frog.[44] Does Freda live in the desert? To solve this, you might reason that frogs usually live by water, so

---

[42] One of Winograd's PhD students, Larry Page, went on to co-found Google.

[43] Minsky wrote in 1974: 'We still know far too little about the contents and structure of common-sense knowledge. A 'minimal' common-sense system must 'know' something about cause–effect, time, purpose, locality, process, and types of knowledge . . . we need a serious epistemological research effort in this area' (Minsky 1979).

[44] This example is taken from (Lenat et al. 1990).

perhaps the answer is no. Cyc handles this sort of query using a similar process, by drawing on hand-coded knowledge from its prodigious memory:

```
IF frog(x) THEN amphibian(x)
IF amphibian(x) THEN laysEggsInWater(x)
IF laysEggsInWater(x) THEN livesNearLotsOf(x, Water)
If livesNearLotsOf(x, Water) THEN ¬ livesInDesert(x)
```

Thus, Cyc agrees that frogs do not live in the desert. Unfortunately, the world is complex and full of exceptions, so codifying human knowledge by hand is nightmarishly impractical. In his satirical travelogue *Gulliver's Travels*, Jonathan Swift parodies the endeavour of assembling the world's knowledge from scraps of information. Gulliver visits the Grand Academy of Lagnado where he finds a professor tending to a machine that generates random sentences in the native language:

> which he intended to piece together, and out of those rich materials, to give the world a complete body of all arts and sciences.

Indeed, whilst Cyc's reasoning about frogs and deserts may appear sound, it could well be wrong. The deserts of Western Australia are home to at least 19 species of frog, most of whom survive by burrowing underground during the dry months, waiting for the rains to fall.

By the early 2000s, computers had become larger and more powerful, and querying algorithms were faster and more efficient. This meant that expert systems—cobbled together with human-curated knowledge bases, search, verification, and quasi-symbolic reasoning processes—began to respond reliably to queries in circumscribed domains. For example, expert systems were developed that supported clinicians in making medical decisions (cognitive prostheses), greatly increasing diagnostic accuracy and potentially saving thousands of lives. However, the ultimate challenge—to respond to open-ended queries about the world spanning any topic or theme—remained elusive.

However, in early 2011, viewers of the TV quiz game show *Jeopardy!* were astonished by the news that one of the players in a forthcoming show would be a computer designed by IBM, pitted against two of the most successful past contestants. *Jeopardy!* is a game show with a twist—on each round, the quizmaster provides an answer and the players have to propose the questions. Competing for cash, players can wager on their replies, placing a high

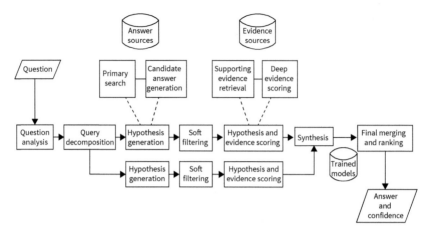

Fig. 3.5 The architecture for Deep QA, which Watson used to triumph at *Jeopardy!* in 2011.

premium on having a well-calibrated sense of confidence about the answers—an area where AI systems have traditionally fallen short. For more than three years, IBM had been working towards this challenge, and their question answering (QA) system Watson had been endowed with an encyclopaedic knowledge base that included all of Wikipedia, reams of newswire, and shelves full of the world's great literary works (Figure 3.5). Impressively, Watson triumphed, beating human rival Ken Jennings, whose unbroken 74-game winning streak had made him the most successful *Jeopardy!* player of all time. Watson took home three times as many points as its opponents and bagged the overall prize pot of a million dollars. However, like other modern systems, it was not inviolable—for example, in answering one question, it gave the impression that it believed that Chicago was in Canada. IBM's hybrid symbolic approach continues to bear fruit, and today they are working on systems that can compete in debating contests.[45]

Thus, over the latter part of the twentieth century, AI researchers entertained both logic- and language-based conceptions of the formal system in which thinking happens. These approaches differed in their neatness (should thinking be governed by rational first principles?) and scruffiness (or should thinking be bounded by what we actually say and see in the real world?). However, they shared the vision that thinking is *symbolic* in nature.

---

[45] See (Slonim et al. 2021). IBM would probably agree that this is a work in progress.

A *symbol* is a representation that refers to an entity in a discrete and arbitrary way.[46] For example, the spoken or written word 'bird' in English denotes that category of animal through a physical medium—a pulse of air or a scratch on a page—that does not bear any iconic (or image-like) resemblance to actual birds.[47] This arbitrariness means that symbols denoting other concepts that share features with birds (like bats) are no more similar to the bird symbol than those denoting different concepts entirely (like bricks). This characteristic of symbolic representations means that they necessarily discard information about the concept they denote. For example, 'birds' of many different shapes and sizes can all be denoted by a single symbol, so that the symbol sheds details about specific features, identities, or contexts that may be important for behaviour (such as whether its referent is a starling or a penguin).

Symbolic AI systems perform mental operations on knowledge. However, the representations that they process bear an arbitrary relationship to the objects and events to which they refer. Unlike in neural networks (and in biological brains), the meaning of items in memory is not signalled by their coding format. Thus, the inference engine cannot use the form or content of the representation to determine how to reason about it. For example, in early theorem-proving systems, inputs were abstract tokens (such as p and q), the meaning of which was entirely external to the system. The theorem provers crunched the proposition of '*if p then q*' in exactly the same way when p and q denote *Aristotle is a man* and *Aristotle is mortal* as when they mean *Aristotle is a goat* and *Aristotle is Scottish*. The computations are unaffected by the nature of p and q, and are instead built into the systems as a set of immutable operations.

Similarly, expert systems encode knowledge, painstakingly gleaned by human researchers and hand-coded into memory. However, like theorem provers, the way in which they reason is blind to the semantic content of the memory representation. Thus, Cyc applies the rule IF frog(x) identically when x is a frog and when it is a bicycle. Symbols are fundamentally arbitrary—this arbitrariness means that they are all equally similar to, and dissimilar from, each other, irrespective of what they represent. Fodor has called this the *formality condition*—that mental processes have access only to formal

---

[46] I take this definition of *symbol* from Peirce. I elaborate in Chapter 4. For a comprehensive introduction, see https://plato.stanford.edu/entries/peirce-semiotics/. Note, of course, that words may not be purely symbolic, in that their sensory properties (phonetics or orthographics) may bear a non-arbitrary relation to their referent. For example, Wolfgang Köhler (whom we discuss below) was the first to document that people exhibit systematic biases in the way they map shapes onto nonsense words, for example reporting that a spiky shape is more likely to be called 'kiki' than 'bouba', an vice versa for a curved shape.

[47] We owe the distinction between symbolic representations (which are arbitrary) and iconic representations (which share features with the represented object) to the philosopher Charles Peirce.

(non-semantic) properties of the mental representations over which they are defined.[48]

For many decades, there were high hopes for purely symbolic approaches to AI. Towards the end of their careers, Newell and Simon received the Turing Award for their pioneering contributions to computing. They used their 1975 award paper to flesh out what they called the 'physical symbol system hypothesis' (PSSH) which states that:

> A physical symbol system [such as a digital computer, for example] has the necessary and sufficient means for intelligent action . . . [and] the symbolic behaviour of man arises because he has the characteristics of a physical symbol system.

thereby asserting a direct link between intelligence and symbolic reasoning in both humans and machines.

Today, however, the era of symbolic architectures has largely passed. Among advocates of contemporary deep learning, they are often dismissed as outdated, and lumped under the slightly patronizing moniker *Good Old-Fashioned AI* (GOFAI). This is mainly because the intervening years have revealed that early symbolic systems suffered a fundamental limitation. This limitation stems from the nature of symbols themselves—because they are fundamentally arbitrary, the information that they carry is established by convention. Symbols thus have meaning imposed upon them by fiat. In symbolic AI systems, researchers simply assert their correspondence to the real world without ever requiring the system to 'know' anything about their environment. For example, researchers chose what p and q denoted—assigning meaning to the symbols from their own (human) semantic repertoire. Symbolic AI researchers thus sidestepped the first of Pylyshyn's two questions ('What do we know?') by denying the systems the opportunity to learn their own symbols from experience. Philosophers usually refer to this as the *symbol grounding problem*.[49] Fodor prefers more colourful language, arguing that the formality condition leads to 'methodological solipsism':

> If mental processes are formal, then they have access only to the formal properties of such representations of the environment as the senses provide. Hence, they have no access to the semantic properties of such representations, including the property of being true, of having referents, or, indeed, the property of being representations of the environment.

---

[48] See (Fodor 1980).
[49] See (Harnad 1990).

Whilst the symbol grounding problem is theoretical, it has important ramifications in practice. For example, when SHRDLU is posed the verbal question 'Is the red cube behind the green pyramid?', this activates a set of symbols in its memory that the researcher has arbitrarily assigned to colours and shapes in the block world. But there was nothing that grounded the meaning of these objects ('green' or 'cube') in the blocks that were physically present in the array. SHRDLU and its fellow symbolic systems did not learn representations from input data. Instead, they had them handed on a plate. This makes symbolic AI systems forever parasitic on human knowledge, grossly limiting their expressiveness and potential for creativity. For example, SHRDLU had a vocabulary of only about 50 verbal concepts and no way of acquiring others, except by researcher handcrafting, so unless the researcher added the symbol 'pink', then it could not express anything about pink blocks. Increasing awareness of the symbol grounding problem led to heightened interest in AI systems that learn their own concepts, rather than purloin those of the researcher.[50]

Nevertheless, this bygone age of symbolic AI laid important foundations for future theories of intelligence. One pathway by which ideas were handed forward was through the development of systems capable of instrumental means-end reasoning and the parallel study of goal-directed behaviour in psychology and neuroscience.

3.5 Mental models

On 7 May 1945, two days before the end of the war in Europe, the director of the Applied Psychology Unit in Cambridge, UK, was cycling past King's College when he collided with an open car door. Thrown from his bicycle, he was struck unconscious by a passing lorry and died later that night. He had just published his first book *The Nature of Explanation*, which married philosophy and psychology to articulate a new theory of the human mind. His name was Kenneth Craik and he was just 31 years old.

Throughout the first half of the twentieth century, psychology had been dominated by *behaviourism*, the school of thought that reduces all psychological processes to the acquisition of habitual links between inputs and outputs. As the war ended, this movement was still in its heyday. In 1950, the radical behaviourist B. F. Skinner wrote an influential article entitled '*Are theories of learning necessary?*', arguing that we should dispense with conjecture

---

[50] See (Garnelo & Shanahan 2019).

about the invisible changes in mental state that occur as learning progresses and instead focus exclusively on the observables—variables manipulated, and data collected—lights, tones, shocks, rewards, and lever presses.[51] But a new era was just around the corner, driven by Craik and other contemporaries. In psychology and philosophy, the theoretical pendulum was swinging away from behaviourist models and towards *mentalist* models of the mind, which proposed instead that thinking itself could be described in the mechanical language of information processing.

In his book, Craik rejected the doctrine that learning relies on stick and carrot alone. Imagine building a bridge, he argued. The notion that the optimal design could be achieved by trial and error is absurd. Instead, it is planned meticulously in advance by an engineer with knowledge of bending moments and force distributions.[52] Laying the foundations for modern cognitive science, Craik argued that human intelligence is grounded in the ability to convert sensory inputs into numbers, words, or other symbols, which, in turn, are the building blocks of thought. He wrote:

> My hypothesis then is that thought models, or parallels reality—that its essential feature is not 'the mind', 'the self', nor 'sense data' nor propositions but symbolism, and that this symbolism is largely of the same kind as that which is familiar to us in mechanical devices which aid thought and calculation.

Craik's radical idea in the *Nature of Explanation* is that the human mind makes its own symbols. He called this process *translation* and argued that it occurs when sensory data are transformed (or 'translated') into symbolic representations that can then be used for reasoning:

> A physical object is 'translated' into a working model . . . comprising words, numbers or other symbols.

This vision of a mental model sounds quite modern.[53] In particular, Craik stated that our internal model is an analogue of the external world it represents (in terms offered by the philosopher Charles Peirce,[54] the model is *iconic*).

---

[51] Two years earlier, Skinner had published a utopian novel entitled *Walden Two*, in which a universal programme of behavioural engineering—implemented via a series of carefully timed rewards and punishments—entrains a community to live together in peace and prosperity.

[52] Tolman offered a comparable example of a man escaping a burning building by considering the hallways, doorways, and exits.

[53] In fact, anticipating the generative models that can be used today for the 'dreaming' of photorealistic faces or almost-bearable music, Craik presciently observed that the basic representation in the 'working model' is a *predictive* one—its role is to attempt to mimic how events actually unfold in the world.

[54] Discussed in Chapter 4.

> By a model we thus mean any physical or chemical system which has a similar relation-structure to that of the process it imitates. By relation-structure I do not mean some obscure non-physical entity which attends the model, but the fact that it is a physical working model which works in the same way as the process it parallels.

This implies that the representational contents are not purely arbitrary but retain their real-world similarity structure—and thus their grounding in experience. Craik was arguing that brain function involves a process of representing objects and events in a mental model that encodes how they interrelate. Today, this might seem obvious. But at the zenith of the behaviourist movement, it was both radical and heretical.

During the 1920s and 1930s, the psychologist Edward Tolman studied the tendency of rats learning to forage for rewards in a maze. In a classic experiment, he first allowed one group of rats to explore the maze freely for several days without reward, before exposing them to a standard operant schedule in which they were rewarded for reaching a specific location. Those rats that had explored the maze previously needed only a handful of rewards to learn to make a beeline for the food ('few-shot' learning), whereas the other group learnt slowly by trial and error. To Tolman—who described himself as a committed behaviourist—this strikingly revealed that learning is not slavishly driven by reward. Rather, during unrewarded free exploration, the rats must have learnt to link chains of states (maze locations) together into a sort of mental map which they could then exploit for faster future reward learning.[55]

These findings led Tolman to embrace the centrality of thinking and reasoning for the study of behaviour:

> Can we, now, shift our point of view and begin to talk about apparently internal subjective things such as thoughts? My answer is that thoughts, or at least the kind of thought with which we are here concerned, can be conceived from an objective point of view as consisting in internal presentations to the organism (on a basis of memory and association) of stimuli not actually present but which would be present if some hypothesized action were carried out.

Tolman built an elaborate theory based on his rodent work, in which mental processes are oriented towards a proximal state (such as a chair) which then, by a relational process driven by stimulus–stimulus learning, is linked to other

---

[55] See (Tolman 1930).

states (such as a table) or affordances (such as sitting).[56] By recursion, this process allows the agent to mentally navigate chains of states, so that, in Tolman's preferred example, a researcher might infer that 'this chair, if kicked out of the way, will conduce to the catching of yonder escaped rat' (this provides a fascinating window into the daily challenges Tolman faced in the lab).[57] He called a full assemblage of states a cognitive-like map, counterpointing it to the metaphor preferred by the behaviourists of brain-as-telephone-exchange:[58]

> [The brain] is far more like a map control room than it is like an old-fashioned telephone exchange. The stimuli, which are allowed in, are not connected by just simple one-to-one switches to the outgoing responses. Rather, the incoming impulses are usually worked over and elaborated in the central control room into a tentative, cognitive-like map of the environment. And it is this tentative map, indicating routes and paths and environmental relationships, which finally determines what responses, if any, the animal will finally release.

Today, 'cognitive maps' remain a topic of fervent study among neuroscientists. Below, we consider emerging theories of how a cognitive map is learnt and encoded in the complex representational properties of neurons in the mammalian neocortex and hippocampus.[59]

Together, thus, Craik and Tolman brought psychology back down to earth. They reminded their colleagues that behaviour is not just an elaborate chain of reflexes—as Skinner proposed. But nor are humans walking logic machines, whose mental cogs and gears compute the truth conditions of propositions, as Newell and Simon later argued. Humans—and maybe even rats—have mental models, but these models have semantic content. The language of thought refers to, and is grounded in, the objects and events that occur in the world.

Across the subsequent decades, this idea gradually seeped into the psychological mainstream. A major advocate of the 'mental models' theory has been Philip Johnston-Laird, whose empirical work has tirelessly reminded us that our reasoning processes are not insulated from knowledge of the world—that in practice, Fodor's formality condition is unmet.[60] People reason more

---

[56] Tolman coined the terms *discriminanda* and *manipulanda* to refer to these states. He in fact was very fond of neologisms, but as far as I know these were the only ones that caught on. He referred to his theory of mental process as the 'sign-Gestalt-expectation' theory, which is a bit of a mouthful.

[57] See (Tolman 1933).

[58] See (Tolman 1948).

[59] See (Behrens et al. 2018) and (Whittington et al. 2020).

[60] See (Johnson-Laird 2010).

accurately when they can harness their knowledge of the world. For example, people are more likely to mistakenly affirm the consequent[61] in the syllogism:

> All oak trees have acorns
> This tree has acorns
> Therefore, this tree is an oak

than in the near-identical alternative:

> All oak trees have leaves
> This tree has leaves
> Therefore, this tree is an oak

which can be rejected by calling upon knowledge that all trees, and not just oaks, have leaves. Similarly, a well-known study from the 1960s confronted participants with four cards, labelled with the letters or digits *4*, *7*, *A*, and *D*, and asked them which cards needed to be turned over to confirm the rule 'if there is an even number on one side, there is a vowel on the other'. Participants tended to overlook that this can potentially be falsified by turning over the D. However, the task can be adapted so that the cards show *beer*, *coke*, *19*, and *35* and participants are told that these represent the age of patrons of a bar and their beverages. Now if participants are asked to verify the rule 'If a patron is drinking a beer, then they must be 21 years or older', they have no hesitation in turning over the *19* card to see if there is 'beer' on the other side—even though the logical inference is identical. As Johnston-Laird says, our mental models are populated with semantic knowledge, so we do not have to rely purely on logic to make inferences about the world.[62]

3.6 Reaching the banana

When the First World War broke out, the German psychologist Wolfgang Köhler had the good fortune to be marooned on a lush volcanic island off the North African coast. He had arrived in Tenerife in 1913 to study the behaviour of apes at the Prussian Academy of Sciences anthropoid research station,

---

[61] That is, more likely to wrongly assert that it is valid.
[62] The original task was from (Wason 1960) and the cheat detection variant was first described in (Cox & Griggs 1982), and later promulgated by Tooby and Cosmides who used it for a theory of intelligent social exchange (Cosmides et al. 2010).

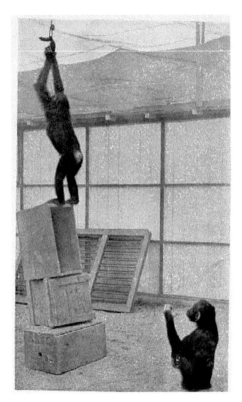

Fig. 3.6 A picture of the chimp *Grande* climbing on wobbly boxes to reach a banana.
From http://www.pigeon.psy.tufts.edu/psych26/images/kohler3.JPG.

and as the war dragged on, he ended up staying 6 years.[63] During that time, he made some striking observations about chimpanzee behaviour, which he described in his 1925 book *The Mentality of Apes*.

Köhler's research question was simple: can animals solve new problems without extensive training? To address this, he first measured whether chimpanzees could reach, on the first try, a coveted banana that they had witnessed being placed behind a barrier. Unlike cats and dogs, who were known to fail on equivalent tasks, the chimps instantly circumvented the obstacle to grab the reward. Upping the ante, Köhler then created scenarios in which a banana could only be attained by scaling a pole, reaching with a stick, or building a rickety tower of boxes. Figure 3.6 shows a chimp known as *Grande* scaling a box mountain of his own construction to reach the prize hanging high above

---

[63] During which time, he may, or may not, have been recruited into German Intelligence to spy on passing naval vessels.

the ground, whilst an admiring friend looks on. Another ingenious chimp called *Sultan* became a master problem-solver, working out (after some rumination) that two short sticks could be joined together to make a long stick, which could then be wielded to knock down an out-of-reach banana. In fact, recent work has shown that quite astonishingly, even birds can display seemingly human-like problem-solving abilities, including the judicious fashioning of tools to retrieve rewards secreted in puzzle boxes.[64]

Köhler's book confronted universal piety in the natural sciences—that the human mind is qualitatively different to that of other species, including our nearest primate cousins. His observations were also decidedly inconvenient for contemporary theories of behaviour. At the time of his chimpanzee experiments, the behaviourist zeitgeist was ascendant—just 10 years earlier, Thorndike had published his famous *law of effect*, which stated that all learning follows from the repeated linking of stimulus and response, and was based on observations of animals escaping puzzle boxes.[65] It was thus perhaps unsurprisingly that on publication, *The Mentality of Apes* was derided as being unscientific and roundly ignored by most of Köhler's colleagues.

But Köhler was on to something. One salient observation was that the chimpanzees did not usually solve problems on the very first try. Often, they first tried out methods that had worked previously and, when these failed, paused to engage in what looked like serious contemplation. They would often, from one moment to the next, spring from contemplation into action, as if experiencing a moment of insight. Seen through Köhler's eyes, the chimpanzees seemed to work out how to reach the banana by *thinking about it*. He described it as follows:

> only that behavior of animals definitely appears to us intelligent which takes account from the beginning of the lay of the land, and proceeds to deal with it in a single, continuous, and definite course. Hence follows this criterion of insight: the appearance of a complete solution with reference to the whole lay-out of the field.

Köhler is claiming that the chimpanzees take into account the whole structure of the problem ('the lay of the land') and form a plan ('a single, continuous and definite course') to reach a solution ('insight'). The audience of the 1920s was not ready for this sort of claim and promptly accused him of anthropomorphizing his subjects. But by the 1950s, 'thinking' had returned to the research agenda with gathering respectability, and Köhler's work was ripe for revival.

---

[64] See (Hunt 1996).
[65] See Chapter 6.

In 1958, three distinguished American psychologists—Karl Pribam, George Miller, and Eugene Galanter—descended on Stanford's Center for Advanced Study for a year-long sabbatical. Three semesters of fruitful discussion led to a book, which they called *Plans and the Structure of Behavior*. The book distilled the meditations of Craik, Tolman, and Köhler into a plausible, mechanistic theory. The theory was grounded in the reality of early AI programs built by Newell and Simon and the emerging principles of cybernetics. It thus built a bridge between early psychological theories of mentation and the nascent field of AI research.

By the post-war era, psychologists and AI researchers had agreed that the ability to reason was a sensible metric for the mind. However, until that point, most focus had been on *epistemic* modes of reasoning. Early theories of thinking were concerned with how the brain determines the validity of a theorem or how to build a system that judges the accuracy of a medical diagnosis. Their currency was truth and falsehood—the hard the hard-and-fast nature of things. Pribam, Miller, and Galanter (PMG) argued that these proposals overlook a vital component: that an intelligent system needs to act. They quote an earlier version of this remonstrance, by Edwin Guthrie:

> Signs, in Tolman's theory, occasion in the rat realization, or cognition, or judgment, or hypotheses, or abstraction, but they do not occasion action. In his concern with what goes on in the rat's mind, Tolman has neglected to predict what the rat will do.

PMG were worried that in focussing on the gap from 'sign to knowledge', Tolman overlooked the step from 'knowledge to action':

> Tolman, the omniscient theorist, leaps over that gap when he infers the rat's cognitive organization from its behavior. But that leaves still outstanding the question of the rat's ability to leap it.

Here, the authors are evoking the dual-process model of cognition that Pylyshyn posits above. Sensory data (signs) are first converted into knowledge—to a world model that encodes their mutual relations ('what we know'). In focussing on this process, however, Craik and Tolman overlook the next question, which is how that knowledge is used to generate intelligent behaviour ('what we do with knowledge'). The criticism was particularly stinging at a time when behaviourism loomed large on the theoretical playing field, because behaviourists considered themselves to have solved the whole 'sign to action' gap with a single construct—the conditioned reflex.

PMG also accused Köhler of overlooking the problem of how mental models lead to intelligent action:

Köhler makes the standard cognitive assumption: once the animal has grasped the whole layout he will behave appropriately. Again, the fact is that grasping the whole layout may be necessary but is certainly not sufficient as an explanation of intelligent behavior.

Instead, PMG called for *instrumental* models of reason. They wanted models that explain how Tolman's rats used their cognitive map of the maze to find the food pellet, and how Köhler's chimpanzees used their representation of how boxes, sticks, and chimp bodies interact physically to reach the banana. Whilst psychologists continued to laud the human powers of abstraction in chess, they were asking for a theory explaining how the Russian grandmaster Mikhail Botvinnik used his mental model of the game to win the world chess championship in the year that they were writing.[66]

In their book, they made a proposal. At the heart of their theory is what they call a 'test, operate, test, exit' (TOTE) unit. Each TOTE unit controls an action, and continuously encodes the degree of incongruity between an actual and a desired state that results from that action, with a command to exit initiated when that incongruity drops to zero. For example, imagine hammering a nail into place: the action (hammer) is executed repeatedly, whilst there is a discrepancy between the current state (nail protruding) and the desired state (nail fully embedded). The theory thus incorporates the basic cybernetic feedback principle that was shared by many theories of motivated behaviour at the time.[67]

In fact, as they wrote, Newell and Simon—emboldened by the recent success of the Logic Theorist—were already attempting to build a model capable of instrumental reasoning.[68] Rather ambitiously named the General Problem Solver (GPS), it was a classical AI system designed to reason about attainment of a distant goal state—such as reaching the banana or checkmating your opponent. It represented each problem as a directed graph that could be mentally traversed by following edges (taking actions) until a desired node

---

[66] Botvinnik is, in fact, a distant relation to the distinguished cognitive scientist (and DeepMind's Director of Neuroscience) Matt Botvinick, who, despite his many talents, claims to have no aptitude for chess.

[67] See Chapter 4. Also, for a modern-day take on TOTE and its relationship to the ideomotor principle, see (Pezzulo et al. 2006).

[68] In fact, PMG cited Newell and Simon's report (which was in press in 1959) in their book and were candid about the extent to which it influenced their thinking.

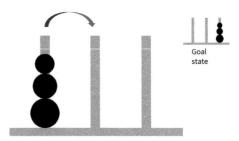

Fig. 3.7 A simplified version of the Tower of Hanoi task.

(or goal state) was achieved. Planning was thus a search process through the graph, constrained by a set of *operators*, which defined the admissible rules by which actions converted from one state into another.

In the earlier Logic Theorist, these operators had been drawn from a limited class defined by the rules of logical calculus. In building the GPS, Newell and Simon envisaged a more general class of operator that enacted open-ended transformations of one state into another—like knowing that fitting a key in a lock would transform a door from open to closed. These general-purpose operators were needed to reason about the sorts of open-ended problems people face in the real world, such as getting your kids to school when your car has broken down. The GPS employed a feedback loop highly reminiscent of TOTE, in which goals were evaluated, methods were executed, and subprocesses were initiated or halted. However, the GPS allowed for the selection of new operators within the execution cycle, such as when inaccurate hammering drives the nail askew and the claw must be used to extract and straighten it.

Newell and Simon applied the GPS to a classical reasoning problem known as the Tower of Hanoi task, in which discs have to be moved between three stacks under the constraint that larger discs never lie underneath smaller ones (Figure 3.7). Adapted to the lab,[69] this is one of a handful of tasks on which PFC patients systematically struggle.[70] The GPS was able to solve the Tower of Hanoi problem, along with 11 other tasks that require reasoning over relatively constrained state spaces. For example, in one toy planning problem, the agent has to work out how to ferry missionaries across a river without leaving any one individual stranded alongside a cannibal, in case they get eaten.[71]

[69] Shallice renamed it the Tower of London task.
[70] See (Shallice 1982).
[71] See https://en.wikipedia.org/wiki/Missionaries_and_cannibals_problem.

However, when the GPS was faced with problems that involved greater combinatorial complexity, it floundered. This is because the number of possible paths through the graph increases exponentially with the number of nodes and edges, making naive search unfeasible for larger problems such as chess. This problem, which is known as the curse of dimensionality, remains possibly the most significant in AI research today. When there are so many alternatives, how can we possibly decide on the best course of action? When anything is theoretically possible, how can we anticipate the consequences of our decisions? How do we avoid the near-limitless cost of inefficient searches, and explore only those pathways that seem the most promising?

In fact, by the time they succeeded at vanquishing a grandmaster at chess some 40 years later, IBM had made strides in electronic computing that were unimaginable in Newell and Simon's day, permitting Deep Blue to process millions of possible pathways per second. But brute computational power is not the whole answer. The legacy of the GPS is that it defined the general framework that our theories still inhabit—planning is heuristic search over structured state spaces, and the secret is to find the right heuristics. The GPS uses a very general heuristic: subgoal reduction, in which progress is tracked towards interim states that form useful waystations en route to the ultimate goal. Deep Blue employed a different type of heuristic, known as alpha-beta search, that is common for two-player zero-sum adversarial games. It involves mentally simulating (and numerically evaluating) the moves of both the protagonist and opponent, but not exhaustively: moves that cannot possibly be better than the current best option are discarded—pruned away.[72] In fact, over subsequent decades, a vast industry of planning algorithms developed, with many of the more promising candidates being deployed to meet impressive real-world challenges.[73] The GPS itself spawned many subsequent architectures, including both direct descendants, such as SOAR, and related systems for means-end reasoning, at least one of which has been deployed to solve a schematic version of the banana problem that Köhler posed to his chimpanzees.[74]

---

[72] Because those moves yield a maximum score for the protagonist that is lower than the opponent's minimum score.

[73] See (Pearl 1984).

[74] See (Fikes & Nilsson 1971). For details of SOAR, see (Laird 2012).

3.7 Your brain as statistician

The world is a confusing and ambiguous place. Uncertainty pervades every aspect of our lives, from the banal to the profound. Was that sneeze the first sign of a nasty bout of flu? Will it rain tomorrow? Does that person like me? Did I study hard enough to pass the exam? Who will win the next football match or election? For both the post-war pioneers of AI research, who lived under the shadow of nuclear annihilation, and for today's generation, who are faced with a global climate emergency, even the very continuation of life as we know it remains in doubt. In order to reason, forge plans, and share information, our mental states encode beliefs about the world. Where states are uncertain, these beliefs can be graded and expressed as probabilities— you might deem the odds of political change at the next election to be 50:50, or grumble that it is *likely*, but not *certain*, that it will rain for your birthday picnic tomorrow.

Systems that deal in hard-and-fast logic are ill-suited to handling uncertainty. We have seen that Cyc, when asked whether Freda the frog lives in the desert, can only answer yes or no. A better answer would be that it is *possible* that Freda inhabits the Australian outback, but more *probable* that she lives in a nice, moist forest glade by a pond. Beginning in the 1990s, a major new current of thought emerged in psychology, neuroscience, and AI research, based around the idea that thinking is grounded in probabilistic inference. This sparked two decades of debate about whether people are capable or clueless when it comes to making inferences in an uncertain world.

If the weather forecast tells you that there is a 70% chance of rain tomorrow, you know exactly what that means. Surprisingly, however, just 400 years ago, neither mathematicians nor lay people understood that events could be assigned numerical probabilities of occurrence. Before the Enlightenment, the predominant view among European thinkers was that the world was fully determinate, with each person's fate decided in advance by an omnipotent deity.[75] In fact, there was no word for *probability* in its modern sense—stating that something was *probable* meant that it had been sanctioned by a reputable authority. This is a quite remarkable lacuna, given the ubiquitous fondness for gambling among the aristocracy of the seventeenth century. However, in the 1650s, the young mathematician Blaise Pascal applied himself to the question of how the stakes should be allocated if a game of chance is prematurely

---

[75] The Jesuits were an exception to this—they believed that each person had free will and was thus accountable for their actions. A nice historical overview is provided in (Glimcher 2004).

interrupted.[76] In doing so, he hit upon a way to formalize probabilities as numbers, and thus laid the foundations for the modern fields of statistics, economics, and machine learning.

A century later, on the other side of the English Channel, a Presbyterian minister and hobbyist statistician called Thomas Bayes stumbled on an insight that would prove to be equally transformative. Bayes identified one solution to the problem of *inverse probability*, or what we can infer about the distribution of a random variable after sampling from it one or more times. For example, if two football teams of unknown quality play a five-match tournament, and team A wins the first match, then what is the most likely final result? Later, Pierre-Simon Laplace elaborated Bayes' insights into their current form, which dictates how an agent should correctly update their belief about a hypothesis h after observing some data d. The hypothesis states that the agent's *posterior* belief in h should be proportional to the product of their *prior belief* in the hypothesis $p(h)$ and the *likelihood* of the observed data under the hypothesis $p(d|h)$. Thus, if you believe a priori that team A has a 60% chance of winning the tournament, and they win the first game, then your posterior belief in team A's victory increases from 0.6 to 0.82.[77]

Bayes' rule thus prescribes exactly how confident you should be in your beliefs after making observations about an uncertain world. It thus provides the basis for a psychological theory of reasoning, in which the units of thought are not hard-and-fast propositions or contentions, but graded degrees of subjective belief. However, whether people do, in fact, reason according to Bayes' rule—and whether mental states can reasonably be said to encode degrees of belief—remains a hotly contested question.

In some settings, people seem to behave naturally like intuitive statisticians. If I ask you: given that a poem has at least 1000 lines, how long is it likely to be? Or given that a person has already lived to 80 years of age, how long are they likely to live? To answer these questions like a statistician, you need to implicitly know the distribution of poem lengths and lifespans and combine this prior with a likelihood term.[78] This is tricky, because poems and lifespans

---

[76] For example, if I bet £10 that a coin will come up heads twice in a row, and you bet £10 that it will not, and after one head has been tossed, the game is interrupted, how should we fairly divide the £20? To us, it is obvious that there is now a 50:50 chance of either outcome, so the money should be divided equally (although my bet was a bit silly in the first place). As a historical note, the Renaissance mathematician Gerolamo Cardano also conducted foundational work on the probability theory from games of chance nearly a hundred years before Pascal.

[77] Formally, $p(h|d) = \dfrac{p(d|h)p(h)}{p(d)}$.

[78] $p(d|h)$ for all $h < d$ will be zero, because (for example) a lifespan cannot be shorter than the age the person has already reached.

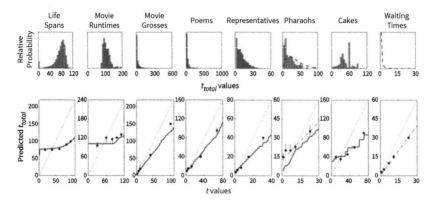

Fig. 3.8 People's predictions for various everyday phenomena. The top row of plots shows the empirical distributions of the total duration or extent, total, for each of these phenomena. The bottom row shows participants' predicted values (dots) and the predictions of a Bayesian model (lines).
Reprinted from Griffiths & Tenenbaum 2006, Fig. 2.

have different distributions—most poems are quite short (say 50 lines), but some, like the *Odyssey*, are of epic proportions, whereas lifespans are approximately normally distributed, but with a skew to the left (Figure 3.8). Thus, if you know that a poem is 1000 lines long, it might easily stretch to 5000, but even if a person has made it to the grand old age of 100, they are unlikely to celebrate a double century. In 2006, the cognitive scientists Tom Griffiths and Josh Tenenbaum posed questions like these (involving movie runtimes, cake baking times, and the durations of Pharaoh reigns) to undergraduate participants, and their predictions matched almost exactly those of an ideal observer with access to the true distributions who used Bayes' rule to compute optimal probabilities.[79]

A large literature in psychology, spanning more than 20 years, has identified numerous other cases—especially in the domains of visual perception and skilled motor control—where people behaved as if they used Bayes' rule to make optimal inferences about the world.[80] For example, we can interpret numerous canonical visual illusions as if people were applying prior beliefs learnt in the natural world, such as the way that luminances change when objects cast shadows, or the frequencies of contours of cardinal and oblique orientation in natural images, to interpret artificial stimuli.[81] This has led to a

---

[79] See (Griffiths & Tenenbaum 2006).
[80] Among many possible references, I strongly recommend this recent book, which makes a convincing argument about Bayesian inference as the computational basis for human intelligence (Gershman 2021).
[81] See (Simoncelli 2003).

vibrant intellectual community focussed on Bayesian explanations for behaviour and brain function.[82]

In the neocortex, neurons tend to carry information about the recent past, and their responses are influenced by interconnected cells with nearby receptivity. In other words, the way the brain works seems to lend itself to integrating priors over space and time with the likelihood that an object or event has occurred. Neuronal signals are themselves stochastic, and their aggregated statistics resemble those of variables in the external world. For example, resting neural activity in the neocortex of young ferrets whose visual experience has been carefully controlled across development matches the long-run average of evoked neural activity, as if spontaneous activity were a prior on evoked signals.[83] Various theories of probabilistic computation have been proposed, including those in which neural ensembles code for probabilities directly or spikes are samples of evidence for particular latent variables.[84] However, it remains unclear whether neural and behavioural signatures of probabilistic computation in humans and other animals, including approximation of optimal posterior beliefs during inference about noisy sensory signals, cannot be equally well explained by simple neural network models.[85]

In machine learning, the use of Bayesian methods has been intertwined with a clarion call for greater focus on systems that infer causality among variables. The most influential voice behind this call is Judea Pearl, a titan of AI research whose career began with the identification of new heuristic tools for classical planning. In the 1970s, Pearl went on to found the probabilistic approach to machine learning. Every student is taught that correlation does not imply causation. For example, imagine that you hear on the news that people who have taken a new medicine are at greatly increased risk of serious illness, leading to indignant calls for its withdrawal. A canny student knows to ask whether it is not simply that more people who are at risk of serious illness have been offered the medicine in the first place. To understand the effect of the medicine, you need to account for the *conditional dependence* among the variables, in this case whether the probability of illness is increased or not conditional on the medicine being given.

In the 1990s, Pearl developed a tool, known as the *Bayesian network*, that modelled variables in a directed graph structure where some variables could probabilistically influence others (but not vice versa), using an approach we

---

[82] For the sake of brevity, I will not go into the lengthy debates that have occurred over whether this theory is useful or indeed falsifiable (Bowers & Davis 2012).

[83] See (Berkes et al. 2011).

[84] See (Aitchison & Lengyel 2017).

[85] See (Orhan & Ma 2017).

now call *belief propagation*. He developed a formal system that he called *do-calculus* to capture the way in which exogenous intervention affected the variables. For example, if smoking causes cancer, but not vice versa, then cancer rates should go up as more people smoke, but conversely, exogenous factors that increase cancer (such as a radiation leak) should not affect the prevalence of smoking. Bayesian networks can thus be used to infer causal structures in data. For example, three variables x, y, and z can mutually affect one another according to at least three different patterns: a chain ($x{\rightarrow}y{\rightarrow}z$), a fork ($x{\leftarrow}y{\rightarrow}z$), and a collider ($x{\rightarrow}y{\leftarrow}z$), where the arrow signals the direction of causal influence. With enough computational resource and good approximation methods, Bayesian networks can thus be scaled up to reason about the structure of complex knowledge systems.

Remarkably, there is evidence from developmental studies that young children reason using the causal principles prescribed by Bayesian networks. In one classic study, a team led by the psychologist Alison Gopnik taught preschoolers that a box (which they called a 'blicket detector') played an engaging melody when activated with an object called a *blicket*. By exposing participants to some objects that activated the machine (e.g. a blue cube) and others that did not (e.g. a red cube), as well as combinations of objects (red and blue cubes together), the team was able to show that children as young as 20 months formed simple intuitive theories about causation, rather than just learning simple associations between event probabilities.[86]

Other studies have revealed that childrens' theories about the world shape the way they explore and learn. For example, Aimee Stahl and Lisa Feigenson showed 11-month-old infants toys that behaved in unexpected ways, for example violating spatiotemporal continuity (a floating car) or object solidity (a ball that rolls through a wall). It is well established that very young infants look by preference at these surprising events, but here the authors showed that infants prefer to play with, and will more readily learn new information about, an object that behaved in unexplained ways. The childrens' subsequent play with the objects even seemed to betray a process of causal hypothesis testing, with infants exposed to the floating car more likely to drop it on the floor (potentially to check if it floats) and those who saw the car apparently drive through the wall more likely to bang it against the table (possibly to verify its solidity).[87] In other words, even very young children can behave

---

[86] See (Gopnik et al. 2001). For other excellent work in causal inference in preschoolers, see (Schulz et al. 2007).

[87] See (Stahl & Feigenson 2015). For the original research on expectancy violation, see (Spelke et al. 1992).

like sophisticated reasoners, consistent with formal frameworks for inferring causation that depend on Bayesian inference.

3.8 Playing Lego with concepts

The classical symbolic approaches that kickstarted AI research in the 1950s have since fallen from fashion. One reason is that by committing to the hard-and-fast constraints of logical reasoning, classical systems did not allow for graded degrees of subjective belief. Bayesian models, as we have seen, rescue our theories of reasoning from this shortcoming, by allowing beliefs to be computed by combining continuously varying probabilities.

However, symbolic approaches to computation have a crucial advantage: they allow for limitless productivity from a limited number of mental primitives. Thus, symbolic representations of complex concepts (like *second cousin once removed* or *fastest sprinter* or *majority of delegates*) need not each rely on a bespoke mental representation. Rather, elaborate concepts can be composed from simpler building blocks by using a set of formal rules. For example, rules describing family relations (cousins share a grandparent; second cousins share a great-grandparent; the 'removal' refers to generational difference) allow us to understand and express any concept of the form *nth cousin k times removed*. Building *fastest sprinter* from transitive rules given by superlatives and comparatives allows us to understand *faster sprinter* or *slowest sprinter*, or even *slower marathon runner*. We can think of a compositional theory of thought as forming concepts from the ground up, similar to a car or a spaceship that might be built from a simple set of tiles, plates, and bricks in a construction toy like Lego™. Compositionality is a powerful principle with the potential to endow computation with great versatility, flexibility, and expressiveness.

The notion that intelligent systems should reason using a composable set of rules motivated the earliest AI systems, in which chains of predicate logic were used to deduce the validity of arguments and theorems. The same idea scaffolded cognitive theories of human intelligence that began to emerge in the 1970s. Fodor famously argued that people reason in a compositional *language of thought*, which he dubbed mentalese. At about the same time, Chomsky proposed that the universal structure of human language arises because people are born with an innate mental grammar that prescribes the rules for generating phrases from their constituent words. Cognitive scientists has long been beguiled by the goal of deriving a simple set of rules that govern the language of thought. But what might these rules be? What constraints might govern the way we think?

This question has been attacked from different angles. Psychologists have attempted to infer the constraints on thinking by measuring the ease or difficulty with which people make inferences under various rule-based systems. One popular idea is that concepts are composed from binary (or Boolean) expressions like AND, OR, and NOT, because the learnability of a concept can be predicted remarkably well from the *Boolean complexity* of the statement in which it is conveyed.[88] The 'complexity' (or incompressibility) of a statement is the length of the shortest computer program in which it can be expressed, which, for Boolean complexity, can be measured in bits. For example, consider the concept '{small AND spiky} OR {small AND [NOT spiky]}'. Because this is equivalent to 'small AND {spiky OR [not spiky]}', it can thus be compressed to just 'small' and expressed with a single bit. However, the concept '{small AND spiky} OR {[NOT small] AND [NOT spiky]}' cannot be compressed any further and thus requires four bits.

Computer scientists have studied the properties of formal languages, in which abstract systems of meaning are built from simple syntactic rules. For example, in a context-free grammar, symbols are combined in a recursive program defined by a production rule of the form $A \rightarrow \alpha$ (which means 'replace the left-hand side with the right-hand side'). Thus, for example, a language comprising the rules $S \rightarrow aSa$ and $S \rightarrow bSb$ can lead to the valid statement *aabSbaa* via recursive application.[89] In 2008, a team led by Noah Goodman proposed a framework for understanding human concept learning as Bayesian inference over a space of syntactic rules within a context-free grammar. Their work was developed under normative assumptions (e.g. a rational agent infers the posterior distribution over rules by using Bayes' theorem) and with simple rules, but when used to predict data from experiments in which participants classified novel category members defined by binary attributes, it did a remarkably good job.[90] The major advance offered by this work is an account of human reasoning that combines the expressivity of a compositional language of thought with the inferential power of probability calculus.

---

[88] Learnability is measured as classification accuracy after a fixed training phase. This relationship held for 41 different types of rule (Feldman 2000). See (Shepard et al. 1961) for earlier work in this vein.

[89] $S \rightarrow aSa \rightarrow aaSaa \rightarrow aabSbaa$. The goal of this research is to understand what can and cannot be computed using simple production rules, and to develop methods for identifying valid exemplars in a formal language.

[90] The paper is (Goodman et al. 2008). The attempt was to capture data from the study by (Nosofsky et al. 1994) and (Medin & Schaffer 1978).

However, whilst this work showed that a particular class of grammar can be used to capture the vagaries of human categorization, it did not attempt full-scale empirical characterization of the primitive operations which give the human language of thought its expressive power. For example, we might ask: is the non-exclusive OR operation a viable primitive? What about the exclusive or (XOR) operation? To address this, we need to measure the human propensity to learn concepts like '{tall AND [NOT green]} OR {NOT [tall AND green]}' and 'tall OR green', and to directly compare the ability of different grammars to account for these empirical data. For example, if XOR is a primitive operand, then we would expect people to learn these concepts with equal readiness.

In a comprehensive study of this nature, Steven Piantadosi trained more than 1500 participants to learn by example 108 different concepts associated with the nonsense word 'wudsy', which could mean something as simple as 'false' or as complex as 'has the same shape as the blue object'. By fitting different models to the data, the authors found that the grammars that best explained human learning included *quantifiers* (such as the operators 'there exists some . . .' and 'for all . . .' as well as 'there exists one or zero'), and that these grammars outperformed both simple and enhanced Boolean grammars. Exercises like this can capture human behaviour in striking ways and offer robust support to the idea that people learn by inferring rules from data.[91]

This framework, known as Bayesian program learning (BPL), uses probabilistic inference to learn the structure of a generative program (or grammar) from the data it generates. Advocates of this approach have hoped that Bayesian methods might offer alternatives to deep learning systems, and perhaps prove themselves to be faster, more flexible, and profligate with data. Consider, for example, the way we write a character by hand. Perhaps we can conceive of each character as generated by a program in which individual strokes and curls are composed on the page to make subparts and parts of each letter, which, in turn, are assembled into words. If so, we might be able to use BPL to learn the generative program, and harness the resulting model to both discriminate new instances of handwritten characters and generate new exemplars.

In 2015, a team led by Brenden Lake and Josh Tenenbaum used BPL to generate new instances of characters sampled from the Omniglot database, a

---

[91] See (Piantadosi et al. 2016). The candidate grammars were based on a formal language called lambda calculus (λ-calculus), developed by Alonzo Church in the 1930s. The same group have developed a programming language called Church for describing stochastic generative processes (Goodman et al. 2014). It is worth noting the caveat that it remains unclear whether the specific grammars found to account best for the data depend on the sets of rules that the authors chose to define the concepts in their experiments.

digital encyclopaedia of the world's writing systems. BPL surpassed human-level performance for one-shot matching of characters from the same alphabet (e.g. matching a single instance of an Ethiopic character to another, rather than to one in Mongolian script), outclassing deep networks that learnt from a large corpus of examples.[92]

Perhaps more impressively, BPL was sufficiently powerful that human participants could not distinguish the generated characters from their original counterparts, so that the system passed a sort of Turing test for visual perception. BPL is potentially a powerful tool, especially for domains involving systems governed by predictable rules of physical or social interaction, where sensible primitives for inference may be readily available. But it is inevitably subject to the critique that researchers have to furnish the relevant primitives for each new problem, meaning that learning about handwritten characters is unlikely to generalize to novel domains, such as modelling ice-skating or Japanese cuisine.[93]

Thus, over the decades, interest in *thinking* as a research problem has waxed and waned in both cognitive sciences and AI research. But there is near-universal accord that being able to reason effectively is a key component of intelligence, and a major contributor to human success both as individuals and as a species. One strong proponent of this view, the psychologist Steven Pinker,[94] has argued that humans have been able to prosper because they occupy a *cognitive niche* which allows them to:

> ... overtake other organisms' fixed defences by cause-and-effect reasoning [...]—to deploy information and inference, rather than particular features of physics and chemistry, to extract resources from other organisms in opposition to their adaptations to protect those resources.

This ability to reason, he argues:

> ... allows humans to invent tools, traps, and weapons, to extract poisons and drugs from other animals and plants, and to engage in coordinated action, for example, fanning out over a landscape to drive and concentrate game, in effect functioning like a huge superorganism.

---

[92] See (Lake et al. 2015). This paper on one-shot learning has been influential but reports higher one-shot error on Omniglot (Vinyals et al. 2017). This paper does slightly better (Santoro et al. 2016).

[93] See (Botvinick et al. 2017) for a critique.

[94] See (Pinker 2010). An opposing view is that we evolved to occupy a 'cultural niche' as a species with superlative social learning (Boyd et al. 2011).

For humans, reasoning from means to end is a basic requirement for tackling the complex puzzles that life throws up. How do I put up this shelf or bake that cake? How do I build this canoe to float, or carve that bow to shoot long and true? How do I express this idea clearly or solve that calculation problem? How do I decide where to live, whom to marry, or how to spend my Sunday afternoon?

Recalling the definition of intelligence given by Legg and Hutter, our human generality is expressed in an ability to solve a multitude of different problems—from baking a cake to winning at chess. According to this view, thus, it is by reasoning—applying mental processes to plan over states and outcomes—that we can consider what will follow from observables, such as the fact that there are eggs in the fridge or that the opponent has lost her queen. Reasoning about states of the world allows humans to devise creative solutions to stubborn problems, imagine counterfactual outcomes, or anticipate important events, even if they are unlikely or far into the future. Indeed, from an empirical standpoint, people who do well on lab-based tests that involve reasoning about verbal propositions, space, or numbers tend also to flourish in the real world—succeeding in school and college and at work. No wonder, then, that we lionize the genius of von Neumann, who could think around mathematical corners, or the of grandmasters of strategic games such as Go and chess, who can anticipate the consequences of a move dozens of turns into the future.

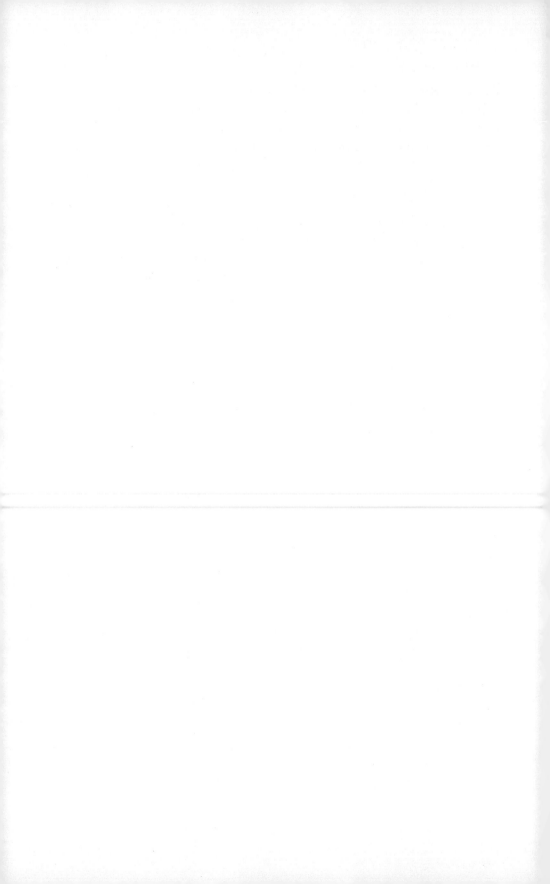

4
The structure of knowledge

4.1 Total recall

Imagine that you had the misfortune to be kidnapped by inquisitive aliens, who whisk you off to their home planet, where they demand that you tell them every single thing you know about life on planet Earth. How many hours would it take? How many alien ring binders would your lifelong knowledge fill? The chances are that even if you have lived all your life on the same street, or generally forget what happened last week, you would still have a lot to recount. Think about how you might organize information for your curious hosts. You might begin by telling them basic facts about the world: the capital cities of Portugal, Norway, and Austria; the dates of Columbus' arrival in Hispaniola, the French Revolution, or the Indian partition; and the names of various species of trees, birds, and flowers. Other aspects of your knowledge are pragmatic. You might know how to make a perfect béchamel sauce, ice skate backwards, play the xylophone, or perform a Maori greeting. Finally, you know a lot of stuff that is hard to verbalize. You might recall a trip to Niagara Falls in winter and bring to mind a view of the great cataract shrouded in ice. You can imagine the face of a long-lost schoolfriend or replay the tune of a favourite Christmas carol in your head. These memories form part of your knowledge about the world too, even if they would be much harder to convey to your alien interrogators.

At the dawn of the AI era, researchers sought to emulate the power of human reason, by building *machines that think*. But in doing so, they stripped away the quintessence of the human mind: that people know stuff. When we see an object, we can recognize it, label it, and know how to use it. When we meet a friend, we recall their name, their relationship to us, and their likes and dislikes. When we read a book or attend a class, we understand the references being made to far-off places, historical events, scientific theories, and cultural practices. Our knowledge about the world is elaborate and intricate. Moreover, it is usefully formatted, permitting us to grasp new concepts, master new fields, conjure sensible intuitions, and make great leaps of creative imagination. Knowledge is integral to intelligence. In this chapter, we will

Natural General Intelligence. Christopher Summerfield, Oxford University Press. © Oxford University Press 2023.
DOI: 10.1093/oso/9780192843883.003.0004

discuss the nature of human knowledge, and ask how it might be possible to build AI systems that learn a rich, conceptual model of the world like humans do. We will consider the promise and pitfalls of building *machines that know*.

Our knowledge is who we are. From the moment we are born, great waves of sensory data wash relentlessly over us. Much of this information is *encoded*— laid down as memory traces in neural circuits. These memories are layered one on top of the other, and are gradually smoothed, sifted, and calcified, until they form the hard contours of what we know. All mental and physical acts—all of our thoughts and behaviour—are filtered through this knowledge of the world. When our knowledge is erased, for example, when dementia creeps tragically upon us in older age, it is catastrophic—we lose our entire identity. The Greek philosopher Socrates famously boasted about his ignorance: he claimed his only true knowledge was how little he knew. However, as a distinguished soldier, father, landowner, and philosopher, who (like other wealthy Athenians) had enjoyed a gilded education in music, poetry, gymnastics, and law, it is likely that he was selling himself short. Even Socrates knew a lot of stuff.

The capacity of human memory is very hard to estimate, but it is undoubtedly very large. In a classic experiment from 1973, the psychologist Lionel Standing showed groups of participants large numbers of photographic slides, each for a few seconds, and requested that they try to remember as many as possible for a later test. One group of five participants were subjected to a particularly gruelling learning phase during which they viewed 10,000 images— totalling more than 15 hours of study. Two days later, they were tested on their recognition memory by being asked to discriminate a subset of 'old' items (those from the training set) from 'new' (those that were not). Extrapolating from their accuracy back up to the full image set, Standing estimated that in the group who had seen the 10,000 photographs, nearly 7000 had been successfully encoded.[1] By far, the most remarkable finding, however, was his observation that the number of successfully recognized items continued to scale lawfully with the size of the training set (Figure 4.1). In other words, the more data we are shown, the more we remember. This suggests that, in effect, the capacity of human memory is theoretically limitless.

How is it possible for the brain to have virtually limitless capacity? One long-standing theoretical problem in computational neuroscience is to identify the maximum number of patterns p that can be stored in a network composed

---

[1] See (Standing 1973). A more recent study has replicated this finding and reported that (quite astonishingly) recognition performance is high, even when foils (competing items) are chosen to be similar to the targets (Brady et al. 2008).

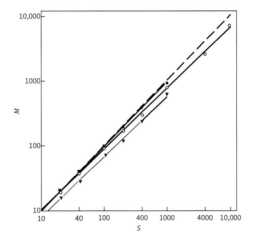

Fig. 4.1 The number of items retained in memory (M) as a function of the number presented for learning (S). The diagonal broken line represents perfect memory. Filled squares: vivid pictures. Open circles: normal pictures. Triangles: words.
Reprinted with permission from Standing (1973).

of n neurons (you can think of each pattern as a unique representation of a single high-dimensional stimulus, such as a photograph). The value of p will depend on the way the information is coded. If we assume no constraints on how information is read in or out, then the theoretical storage capacity of the network is immense. For example, if neurons encode a single bit (they can be either on or off), then $p = 2^n$. Thus, even with just ten neurons, you can already encode a thousand different patterns; with 250 neurons, p is greater than the number of atoms in the universe.[2] In practice, however, the way the network stores data depends on the computations that underlie memory formation.[3] An example of learning rule is Hebb's principle that neurons receiving coincident input strengthen their connections. Under this assumption, one popular class of network can be shown to store at least $p = n/2\log_2(n)$ patterns, which typically means that p is somewhere between 1% and 10% of n. This is a more modest capacity, but still large when you consider that the adult neocortex houses about 16 billion neurons. In fact, under reasonable assumptions, it is possible to recreate Standing's results and mimic his scaling law with a network comprising just a few hundred neurons.[4]

[2] $2^{10} = 1024$.
[3] And the order in which it is encountered, and many other factors.
[4] See (Androulidakis et al. 2008).

Our memories can be rich and vivid. In mammals, one part of the brain that is very important for storing elaborate and detailed information about the past is the temporal cortex. In the 1950s, the neurosurgeon Wilder Penfield used electrodes to stimulate specific points on the lateral temporal lobes of patients undergoing surgical treatment for epilepsy, whilst asking them to verbalize their experiences. Here is an excerpt from his report referring to a female patient:

> After a point in her temporal cortex had been stimulated, she observed with some surprise, 'I just heard one of my children speaking.' Then she added, 'It was Frank, and I could hear the neighborhood noises.' When asked, she explained that by neighborhood noises she meant such things as automobiles passing in the street.

Other patients reported vividly hearing orchestral music or songs they knew from the radio, with one patient humming along to the tune evoked by stimulation.[5] More recent studies have electrically stimulated portions of the temporal lobe that are known from neuroimaging studies to be sensitive to visual stimuli. For example, stimulating a ventral temporal region that is sensitive to images of scenes elicited hallucinations comprising complex visual topographies, such as a train in a station seen from a first-person perspective. Stimulating a face-sensitive cortical region provoked perceptual distortions in which the researchers' faces morphed into those of other people. These experiments suggest that localized portions of the cortex code for the past in rich and cohesive ways that can be relived in glorious sensory detail when the relevant population of neurons become active.

Most people report that memories vary in the level of detail they evoke. For some, however, they can take on almost tyrannical levels of precision. A handful of individuals exhibit a strange syndrome known as hyperthymesia, which allows them to accurately recount personal events from the distant past in astonishing detail. The first hyperthymesic patient to be identified, known as AJ, can recollect the events of almost every day from the age of about 11. For example, when asked (without warning) about 27 April 1994 (more than 10 years before the date of testing), she replied:

> That was Wednesday. That was easy for me because I knew where I was exactly. I was down in Florida. I was summoned to come down and to say goodbye to my grandmother who they all thought was dying but she ended up living. My Dad and

---

[5] Importantly, patients were not simply confabulating, because they reported 'nothing' after an unexpected sham stimulation event.

my mom went to New York for a wedding. Then my mom went to Baltimore to see her family. I went to Florida on the 25th which was a Monday. This was also the weekend that Nixon died. And then I flew to Florida and my dad flew to Florida the next day. Then I flew home, and my dad flew to Baltimore to be with my mom.

A.J. reliably kept a personal diary throughout her life, allowing researchers to verify the accuracy of her reported memories. Since the original 2006 publication detailing her remarkable abilities,[6] several other patients with putative hyperthymesia have been identified worldwide. One celebrated case is that of Franco Magnani, who emigrated to America from his native village of Pontito, Italy, in the 1940s. Years later, he suffered an illness during which he experienced overwhelmingly vivid dreams of home, and afterwards, he discovered an ability to paint—in astonishing detail—images of Pontito, where he had not set foot for over 20 years.[7]

In his short fable entitled *Funes, el Memorioso*, the Argentinian novelist Jorge Luis Borges describes a young man with an extreme case of hyperthymesia. Funes can precisely recall everything that he has ever encountered. The narrator recounts his remarkable powers of perception and recollection:

> We, at one glance, can perceive three glasses on a table; Funes, all the leaves and tendrils and fruit that make up a grape vine. He knew by heart the forms of the southern clouds at dawn on the 30th of April, 1882, and could compare them in his memory with the mottled streaks on a book in Spanish binding he had only seen once.

Funes can thus perfectly remember the shapes of clouds, the exact sound of words in a foreign language, or the precise pattern traced by flames from a fire, even years after they occurred.

In a network of neurons, recall can be improved by reducing the overlap between memories. Intuitively, if two experiences evoke overlapping patterns of neural activity, then the systems reading information out from memory might confuse one with the other. Conversely, if you store memories with two distinct, non-overlapping traces, then they are less likely to interfere, and more likely to be accurately recalled. A coding system that minimizes overlap between memories is often called a place code or a localist code. A localist coding scheme operates like a system of pigeonholes, into which information

---

[6] See (Parker et al. 2006).
[7] The late great neurologist Oliver Sacks wrote about Franco Magnani in an article for *The New Yorker* in 1992.

can be placed and from which it can be retrieved intact. In the most extreme version of a localist code, each of n neurons responds to just one pattern p, so that there is no overlap in neural signalling. Neuroscientists slyly refer to theoretical neurons that have a one-to-one relationship with real-world entities as 'grandmother neurons', as their existence implies a neuron somewhere in your brain that is reserved for your grandmother.[8]

In Borges' tale, Funes encodes information in his prodigious memory using a localist code. Each experience is stored in a unique slot. Thus, he can distinguish the shape of the clouds on 30 April from that on 29 April because he has a separate memory for each event, rather than merging them together into a common representation. We can imagine his memory like the hard disk of a computer, allowing uncorrupted read/write operations to unique addresses in memory. This principle is visible in the bespoke counting system that Funes invented, in which each number is denoted by a unique and arbitrary word or phrase (e.g. 7013 is 'Máximo Pérez', whereas 7014 is 'El Ferrocarril'). Unlike the counting systems that most humans use, where the number word can be used to infer the cardinality, Funes' system uses random signs that ignore how numbers are related. For example, unlike our decimal system, its number words offer no clues that 7013 and 7014 bear the same adjacency relation as 7014 and 7015. It is as if Funes' brain consists entirely of grandmother neurons.

Funes' capacious memory might sound like a blessing. But storing information in this way has a serious drawback. Although he can recollect minute details about each experience, Funes cannot work out how his experiences relate to one another. As the narrator of Borges' tale recounts, Funes remembers the *specific* but cannot understand the *general*:

> Funes was, let us not forget, almost incapable of ideas of a general, Platonic sort. Not only was it difficult for him to comprehend that the generic symbol dog embraces so many unlike individuals of diverse size and form; it bothered him that the dog at three fourteen (seen from the side) should have the same name as the dog at three fifteen (seen from the front).

Because his memory consists of an infinite series of slots, it needlessly partitions experiences. Funes forms separate representations of dogs encountered at one instant or another or seen from one viewpoint or another. His memory

---

[8] The use of this term, now ubiquitous in neuroscience, began as a joke—told in a class that Jerry Lettvin taught at the MIT in the 1960s—about the consequences of removing the cells coding for 'mother' in the mother-obsessed character in the Philip Roth novel *Portnoy's Complaint* (Gross 2002).

is endlessly fragmented, and so its content is stripped of *relational structure*— it conveys no information about how the world is organized. Even real-world hyperthymesics sometimes report that their excessively precise memories are burdensome and intrusive, and do not help knowledge to be arranged in useful ways. For example, A.J. was unable to use her powerful recall to do well in school, where her academic performance was no better than average, even in disciplines that required significant levels of rote learning.

This tells us that knowledge is more than a list of facts and experiences. For a memory system to be effective, capacity matters less and organization matters more. Imagine a company that owns a giant warehouse but stores goods in random locations. No matter how large the store, or how plentiful the goods, the distribution system will be catastrophically inefficient. What is needed is a method for organizing the repository. It is the same in a memory system. Our memories need to be laid down in a well-structured fashion, so that they can be retrieved in ways that are useful for ongoing behaviour.

Correspondingly, intelligence is only possible because the world has structure. In a wholly random world, there is nothing to learn—each action is as good or bad as any other. Intelligent agents need to learn structure in order to take coherent actions, infer what is true, predict future events, and achieve their goals. The question that has historically divided AI researchers is how agents should acquire this structure. For most of the twentieth century, most researchers believed that the key to intelligence was thinking deeply. The symbolic AI systems discussed in Chapter 3 did not learn structure from the environment. Instead, any structure in their computations was imposed by hand. AI researchers believed that 2000 years of philosophy had provided answers to the deep questions of how reality was organized, and so they simply uploaded those principles directly into the minds of artificial agents. They knew that given the proposition *if p, then q*, if p was true, then q was unarguably true too, so they built machines that operationalized this logic in computation. These agents did not need to learn about how the world was structured, because their creators had already endowed them with plausible primitives of thought. However, the agents they created were disconnected from reality. Their representations were empty tokens like p and q, which it was left to the researcher to imbue with meaning. Reality, it turned out, is too messy for the clean contours of pure logic.

The alternative is to build AI systems that learn their computation from the world. This idea forms the basis for the connectionist or 'parallel distributed processing' (PDP) movement, which began in the 1970s and has since morphed into the deep learning revolution which is powering the march of technology in the twenty-first century. The main tool on which this approach is founded—the deep neural network—draws its power from an ability to learn about how the world is structured. Unlike Funes, neural networks learn representations of objects and events, the similarity of which—expressed in patterns of activity across processing units—reveals how they relate to each other. The latest incarnations of these models, which learn to perform tasks directly from atoms of sensory experience (such as the pixels of an image or video), are able to ground computation in the natural world, just like biological systems. Rather than being gifted mental operations from a benevolent creator, this class of AI system acquires its computation from the world, allowing it to predict sensory properties, estimate the value of action, and derive optimal policies for intelligent behaviour.

4.2 Perceptrons in space

The Bronx High School of Science is an island of academic excellence sitting amid one of the most economically deprived neighbourhoods in New York City. It boasts eight Nobel laureates among its alumni—a record unmatched by any other secondary school in the world. In the 1940s, two pupils graduated just a year apart,[9] who would go on to shape the history of AI research. In the 1950s, they forged an intellectual rivalry that embodied the twin research approaches that continue to divide the field. Their disagreement focussed on the relative merit of building machines that *think* and machines that *know*.

One of this duo was Marvin Minsky. As we have already heard, in the 1950s and 1960s, Minsky was busy building classical reasoning architectures in the newly inaugurated MIT laboratory for AI. The other was a psychologist by the name of Frank Rosenblatt, who was working at Cornell Aeronautical Laboratory in upstate New York. Rosenblatt's work was heavily inspired by an emerging understanding that the brain consisted of networks of neurons, the connections of which were gradually learnt by experience. In 1958, he unveiled the perceptron,[10] a simple computational tool that would end up being the progenitor of all modern neural networks.

[9] Minsky in 1945, and Rosenblatt in 1946.
[10] Many authors are tempted to capitalize the name. Rosenblatt did not agree. He wrote: 'it is only with difficulty that its well-meaning popularisers can be persuaded to suppress their natural urge to capitalize the initial "P". On being asked, "How is Perceptron performing today?" I am often tempted to respond, "Very well, thank you, and how are Neuron and Electron behaving?"'

The perceptron is a model of a neuron, not of an entire brain. It embodies a very simple idea: that outputs should be a linear weighted sum of inputs. Imagine you are faced with a tricky decision like choosing a rental apartment based on various attributes: square footage, distance to the city centre, and monthly rent. Depending on your preferences, some factors might carry more weight than others. For example, if you are on a tight budget, perhaps cost is the most critical variable. A sensible way to make your choice is to add up the factors, weighted by their relative importance to you, and compare the result to a numerical criterion (accept vs reject). In linear algebra, this is achieved by taking the (inner) product of an input vector x and a weighting vector w, before binarizing the output according to a threshold. This is exactly the computation that a perceptron performs.

Rosenblatt had two seminal intuitions. The first was a hunch about how the perceptron weights could be adjusted by experience, permitting the network to learn by itself. Rosenblatt used the relationship between a desired and an observed output to adjust the weights w fractionally in proportion to the inputs x which, when repeated in small increments, often led the network to converge towards a desired outcome.[11] For example, imagine that you show me a list of apartments (observations), along with your decision to rent or not (supervision signals). With enough examples, I should be able to infer the relative weights you place on size, location, and rent. This allows me to make a good stab at predicting whether you will like any future apartment or not.

The second was the idea that many perceptrons could be wired together in series, just like banks of neurons are connected in the brain, to solve more complex problems. Rosenblatt speculated that whilst the perceptron was simple, its potential was huge—because it was able to learn entirely by itself and there was virtually no limit to what it could do if sufficiently scaled up. Perhaps unwisely, he enthused about his far-flung hopes to journalists from *The New York Times*, who quoted him as claiming that a perceptron could one day be blasted into space and sent to explore other planets in our stead.[12] The hype that accompanied his claims has since greatly undermined Rosenblatt's credibility, although it is clear that he was actually more interested in building a model of biological intelligence than AI.[13]

---

[11] In fact, unlike later methods, Rosenblatt's approach did not have convergence guarantees.

[12] 'New navy device learns by doing', *New York Times*, 8 July 1958.

[13] In his 1961 book *Principles of Neurodynamics*, Rosenblatt later wrote: 'the perceptron program is not primarily concerned with the invention of devices for "artificial intelligence", but rather with investigating the physical structures and neurodynamic principles which underlie "natural intelligence". A perceptron is first and foremost a brain model, not an invention for pattern recognition.'

Rosenblatt's ambitions for the perceptron were misplaced. Whether he was wrong about the principle—that learning systems can be scaled towards superintelligence—is still controversial. But everyone agrees he was wrong in practice, because the perceptron suffers from a fundamental limitation. Its integration rule is linear (the output is just a weighted sum of inputs), and so the network is limited to learning linear mappings between inputs and outputs. This grossly limits the range of problems it can solve.

To understand why, consider a perceptron that receives a scalar input. This might denote, for example, the size of an object compared to a standard. If the task is to decide whether the object size is *greater than* the standard, then this can trivially be solved by a linear network, which simply has to threshold the value after appropriate weighting.[14] However, if the objective is to indicate whether the object is *more similar to the standard* than some criterion, then a perceptron will fail. This is because similarity is a non-linear (quadratic) function of the input value—it starts small and gets larger, but then (as the object exceeds the standard) becomes small again.[15] Thus, there exists no weight that will allow a linear mapping from input to output. The implications of this tiny example hold in the more general case. Unfortunately, most of the problems that Rosenblatt imagined a neural network would soon be able to solve—such as labelling objects or translating between the world's languages—involve non-linear mappings, which cannot be learnt by his perceptron.

The other player in this drama Marvin Minsky had also begun his career by toying with machines that learnt for themselves.[16] However, his explorations had largely come to nothing. Minsky thus believed that as a tool for building intelligence, his former schoolmate's idea was dramatically limited. In 1969, together with his MIT colleague Seymour Papert, he wrote a book saying exactly this. The book had a devastating effect on the nascent field of neural network research, sending it into recession for at least a decade. In fact, by the time the book was published, Rosenblatt—buffeted by a controversy he had not courted—had already pivoted to studying a very different (and slightly esoteric) topic—the impact of transplanting brain matter from trained to naive rodents. Tragically, he was killed in a boating accident just a few years later.

However, a vital intellectual seed had been planted. By the 1980s, several people had independently worked out a learning rule that allowed neural

---

[14] In this case, the weights would be adjusted to a value commensurate with the chosen size criterion.

[15] Because it is greater when both inputs are low or both inputs are high, but not otherwise.

[16] During his PhD and early career, he built the Stochastic Neural Analog Reinforcement Calculator (SNARC).

networks to acquire non-linear mapping functions. This permitted the optimal weights to be found in networks composed of multiple layers, with non-linear activation functions—the precursor to modern deep learning. This rule, which became known as backpropagation, allowed the gradients of weight adjustment to be calculated in a chain that flowed backwards from the output to the input. Paul Werbos, whose 1974 PhD thesis is the most often cited (if not the first) reference for backpropagation, claimed to have dreamed up the idea after reading about the backward flow of subconscious reasoning in Freud's psychodynamic theory. Although the term would not be popularized for several decades, the *deep neural network* was born.[17]

Like Rosenblatt, many of the founders of the connectionist movement were psychologists by training. This affinity was natural—unlike classical AI architectures, neural networks look like brains (consisting of neurons wired together) and they learn gradually by experience (like human infants). Most importantly, however, neural networks learn how the world is structured, because like biological systems, their neural codes conserve the similarity among inputs. Their memory systems, thus, are ripe for acquiring the knowledge that underlies intelligent behaviour.

Representational theories of the mind state that the brain encodes the world in microcosm. Cognitive scientists often use the term *schema* or *concept* to refer to a set of experiences that evoke a common mental state. This mental state itself is referred to as a *representation*.[18] If you have read the *Harry Potter* novels, you will have formed a representation of *Crookshanks*, which helps you recognize the bandy-legged ginger cat with superlative intelligence owned by Hermione Granger. Crookshanks has an unusually squashed head, which is one of many features that distinguish him from Mrs Norris, the scrawny, yellow-eyed cat belonging to the Hogwarts caretaker Argus Filch. However, Crookshanks and Mrs Norris also have some things in common. They are both felines, they are both quite clever, and they both live at Hogwarts. These properties are not shared by other pets who feature in the books, such as Fang, the cowardly boarhound that belongs to the groundsman Rubeus Hagrid.

In the wizarding world, just like in the natural world, entities are structured according to a hierarchy of generality. *Crookshanks* is just one instance of *cat*, which is just one instance of *animal*, which is just one instance of *thing*. Thus, for an agent to be able to distinguish between the two Hogwarts cats, it needs

---

[17] Technically, Rosenblatt's original network was 'deep' too, in that it comprised multiple layers. However, given that it is possible to express multiple sequential linear operations as a single linear operation, the number of layers did not widen the class of problems it could solve.

[18] Or sometimes, interchangeably, the computations by which the mental state is produced.

representations of *Crookshanks* and *Mrs Norris* that are uniquely activated by their corresponding referent.[19] However, to know that Crookshanks and Mrs Norris share certain properties, it is useful to have a more general representation, such as *cat*. Thus, representing information hierarchically is useful both for grouping things together (via general representations) and for telling things apart (via specific representations).

For neuroscientists, mental representations are expressed in patterns of activity across a population of neurons. Information about how the world is structured is reflected in the similarities and differences in this neural activity. For example, Crookshanks and Mrs Norris would evoke similar, but not identical, patterns of activity in a population of neurons, whereas Fang would induce an activity pattern that is quite different from both of them. A useful tool for analysing patterns of neural activity is known as a *representational dissimilarity matrix* (RDM). The representational dissimilarity between two objects or events can be measured by calculating the distance between the activity patterns they evoke across a neural population.[20] An RDM is a matrix of size $p \times p$ that encodes the distance between the neural activity elicited by each of the p patterns and every other pattern: a rich description of how the network activity reflects the structure of the world. If each pattern that the agent encounters is encoded in a unique slot, for example by a tailored grandmother neuron, then the RDM will have zeros on the diagonal, and a constant value elsewhere. An RDM from Funes' memory looks like this. It carries no information about the structure of the world, because it just indicates that each state is identical to itself, but equally different to everything else. However, if the representational dissimilarity among neural patterns elicited by stimuli matches their differences in the real world, then a memory system is encoding natural structure.

Knowing how the world is structured allows agents to *generalize* knowledge. Generalization is the ability to make accurate predictions about new, unfamiliar experiences. Dealing with novelty is critical in the natural world, because each event across our lifetime is different, however subtly, from every other we have previously experienced. This is what the Greek philosopher Heraclitus meant when he proclaimed that no man steps in the same river twice. That river is time, and it runs inexorably forward, meaning that no instance is ever precisely repeated. Each pattern of sensory stimulation is new, all percepts are uncertain, and all meaning is fundamentally ambiguous.

---

[19] In other words, a population of neurons for which the two pets evoke different patterns of activity.
[20] For example, by calculating the Euclidean distance, or one minus the correlation distance.

However, this ambiguity can be resolved if we know how the world is structured.

In natural environments, sensory signals are highly patterned in space and time. In the visual domain, colours and textures that are present in one part of the visual field are often present in nearby locations. When taking in a view of a park on a cloudy day, the grass (green and spiky) tends to be at the lower portion of the visual field, and the sky (grey and fluffy) in the upper portion. By knowing that the sky is grey on the left of the image, you can predict with reasonable accuracy that it will be grey on the right of the image too. Percepts are also autocorrelated in time. If you look up from where you are reading this, you will probably find that the overall context—the clock ticking on the wall, the cat asleep on the sofa—has not changed much over the past few minutes. So you can predict that they will still be the same in a few moments' time. Generalization also allows us to infer the properties of new objects. If we have learnt a concept of *cat*, then Crookshanks and Mrs Norris evoke a common patterns of neural activity. This means that a new Hogwarts pet that elicits a similar activity pattern (such as Fuzzclaw)[21] is also likely to be a cat. We can thus predict that it will share properties with Crookshanks and Mrs Norris, such as *being clever* and *enticed by fish*. Because the world is structured, we can make predictions about new experiences. We can use the past to deal with both the present and the future.

This was Rosenblatt's fundamental realization. Building systems that can generalize opens the door to a new class of AI: one that can deal with the ever-changing world that we inhabit, where no two experiences are ever exactly alike. Symbolic AI systems had a memory that comprised a series of unrelated slots. This meant that when faced with novel inputs—like when pink blocks were added to the SHRDLU's blockworld—their brains had to be manually expanded, with new slots added by hand. An agent that does not learn structure will, like Funes, live in a mentally fragmented world, in which everything is dissimilar to everything else. Borges understood this. His narrator writes:

> To think is to forget differences, generalize, make abstractions. In the teeming world of Funes, there were only details, almost immediate in their presence.

Funes' understanding of the world is crippled by a failure to grasp generalities. If each stimulus evokes a unique activity pattern—one that is equally dissimilar to every other pattern—then all knowledge of how the world is

---

[21] Technically, it is unclear whether Fuzzclaw, who belonged to Rowan Khanna, actually resided at Hogwarts.

structured is discarded and it will be impossible to generalize. By contrast, neural networks can form capacious new memories as the parameters in the network gradually change to map inputs onto desired outputs.[22]

Interest in neural networks continued to grow across the 1980s and early 1990s. Perhaps chastened by Rosenblatt's folly, enthusiasts mostly avoided grandiose claims about the power of AI, focussing instead on connectionist models as theories of human psychology. There was a waning in interest in neural networks towards the start of the millennium, but as discussed in Chapter 1, since 2006, it has come roaring back in the form of the deep learning revolution. Modern deep networks can learn to recognize objects from pixels alone, like human infants do.[23] This has opened new doors to understanding how knowledge is formed, and reawakened a fascination with the idea that there exist common design principles for artificial and biological brains.

4.3 Maps in the mind

If you have visited Paris, France, you probably returned home with a treasury of memories: the idyllic glint of sun on the water as you strolled along the banks of the Seine, or that withering glance from the waiter when you foolishly ordered a glass of Merlot with your Coquille Saint Jacques. But how should we characterize your knowledge of Paris? Asked to explain the *what*, the *where*, and the *when* of Paris to alien anthropologists, how would you even begin?

As we have seen, an effective memory system retains the natural structure of the information it encodes. However, there are many different ways in which facts and experiences from the real world can be formatted. After visiting Paris, you can mentally replay episodes from cafés and cobbled streets. But during your *séjour*, you will also have learnt new names of people, places, and things: *Georges Pompidou*, *La Place des Vosges*, and *Le Passe Navigo*. You might have gathered how Paris is arranged spatially, with its *arrondissements* coiling lavishly around the city in a numbered spiral. You negotiated its labyrinthine transit map, with fast regional train routes intersecting a tangle of underground and elevated metro lines from *Boulogne* to *Bastille*. Your knowledge of Paris encompasses its extrinsic relationships. You may also know that if French cities were sorted by population, Paris would be at the head of

---

[22] A useful distinction is to think of neural networks as *parametric* models (where the representations are governed by the values of their parameters), rather than as non-parametric models (where the representations are crafted by hand).

[23] In fact, this 'end-to-end' learning was one of Rosenblatt's original goals for the perceptron. Alas, object labelling is a largely non-linear problem.

the line, boasting nearly triple the headcount of its fierce rival Marseille. You might associate Paris with other European cities like *Vienna* and *Rome*, but perhaps not *Helsinki* or *Mumbai*, which lie at more geographically or culturally distant junctures. Each of these memory formats provides a unique slice through how facts and experiences about Paris relate to one another.

It was Tolman who first proposed that we can think of memory as a mental map. Tolman focussed on spatial maps that signal the geography of landmarks, waystations, and routes in Euclidean space. But there are many different relational patterns in our knowledge. There are feature maps that chart the physical likenesses among people and things, and episodic maps that encode the relations between autobiographical events. There are also more abstract conceptual maps, like the ones that chart how cities interrelate on the axes of urban sprawl, architectural grandeur, or political clout. Maps differ in their dimensionality. The axis of French city size, headed by Paris, lies on a single dimension, and the Cartesian map of the metro system, with Châtelet at its centre, is a two-dimensional manifold. Other maps are high-dimensional, like that charting the historical ties between politicians and palaces or that documenting your Parisian visit itself, weaved together from memories of boulevards and brasseries that were linked in space and time. Each of our mental maps embeds a dense web of associations that specifies how everything we know is related to everything else.

Sensory data arrive to the brain in a relentless, massively detailed, multimodal input stream. Our sensory systems mine data from this stream, sorting it in meaningful representational units. These units form the building blocks for our mental maps, which collectively make up our knowledge—our model of the world. It was Craik who first argued that to be useful, our internal models should be organized to match the external world. But there are many different ways to carve up natural experience into a mental model. What are the different formatting constraints on our mental maps? How is incoming information selected, sorted, and indexed to form those mental building blocks? Previously, we discussed the shortcoming of purely symbolic AI systems, that their representations are not grounded in the external world. Neural networks have the opposing problem—there are an infinity of possible ways in which mental representations could be grounded, and so how do we choose which formatting to adopt? What should our mental representations *refer to*? Along which conceptual axes should our maps be formed, and how are they combined to support thought and action?

Writing in the nineteenth century, the philosopher Charles Sanders Peirce founded the modern field of semiotics by prescribing three ways in which signs relate to their referents. He called these relations *iconic*, *indexical*, and *symbolic*. Iconic relations are likenesses: a photograph is an iconic representation of the scene it portrays. Indexical relations are those that arise when a shared context is created between sign and reference. This can be through an overt act (like when I point to something, or otherwise single it out) or passively (as when a murderer, victim, and witness mutually index one another in the context of a crime). Symbolic relations denote otherwise arbitrary links which are agreed by convention, such as between an object and a verbal label. The word 'cat' is an arbitrary symbol that we use to refer to domestic felines.

Peirce was writing long before the advent of cognitive science, but his tripartite theory can be usefully repurposed to consider how mental representations are grounded. Some are grounded in physical likenesses. The activation of an *iconic* mental representation depends on physical similarity. For example, a neuron that responds to a cricket ball might also activate to a Gala apple, because they are approximately the same size, shape, and colour. Other representations are grounded by indexicality: the association between a cricket bat and ball is not forged by physical resemblance, but by the fact that in the natural world, they are linked by a shared context in space and time—they are found together in the kit bag. Finally, some representations are grounded in shared convention or culture. A cricket ball and a snowboard rarely co-occur, as one is used on a well-tended lawn in summer, and the other on the ski slopes in winter. But they are grounded in a category that humans agree to denote as *sport*—they both have the latent (or unobservable) property of being items of sporting equipment.[24] As we shall see, the human brain forms representations that are grounded in all three of these ways, as well as learning some more exotic classes of concept.

Early adopters trained neural networks on arbitrary mappings between verbal labels. Networks learnt to encode the hierarchical semantic structure that relates words denoting objects (*rose*), categories (*flower*), and properties (*has petals*). In fact, it is a poorly kept secret that the pioneers of connectionism used the same sleight of hand as proponents of symbolic AI: input and output patterns were non-overlapping (one-hot vectors),[25] so that patterns for

---

[24] One latent property has been deemed so significant that it forms the basis for a whole subfield in machine learning. This property is a proxy for the survival value for the agent of experiencing an event or acquiring an object, and is usually called *reward*. The framework of RL assumes that learning to maximize reward is a necessary, or even sufficient, condition for intelligent behaviour. It is discussed in Chapter 6.

[25] In a one-hot vector, one unit has a value of 1 and other inputs have a value of zero. If each input is denoted by a unique one-hot vector, then all inputs are equally dissimilar to one another.

rose and *daisy* and *spaniel* were all equally dissimilar. Thus, although we are taught to think of connectionist models as a counterpoint to symbolic AI, in Peirce's terms, early neural networks were 'symbolic' models, because the inputs and outputs were hand-labelled by the researcher. This choice was driven by necessity. The computers of the 1980s were too puny to process natural images or speech in all their high-dimensional input complexity. However, this meant that unlike their modern counterparts, these networks were not ultimately grounded in natural sensory signals.

Instead, it was the supervision signals that taught the network the structure of categories and properties. Early networks learnt concepts that were grounded in the teaching signals provided by the researcher. The most efficient way for the network to map inputs like *spaniel* and *pug* onto properties such as *likes walks* and *goes woof* is to acquire a concept that we would recognize as *dog* in its hidden layer. In fact, given the hierarchical structure of the objects and categories on which the network was trained (e.g. that both cats and dogs *have fur*, but only dogs *like walks*), the network learnt well-structured representations in its hidden layer. They can learn distinctions that are fine (spaniel vs pug), intermediate (cat vs dog), and coarse (plant vs animal), all from the same data, encoding them in a semantic hierarchy of generality that mimics human conceptual learning.

Early excitement around neural networks was spurred on by the finding that their learning follows a human-like developmental trajectory (Plunkett & Sinha 1992). For example, neural networks show *progressive differentiation*, acquiring coarse distinctions before fine ones, just like children distinguish *dog* and *cat* before *spaniel* and *pug* (Keil 1979). Networks gradually learnt to generalize, just like human children do. For example, after learning that a rose *has petals* and is a *flower*, they could infer that because a daisy has petals, it is probably a flower too. Both children and neural networks learn with distinctive pathways, in that periods of rapid progress are followed by plateaus of relatively static performance. During some stages, both children and neural networks maintain stereotyped illusory beliefs, such as the fact that worms must have bones,[26] which are gradually erased as training converges. Without being explicitly programmed to do so, thus, neural network models make a similar staccato progress towards understanding the world that people do. Recent work has studied the formal properties of learning in deep networks, providing explanations for these phenomena that are couched in terms of the mathematics of gradient descent.[27]

---

[26] Because they are animals, which mostly have bones.
[27] See (Saxe et al. 2019).

Powered by modern computers, deep networks today can process data from the ground up. In each processing cycle, hundreds, or even thousands, of pixel values from a photograph or video stream are fed directly to high-dimensional input layers. This allows neural networks to learn and generalize representations from naturalistic sensory data, and thus to solve real-world challenges, such as biometric facial identification or automated vehicle licence plate recognition. This opens the door to representations that are grounded in physical likeness (iconic concepts), spatiotemporal contiguity (indexical concepts), or arbitrary categories trained with supervision (symbolic concepts). It also raises the empirical question of how representations in deep networks are formed in practice, and the normative question of which constraints will allow rich conceptual knowledge to emerge. How can we build AI systems that can grasp abstractions that only humans currently understand?

The first forays into these questions began in the early 2000s, when deep networks started to show leaps and bounds on supervised classification of handwritten characters (such as MNIST[28]) and natural objects (ImageNet). This invited researchers to dig into their hidden layers and perform the sorts of experiments familiar to neuroscientists: to probe the inner workings of their virtual brains by measuring their representational properties. This naturally led to the question of whether these neural codes resemble those in biological systems. Can we treat deep networks not just as tools for engineering accurate predictions, but also as generalized theories of representation learning for the neural theory?

Intriguingly, the brains of humans and deep networks exhibit striking similarities. When trained with supervision on benchmark tasks, such as ImageNet, supervised deep convolutional neural networks (CNNs) form visual representations that resemble those in neural data recorded from humans and other primates. This result is obtained in various ways, but perhaps the most compelling is the comparison between RDMs from neural activity patterns in the visual cortex[29] and those from ensembles of network units (Figure 4.2). The primate and network RDMs—viewed side by side—show striking commonalities. In fact, some researchers have set sterner tests of this correspondence, by using advanced deep learning methods to predict how neurons should respond to unusual stimuli, or using networks to estimate how long it should take a monkey to classify an image with a potentially ambiguous class label.[30] This suggests that there are overlapping principles by

---

[28] The 'Modified National Institute of Standards and Technology database'.
[29] In either functional magnetic resonance imaging (fMRI) signals or multi-electrode recordings.
[30] See (Bashivan et al. 2019) and (Kar et al. 2019). In general, the work of Jim DiCarlo's lab has been visionary in tackling this problem.

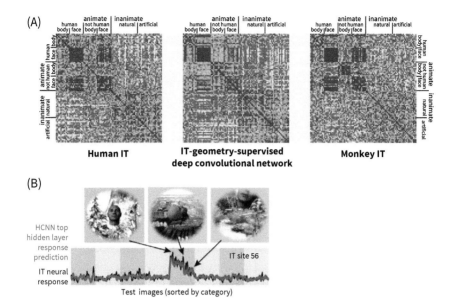

Fig. 4.2 Examples of correspondence between neural representations formed in deep networks and biological brains.

(**A**) Representational dissimilarity matrices (RDMs) signalling the dissimilarity in neural code between each stimulus and every other stimulus for human BOLD signals (left panel), deep convolutional networks (middle panel) and monkey IT cortex (right panel). Warm colours are areas of greater dissimilarity; cool colours are areas of greater similarity.

Reprinted from Khaligh-Razavi and Kriegeskorte 2014.

(**B**) Average response to images sorted by category (black) and equivalent response in a performance-optimized deep neural network.

Reprinted with permission from Yamins et al. (2014).

which object recognition occurs in primates and CNNs—for example, that the degree to which they think that roses and daisies, or dogs and flowers, or animals and tools are related to one another is roughly the same as in biological brains. For neuroscientists, this has raised hope that deep networks are on a path to crack the problem of generalization for naturalistic vision, in which objects are recognized under novel combinations of position, pose, and illumination.

Decades of scrutiny have taught us that neural coding in the visual cortex respects a hierarchy of complexity. This hierarchy unfolds along the neural highway linking the visual cortex and temporal lobes, colloquially known as the ventral stream. At the outset of this pathway is area V1, just two synapses from the retina,[31] where neurons respond preferentially to basic elements of a scene, such as oriented edges or texture primitives, within a tightly confined spatial window. Thus, one neuron might fire to a contour tilted at 45° in its preferred aperture, and but not to a vertical edge, whereas another neuron might respond in a converse fashion. At subsequent stages of processing, neurons prefer simple shapes and rudimentary objects; delving deeper into the temporal lobe, they fire to complex stimuli such as cars, faces, animals, or entire natural scenes, irrespective of where they occur in the visual field. These are the temporal lobe regions where intracranial stimulation provokes mind-bending hallucinations of people and places that materialize from nowhere in the middle of the operating room.

The coding patterns formed in deep CNNs trained to label images obey a similar principle. Early layers form simple filters for tilt and spatial frequency, akin to those in area V1, whereas deeper in the network, we observe units that code for high-level categories and concepts—just like in the primate ventral stream. For example, reverse engineering the selectivity of CNN neurons identifies units that prefer faces, tools, or alphanumeric characters, even though these labels do not exist in the ImageNet data set on which it was trained.[32] This means that CNNs learn, from natural signals alone, a hierarchy of generality that allows them to make both coarse and fine distinctions, acquiring visual codes that allow them to lump and split the world according to semantic necessity—just like biological brains.

How is it then that deep networks learn human-interpretable semantic structure from just a handful of computational tricks and a million parameters? Where are these neural codes grounded? One clue comes from the fact that meaningful representations can be read out from deep CNNs, even before any training has occurred, when weights are still initialized to random values.[33] This might sound implausible at first: how can neural networks seemingly exhibit representations of *rose* and *spaniel* without being trained to distinguish dogs from flowers, and with recognition performance that is no better than chance? The answer is that the sensory signals naturally contain structure which is related to their meaning, because objects that belong to common categories often look alike. Thus, neural systems can form iconic representations even without being trained on symbolic information, such as matching to verbal labels via supervision.

---

[31] Visual area 1 or Brodmann's area 17, the first cortical waystation for most visual information.
[32] See (Yosinski et al. 2015).
[33] See (Yamins et al. 2014).

This physical resemblance is not always expressed at the level of local patches of pixels—for example, if viewed through a small aperture, roses, daisies, and spaniels may all seem quite different. However, natural scenes are themselves hierarchically structured. Shapes are made of lines and edges, objects are ensembles of shapes, and scenes are arrays of objects.[34] The natural sensory hierarchy affords many distinct levels at which images can resemble one another. After accounting for the high-level interactions among features, such as the common juxtaposition of stem and petals, roses are more physically similar to daisies than to spaniels.[35] We can see this by looking at the RDM computed from patterns of activation in the deeper layers, which is structured in a semantically coherent way, even before the network has been trained. By wiring up the network to gradually express these interactions through successive computation, activity in deeper processing units reflects the similarity among higher-level concepts such as flowers and dogs.

In both brains and CNNs, much of the connectivity needed to achieve this is present at birth. Biological sensory systems start out in life with a hierarchical wiring diagram dictated by the genes, which mandates that cells coding for an adjacent retinal territory project to common neuronal targets in the subsequent layer. Thus, neurons in the deeper reaches of the visual system have a wider purview of the visual field by virtue of all the lower neurons that project to them, just like a general has the broadest oversight of the battlefield from the information that percolates up the military hierarchy, via dispatches from colonels, majors, and captains. In CNNs, a similar pattern of converging connectivity (and expanding receptivity) is also crafted directly into the network by the researcher. It is a core architectural motif that each layer receives inputs from a subset of units in the layer below with adjacent local receptivity, so that like biological systems, a CNN represents a spatial hierarchy of filters.

For systems wired up in this way, visual recognition resembles a well-known parable in which blindfolded men attempt to recognize an elephant. Each man receives information about a distinct body part—the trunk, the ear, the leg, or the flank—and confidently (but wrongly) infers that the object is a snake, a fan, a tree trunk, or a wall. The representations of early visual neurons are like the reports of these men: they signal the parts of an object but fail to grasp the whole.

---

[34] In fact, early models imagined that vision literally involved constructing mental objects from geometric primitives called geons (Biederman 1987), much like proponents of symbolic AI believed that reality was built from AND, OR, and NOT.

[35] Except perhaps when viewed from a very unusual angle. Images with unusual views would mostly be pruned from image data sets. Note that this was not the case for early connectionist models, in which the inputs *rose*, *daisy*, and *spaniel* were orthogonal (non-overlapping) one-hot vectors, so they were all equally unalike, obliging the network to learn structure from supervision, and not the inputs.

However, an overseer receiving these reports can infer the presence of an elephant, like higher neurons in the temporal lobe can recognize objects from the combined outputs of neurons at earlier stages. Critically, if you swapped the men around, their individual reports would differ radically, but the elephant could still be inferred; just like if you altered the view of a rose, individual pixels would change, but it would still be recognizable from the presence and relation of a stem and petals. This is why neurons at higher stages are invariant to the minutiae of low-level stimulation. The simple fact that neurons in deeper layers have access to interacting throughput from earlier layers, coupled with the intrinsic structure of the world, is enough for a hierarchy of generality to emerge in a deep neural network.

These observations tell us that the neural wiring diagram in both biological and artificial sensory systems is pre-engineered to encode information in a well-organized fashion, in particular by capitalizing on an existing input structure. Returning to the warehouse example, if imports arriving from the four points of the compass are housed in corresponding storage zones located in the north, south, east, and west of the warehouse, then it will be considerably easier to sort them for distribution. Even more usefully, if patterns of imports that tend to arrive at once—chassis from the United States, tyres from Italy, and engines from France—are stored in the same place, then it is easier to ship them out together. The way the switches are set help memory systems store information in a useful format.

However, it is important to note that good connectivity is only the start. Ultimately, external supervised training is eventually needed for successful object labelling. It is not enough to store tyres and chassis and engine together—you need to know to which car manufacturer to ship them. Supervised training maps the representations onto the correct output labels (the stem-and-petals pattern onto *flower*), so that the network outputs are interpreted correctly. But in neural networks, supervision also sculpts the representations themselves. Although seemingly sensible coding patterns can emerge, even in randomly initialized networks, training with supervision makes deep networks more human-like. In fact, careful analysis has revealed that those CNN variants that achieve the highest accuracy on benchmark challenges, such as ImageNet, are those that learn the most biologically viable visual representations for the challenge stimuli.[36] This implies that the neural codes we form in the visual cortex are massaged by the words we have learnt to

---

[36] Under the assumption that hidden layer activity is a affine fit of neural activity (obtained in cross-validation).

refer to concepts. For example, penguins, ostriches, and swifts look very different but are all birds; our semantic knowledge of their relative position in the Linnean taxonomy moulds their neural similarity into a common schema for *bird*, even though they differ radically in size and shape. The way we perceive the world is shaped by the verbal labels we use to describe the objects and events that we encounter.[37]

4.4 Deep dreams

In November 2019, the UK think tank Future Advocacy[38] released a video in which political rivals Jeremy Corbyn and Boris Johnston made compelling cases for how the public should cast their votes in the forthcoming general election. Remarkably, however, neither leader took the opportunity to canvas votes for themselves. Instead, each advocated for the opposing party, turning the usual political consensus inside out. Unfortunately, however, the video was not a harbinger of some gentler new era of political bipartisanship. It was a fake—and a remarkably authentic one. Future Advocacy released the video with the specific intent of alerting the public to the threat posed by so-called *deep fake* photos and videos, which are media content synthesized to distort or misrepresent reality, that can be used maliciously for political advantage or for other nefarious purposes.

A branch of deep learning, known as *generative modelling*, has made this possible. Generative models are trained to *infer the causes* of their input data. The central intuition is that whilst input signals are high-dimensional and varied, they are often generated by just a handful of semantically meaningful variables.[39] For example, imagine a data set consisting of photographs of apples. Apples can be larger (Fuji) or smaller (Crab), and redder (Gala) or greener (Granny Smith). There are an infinity of possible apples, but they all lie within the bidimensional space defined by apple colour and size. A generative model learns to encode these latent factors—the axes of the map of pomological space—by predicting the high-dimensional training data. Having successfully done so, the model can be inverted to generate—or 'imagine'—new synthetic images, for example those comprising apples defined by a particular size and

---

[37] As discussed in Chapter 2.
[38] See https://futureadvocacy.com/. See https://www.youtube.com/watch?v=EkfnjAeHFAk.
[39] With other variation being considered a nuisance.

colour (i.e. position in latent space).[40] It can even be used to generate new apple varieties that do not exist—deep fake apples, if you like.

One successful tool for generative modelling is known as a variational autoencoder (or VAE). An autoencoder is a class of generative model that learns to reconstruct the very data that it receives as inputs, in a process often called self-supervision.[41] At first glance, this sounds nonsensical—if the inputs are already available, then what is to be gained by reproducing them? The secret, however, is that the network encodes the signals onto a *bottleneck* layer with reduced capacity (fewer processing units). For example, if a VAE were trained on images of apples with just two bottleneck units, it might learn to embed each image in a space whose axes are size and colour. This encourages the network to reconstruct apple images that live within the space of small-to-large and red-to-green that the network has experienced—to learn a good compression of the data. In a VAE, the semantic interpretability of the concepts learnt is enhanced because the network is additionally encouraged to form latent factors which are as unrelated as possible, through a separate cost term for *disentanglement*.[42] One variant of this architecture known as a β-VAE, has been used to learn human-interpretable factors from natural images, such as data sets of faces, vehicles, or chairs. For example, when trained to reconstruct face images, it acquires latent units (those in the bottleneck layer) that code for age, gender, hairstyle, and affective expressions such as happiness (smiling or frowning) (Figure 4.3).[43]

To probe the latent variables that the network has learnt, we can intervene virtually, by setting the latent units to values of our own choosing and running the model in reverse to decode (or generate) predicted sensory signals. For example, we can systematically clamp a single latent unit to a series of continuous values, and thus generate a sweep of imagined face images that vary on a single latent dimension, such as young to old, fringy to bald, or happy to sad. The factors can also be recomposed in interesting ways for imagination

---

[40] In fact, to generate astonishingly photorealistic synthetic faces, an extra trick is used, whereby one network is trained to generate images, and another to discriminate between the generated data and the training data. The first network is encouraged to try and trick the second. This is called a generative adversarial network (or GAN) (Goodfellow et al. 2014).

[41] That is, to produce outputs that are as similar as possible to the inputs. There is some confusion over the terminology. Methods for learning the latent factors in data (e.g. like principal or independent component analysis (PCA or ICA)) have traditionally been referred to as 'unsupervised'. The term self-supervision is usually reserved for methods that construct an auxiliary loss from the data (such as predicting one patch from another). For simplicity, we only use the latter term here.

[42] See (Higgins et al. 2016). The β-VAE increases the pressure to disentangle, which helps learn unrelated factors from data.

[43] What makes a 'good' compression is inevitably somewhat subjective. If the researcher has created the data set with a small set of factors, then a good compression might recover these. But the researcher's intuitions about the independence of the factors they have used might be wrong. For example, if all green

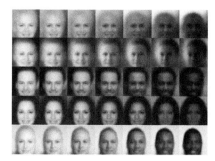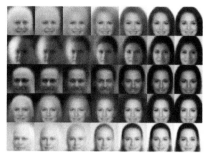

Fig. 4.3 Images generated by systematic activation of latent units in a β-VAE. Left units encode ethnicity; the right unit encodes age/gender.

and mental simulation. For example, if you have learnt disentangled neural codes for facial age, gender, and affect, then you can imagine Greta Thunberg as an angry old man or Donald Trump as a happy young woman. You can generate a video with Boris Johnson mouthing Jeremy Corbyn's words, or vice versa. Beyond the domain of faces, a β-VAE trained on videos of first-person movement through a virtual maze can be adapted to reimagine new scenes from environmental building blocks such as walls, doors, and furniture, as if it had learnt key latent factors that make up our carpentered world.[44]

The success of generative models tells us that by compressing and orthogonalizing transformed sensory signals, we can learn rich concepts from sensory data alone.[45] Embedded in the streams of sensory information that we receive are deep patterns expressing semantically meaningful variables. Generative models trained with photographs of faces can learn the concept of age—that some faces are fresh and youthful, and others are wizened with time. Trained on furniture, they learn that there exists a low-dimensional manifold of chair shapes—on which *stool*, *pew*, and *sofa* are all unique points. This even allows them to creatively remix these concepts to imagine new furniture items, such as a plush church pew without a backrest. Thus, generative models allow us to form highly structured and semantically interpretable maps of how features and objects in the world relate to one another.

---

apples are mottled, whereas red ones are not, then being mottled might not be a factor in itself. In the natural world, we do not know what the generating factors are, so good compressions are those that we can interpret.

[44] See (Higgins et al. 2017).

[45] Here, we focus on visual data, which have been explored most extensively. Vision is the dominant modality for primates, with up to 30% of the cortical real estate devoted to visual perception in humans, and 50% in the macaque, which is the non-human primate whose visual system has been studied in greatest detail.

The idea that the natural world offers up its abstractions from sensory data alone echoes a long-standing theme in developmental psychology. Even before they learn language, children seem to understand what objects are. They sense how objects interact physically and know how they can be grouped. Infants as young as 12 weeks can perceive object boundaries, fill in occluded object parts, and predict when objects will move or come to rest.[46] They can also discriminate basic visual categories, such as shapes (squares and triangles) and animals (birds and dogs).[47] Babies thus rapidly begin to make sense of what William James famously called the 'buzzing, blooming confusion' of sensory experience, and they do so largely without the help of verbal labels.

Recently, researchers have started to gather large-scale data sets documenting the visual experience of human infants, for example by embedding a coin-sized camera in a beanie that is constantly worn as the babies go about their daily lives.[48] Capitalizing on one such data set comprising tens of thousands of headcam images, a team of researchers at New York University asked whether a generative model in principle allowed the formation of high-level object categories from naturalistic sensory experience. After training, the representations learnt by the model could be mapped linearly onto high-level object categories from a labelled problem set focussing on toys[49] (such as *cat*, *spoon*, and *helicopter*). This implies that self-supervision is, in theory, sufficient to allow the formation of high-level concepts, even when explicit object labels are unavailable.

Evidence from neuroscience suggests that the computations carried out by generative models, such as the VAE, explain how representations are formed in biological brains. Generative models imply the existence of low-dimensional neural codes—that neurons will represent complex inputs with as few factors as possible.[50] In fact, the idea that single neurons code for the latent generative factors first found voice more than 20 years ago,[51] when it was shown that when monkeys are trained to discriminate unusual shapes—closed curves with prominent bulges and wiggles—inferior temporal cortex (IT) neurons respond

---

[46] See (Spelke & Kinzler 2007).

[47] As demonstrated by studies in which viewing preferences are measured after sensory habituation. The infant is exposed to one category (e.g. dogs), and then given a choice between exemplars from that category (e.g. more dogs) or a new category (e.g. birds). Infants usually prefer to look at novel objects, and so (for example) the fact that they choose to look at birds suggests that they can tell dogs and birds apart by this age.

[48] For example, the SAYCam data set from Michael Frank's laboratory at Stanford (Sullivan et al. 2020) or the Homeview data set from Linda Smith's laboratory at Indiana (Clerkin et al. 2017). One interesting finding is that children's visual experience changes with time in stylized ways as they first learn to sit up, crawl, and then walk, with the different stimuli and viewpoints they experience. Thus, learning about the visual world according to a natural curriculum may help the emergence of visual cognition.

[49] The ToyBox data set (Wang et al. 2018b).

[50] For example, in the VAE, with as many dimensions as there are units in the bottleneck layer.

[51] See (Op de Beeck et al. 2001).

to the two principal stimulus-generating factors. In other words, IT neurons are tuned to locations in the mental map of frequency and amplitude of curvature variation.[52] In newer studies, the tuning properties of IT neurons to faces were shown to correspond to the latent factors learnt by a β-VAE, which was trained to reconstruct faces from the same data set.[53] The implication is that brains may share computational motifs with self-supervised models, allowing them to learn factorized, low-dimensional representations of input data. This allows the brain to parse the world into abstract visual concepts, even if these are several processing stages away from the low-level pixels that make up the input data.

In a vanilla CNN, such as AlexNet, signals travel forward through successive network layers as input pixels are gradually mapped onto object labels. Generative models, however, allow information to flow both forward and backward through the network. The forward flow occurs as inputs are *encoded* onto latent units to compress the signal, and the backward flow as the latent signals are *decoded* back into the input space to reconstruct the image. This bidirectional passage of information is also a key feature of biological sensory systems. In fact, in the primate visual system, backward connections may outnumber forward projections by a ratio of 10:1. The stereotyped exchange of neural signals with both lower and higher processing stages is baked into the canonical microcircuit for granular cortex, which specifies how efferent and afferent signals flow to and from each of the six cortical laminae[54] (Figure 4.4). Biological vision is thus often described as being jointly guided by both *top-down* (backward) and *bottom-up* (forward) signals.

Neuroscientists have long suspected that the role of top-down neural signals is to predict the sensory world. Biological brains seem to be exquisitely sensitive to whether an observed signal is likely or unlikely. When a stimulus is expected, its corresponding neural pattern builds up in advance of presentation, as if the brain were anticipating what is to come. By contrast, when a stimulus occurs out of the blue, its neural pattern is expressed more powerfully, as if the brain were caught off guard. Neural activity is thus constantly up- and downregulated in an economy of expectation and surprise. These observations have spawned wide-ranging theories that have argued that making predictions is the basic function of intelligent systems or that the ultimate goal of the nervous system is to avoid surprise altogether.[55]

---

[52] See (Cortese & Dyre 1996).

[53] See (Higgins et al. 2021).

[54] This article provides a nice overview (Bastos et al. 2012).

[55] See (Hawkins 2004). The latter point, associated with Karl Friston, has been made with a mixture of poetry and pomposity (Friston 2013). For one of many ripostes, see (Sun & Firestone 2020). As mentioned in Chapter 1, this is perhaps the closest we have got to general theories in psychology.

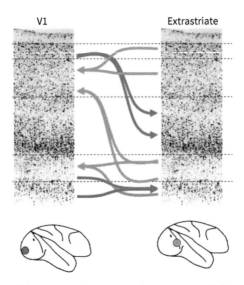

Fig. 4.4 A schematic of the connection patterns between cortical stages in the primate visual cortex. Dashed lines show the boundaries between layers.

Neural evidence for predictive signals abounds in biological brains. For example, if you present an image comprising a non-descript blob on a pair of realistic shoulders, the human brain interprets it as a face, even if it has no visible features—and face-sensitive regions of the visual cortex respond accordingly (Figure 4.5).[56] In one inventive study, the brains of human participants were scanned whilst they viewed naturalistic photographs that had one quadrant blanked out. The authors then used multivariate analysis methods to show that it was possible to decode the contents of the photographs from voxels in the visual cortex that were spatially selective for the missing quadrant. Because these voxels received no bottom-up visual signals, the successful decoding was most likely due to predictive signals that allowed the brain to 'fill in' the missing quadrant with plausible information about the photographs, offering a pleasing demonstration of how the human brain predicts the world.[57]

In neuroscience, the idea that the brain is a generative model has a long pedigree, dating back to at least Helmholtz.[58] One modern variant of this theory, called *hierarchical predictive coding*, proposes that predicted and observed signals collide at each successive processing stage, with the former

[56] See (Cox et al. 2004).
[57] See (Smith & Muckli 2010).
[58] Hermann von Helmholtz: see https://en.wikipedia.org/wiki/Hermann_von_Helmholtz.

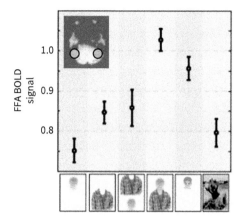

Fig. 4.5 BOLD responses in the fusiform face area (shown in inset) to several conditions, including faces and non-faces in a face context. FFA, fusiform face area.
Adapted with permission from Cox et al. 2004.

'explaining away' the latter via a process of subtractive normalization.[59] This means that each processing layer receives predictions (from above) and observations (from below) but, in turn, only passes forward that part of the bottomup input that *remains unexplained* by the top-down signal (the *prediction error*). This latter claim explains why surprising events elicit large neural transients, because they are associated with more substantial prediction errors.

If I ask you to think of a zebra, your mental image probably contains some impressive detail—the distinctive markings, equine form, black snout, and spiky mane. But whilst you can probably imagine its stripes in some detail, can you count them? Most people report that they can't. This illustrates the fact that when we imagine the sensory world, our predictions are somewhat impressionistic—rarely detailed right down to the level of photographic pixels. This is different from generative models like the β-VAE, for which reconstruction error is computed in the native space of the training images themselves. One merit of hierarchical predictive coding is that the contrast between expectation and observation is computed separately at each level of abstraction. This means the model can compute zebra expectations in the abstract space defined by stripiness and horsiness, not in terms of the precise phase or orientation of the black-and-white stripes on its hide. More generally, in predictive coding for vision, the job of predicting the scene is partitioned over the visual hierarchy, so that high-level neurons predict objects, mid-level

---

[59] See (Rao & Ballard 1999).

neurons predict shapes, and low-level neurons predict lines. The network is thus relieved of the burden of reconstructing every atom of a visual scene.

A significant new development in machine learning draws on this intuition,[60] and has adapted it to beat various benchmark tests for object recognition. The idea behind *contrastive predictive coding* (CPC) is to cut a visual scene up into random overlapping patches, and to use information about past patches to predict whether the next patch comes from the same or a different image.[61] The idea that a scene is taken in sequentially, in discrete segments, is, of course, reminiscent of another biological motif—that we sample a scene by moving our gaze to repeated points in succession, by making saccadic eye movements.[62] Critically, however, and just like in biological predictive coding, the network is not obliged to reconstruct every pixel but instead has to predict whether this is the right sort of patch for the image, given its high-level statistics. In this sense, it is obliged to do something very similar to participants in the missing quadrant study—given a partial view of a scene, it infers what is absent. CPC has proved remarkably successful. It learns semantically meaningful visual concepts, even from largely unstructured image data sets such as ImageNet, as shown by the interpretable response properties of single neurons—that learn to code for birds, human faces, vehicle wheels, and mountains. Linear decoding from its representations was sufficient to beat the 2019 state-of-the-art classification accuracy on ImageNet by nearly 10%, a significant leap forward at the time.[63]

Generative modelling allows networks to learn the factors from which the visual world is built. By identifying the deep structural patterns by which image pixels covary across a data set, they can learn meaningful high-level concepts from sensory data. When trained on faces, the β-VAE learns a concept of age because buried in the pixels themselves, there is a latent factor whose activity denotes whether a face is young, middle-aged, or old. This is impressive, but compared to the breadth and scope of human knowledge, it only begins to scratch the epistemological surface. Human knowledge is spread across multiple different mental maps, each charting a different aspect of the relations among objects and events. We know that the Eiffel Tower is tall and approximately triangular in shape—physical characteristics that can be learnt from visual data. However, we can also mentally place it next to the

---

[60] In fact, predictive coding is an old idea in signal processing, dating back to the 1950s (Elias 1955).

[61] CPC can, of course, be used with auditory stimuli too—just replace 'image patch' with 'auditory segment'.

[62] Saccadic control is largely a hallmark of primate vision, although other species may orient their eyes to sample visual information in more limited ways.

[63] See (van Oord et al. 2019).

Champ de Mars, in the 7th Arrondissment; we know that it was constructed in the nineteenth century, is made entirely of iron, and was the tallest building in the world until 1929 when it was surpassed by the Chrysler Building in New York. How could machines ever acquire knowledge like this?

4.5 When there is no there, there

In the early 1990s, a patient known as R.M. had the misfortune to suffer two strokes in quick succession, leaving him with a spate of nasty headaches. A magnetic resonance imaging (MRI) scan revealed an unusual pattern of brain damage: symmetric, bilateral lesions to the posterior parietal cortex (PPC) (Figure 4.6). The PPC lies at the back of the brain, just above the visual cortex, and is thought to be involved in selective attention, sensorimotor integration, and control of eye movements. At first, it was not clear exactly what R.M.'s difficulties might be. He fell within the normal range on standard tests of visual function, such as those quantifying acuity, contrast sensitivity, colour and shape perception, and ability to segment figures from the background. However, R.M. had some unusual deficits. If you showed him an object, he could name it. But if you showed him two objects, he seemed to be unsure what they were—or even that there were two of them. He could read single words fairly well but struggled with sentences. He could identify single faces but was confused by a crowd. His depth perception was poor: he was unable to tell you how far away an object might be or which of two objects was nearer. Most aspects of his language and cognition were normal, but he was very spatially disoriented and needed help getting to the hospital for his regular check-ups at the neurology clinic.

Patient R.M. had a rare neurological disorder known as Bálint's syndrome. One of the cardinal symptoms of Bálint's syndrome is *simultanagnosia*, which is an inability to perceive more than one object at a time. Thus, if you showed patient R.M. an image of a cat, he could tell you it was a cat. But if you showed him a cat and a dog, he could not tell you which was which. Nor could he tell you which was larger or how many animals there were on the screen. The existence of patients with Bálint's syndrome tells us something quite remarkable: that the brain has evolved specific regions that help us understand how objects relate to each other in visual space.

Figure 4.7 shows Camille Pissarro's famous canvas *Boulevard Montmartre*. Painted in 1897, it depicts the great thoroughfare that traverses Paris from *Arc de Triomphe* in the west to *République* in the east. Pissarro was a

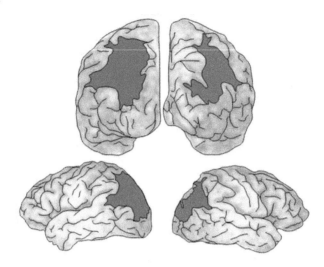

Fig. 4.6 Bilateral lesions to the posterior parietal cortex resulting in Bálint's syndrome. Reprinted with permission from Robertson et al. 2003.

pivotal figure in the movement of impressionist painters that flourished in nineteenth-century Paris. The impressionists were the radicals of their age. They rejected the dull, well-mixed tones, photorealistic styles, and historico-religious themes that were sanctioned by the influential *Académie des Beaux-Arts*. Instead, they experimented with landscapes and cityscapes, examining the interplay of movement and light between scene elements. They broke with traditional compositional pieties which demanded that a painting has an obvious subject in the foreground. Instead, the background was often the focus—trees bending in the wind, the sun on the water, or houses dotting a hillside. The impressionists' goal was to capture the *impress* of the scene on the viewers' mind. To achieve this, they trained their painterly gaze on the world just as we see it every day, producing richly textured and layered urban and rural scenes that portrayed people going about their daily lives.

The impressionists realized that visual meaning is located in the relations between objects, people, and places. Plane trees frame the entrance to a village. Children throw snowballs in the shadow of a house. Carriages scurry down a muddy highway at dusk. A horse stands patiently before a hay cart. Similarly, when recalling (or imagining) a visit to Paris, your mental images are not of isolated objects. They are like a Pissarro canvas—they feature bustling pavements and busy cafés and lights twinkling all over the city at dusk. By contrast, the photos that make up the ImageNet data set, which are so widely used in visual recognition challenges, are quite bizarre. Like the carefully framed

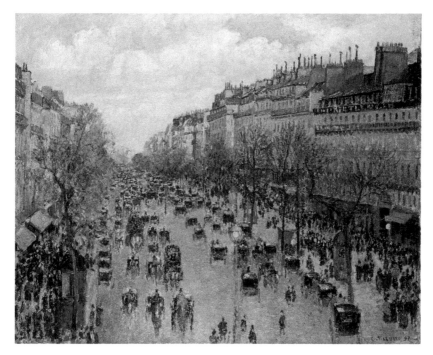

Fig. 4.7 The impressionists understood that perception depended on the relations between elements of a scene.
Boulevard Montmartre by Camille Pissarro (1897).

portraits favoured by the nineteenth-century *Académie*, most have a single, obvious subject—*lighthouse* or *labrador*. This allows them to be readily associated with a simple word or phrase, for labelling or captioning challenges. But for the most part, our visual world is not like that. It is the juxtaposition of elements that discloses the meaning of a visual scene.

Patients with Bálint's syndrome teach us that visual structure is not perceived directly. Instead, scenes are mentally constructed, with each element allocated to its relative location on a sort of mental canvas.[64] In humans and other primates, one important locus for this canvas is the PPC.[65] When healthy people see a cat and a dog side by side, they allocate the cat and the dog to two separate positions on the canvas, which allows them to identify, distinguish, and count them. But without the canvas, objects fall catastrophically

---

[64] From a psychological perspective, a *scene* has been defined as 'a semantically coherent . . . view of a real-world environment comprising background elements and multiple discrete objects arranged in a spatially licensed manner' (Henderson & Hollingworth 1999).
[65] And probably the hippocampus. See below.

on top of each other and cannot be mentally untangled. In patient R.M., this is revealed by a classic psychological test in which two alphanumeric characters are presented in different font colours at distinct locations on a screen.[66] If this image is flashed tachistoscopically, disappearing after milliseconds, then even healthy people will occasionally *misbind* the colours and shapes, reporting a red X and green A when, in fact, the A was red and the X was green. But R.M. exhibited these misbindings on 33% of trials, even when allowed to inspect the array for up to 10 seconds. Without a mental canvas, the shapes and colours cannot be separated into their spatial locations—red A on one side, and green X on the other. They are all just a confusing jumble of shapes and colours. R.M. himself explains this when asked to describe his visual experience:

> When I first look at it, it looks green and changes real quick to red. I see both colours coming together . . . When I look at it, it is an A. And sometimes I see a shadow of it [. . .] It looks like one letter is going into the other one. I get a double identity. It kind of coincides.

Bálint syndrome patients have no mental canvas, and so their visual space has no extent. To quote the neuropsychologist Lynn Robertson, who worked with R.M. for several years—it is as if for these patients, 'there is no there, there'.[67]

The meaning of a natural scene is disclosed by the relations among its elements. Consider the set of cartoons shown in Figure 4.8. All four panels show a man and a car. But the way we interpret the scene is entirely different in each case. On the left, the man is *inside* the car, whereas on the right, he is *outside*. In the upper panels, the man is *smaller than* the car, whereas in the lower panels, he is *larger than* it. This leads to a range of possible scenarios, in which the man is driving, or has broken down, or is riding in a child's go-kart, or is toying with a model vehicle. Yet if you were to train AlexNet on images such as these, it would simply label them all with 'man' or 'car'. The subtle meaning conveyed by the relations among elements would be lost.

Since the 1980s, neuroscientists have argued that the primate brain has evolved two distinct pathways for visual processing. We have already met the *ventral stream*, which runs along the underside of the brain from the visual

---

[66] See (Treisman & Schmidt 1982). The term illusory conjunctions is often used to describe this phenomenon.

[67] The original quote is attributable to Gertrude Stein and occurs in a very different context—she is talking about Oakland, California. See excellent papers by Lynn Robertson on this topic (Friedman-Hill et al. 1995; Robertson et al. 1997).

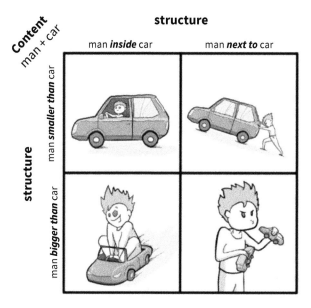

structure

Content
man + car

man *smaller than* car

man *bigger than* car

structure

man *inside* car

man *next to* car

Fig. 4.8 Interpreting a scene relies on the relations between its constituent objects.
Drawings by Hannah Sheahan.
From https://psyarxiv.com/zfxj2/

cortex to the temporal lobes. Here, objects are untangled from their context by
successive layers of neurons whose feature receptivity gradually narrows, but
whose spatial selectivity broadens until information about object location is
almost totally discarded. This pathway forms neural representations of complex features and objects, such as neurons that code for *car* or *man*—including
specific types of car or identities of man—in a way that is mirrored in deep
convolutional networks. In the primate, however, the ventral stream is accompanied by a parallel pathway that starts in visual regions and heads up along
the dorsal side of the cortex towards the PPC. On this *dorsal stream*, neurons
care less about *what* an object is and more about *where* it is.

Dorsal stream neurons, including those in the PPC, become active when a
salient object or feature occupies their preferred spatial location. The frame of
reference for spatial coding in the dorsal stream is centred on the self, so that
the neural population encodes locations in which objects can be grasped or
fixated with the gaze. In fact, the same neurons become prominently active
in the milliseconds before a reaching movement or saccade is made to their
preferred location in space. The cells are thus both active when a location in
space is earmarked by a prominent sensory stimulus or tagged as a probable

location for future action. Neuroimaging studies, which can chart brain activity at the regional level, have shown that directing attention to different locations evokes topographically coherent changes in PPC BOLD signal that generalize across tasks involving attention, working memory, and intention. In other words, the PPC may function as a generalized *priority map* of local visual space, signalling where we will direct attention in the visual world.[68]

By representing space in self-centred coordinates, the PPC is well placed to encode relations among objects. Imagine a rectangular sheet, laid out on the floor. We can dot the sheet with well-spaced objects—a book, a mug, a comb, and a watch. This is like mental representation in the intact PPC. Now imagine that I gather up the sheet, holding it on each side—the objects will all fall higgledy-piggledy into a central well. There is now no space, and so the objects are jumbled up and hard to individuate. This is what R.M. experiences. Now imagine what happens if I pin the sheet at its midpoint on the top and bottom, and just lift up one-half. The objects on that side—perhaps the comb and the mug—will slide down to the midline, coming to rest on the opposing side. This is similar to the experience of patients who have PPC damage in just a single hemisphere, who display a well-known pathology known as unilateral hemispatial neglect. When asked to draw a multielement array, patients either ignore objects contralateral to the lesioned side or crowd all the objects onto the intact side of visual space, as if their mental representations had slid down to the other side of the sheet. This phenomenon is known as allochiria (Figure 4.9).

Deep networks are often accused of lacking robustness. According to their critics, they slavishly spit out object labels but fail to grasp the deeper meaning of a scene. For example, in a recent critique of deep learning methods, Brenden Lake and colleagues highlighted the photo/caption pairing shown in Figure 4.10. A deep network catastrophically fails to grasp the meaning of an image.[69] These sorts of failure might be explained if networks fail to process how scene elements relate to one another: the juxtaposition of roaring waves, stricken building, and gritty determination on the faces of the fleeing people. Similarly, a vanilla CNN would fail to grasp the deep conceptual symmetry between the two scenes shown in Figure 4.11, in which a family are precariously balanced on a motorbike, or a litter of kittens on the resident dog. AlexNet may be a plausible model of the ventral stream—like R.M., whose ventral stream is intact, it can recognize and label lone objects. But because it lacks a dorsal stream, it has no sense of space. It cannot understand how scene

[68] See (Jerde et al. 2012). Also (Bisley & Goldberg 2010) provides a very nice review.
[69] See (Lake et al. 2017).

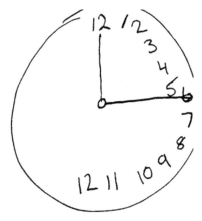

Fig. 4.9 An example of a drawing by a patient with Allochiria.

elements conspire to inject an image with meaning. Standard deep networks are thus like Bálint syndrome patients.

So what are the relations among objects that an intelligent agent needs to grasp? Is there a grammar for understanding visual scenes? In early twentieth century, not long after the heyday of impressionism, the *Gestalt psychologists* wrote down a set of axioms for understanding the world in terms of global configurations, rather than local elements.[70] Canonical Gestalt principles include similarity (are the elements the same?), proximity (are the elements close together?), connection (are the elements joined?), and continuity (are the elements aligned?). The spatial grammar that defines a visual scene might also include information about the number of copies of each element ('four cats') and their relative position to other objects ('a dog') given by basic prepositions ('on top of'). Their idea is that mentally constructing a percept surfaces more explicit information than is conveyed by the elements alone. Perception, the Gestaltists argued, is more than the sum of its parts (Figure 4.12).

These are, of course, precisely the sorts of aspects of a visual scene that standard deep networks like AlexNet fail to recognize. If you present a scene with four cats, the network does not know that there are four, rather than three or five. Instead, it just becomes more confident that there are cats in the image, because evidence is aggregated over multiple cat filters. In fact, standard deep networks are very poor at learning to count objects, unless

---

[70] Among these was Wolfgang Köhler, whose work on insight we discussed in Chapter 2. Recall his theory that the monkey has to 'grasp the whole layout' to solve the puzzle—a very Gestalt notion.

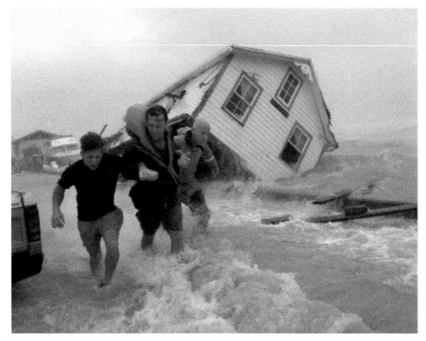

A group of people standing on
top of a beach

Fig. 4.10 Example of inappropriate image captioning by a deep network due to failure of scene understanding.
From Lake et al. (2017).

(A)   (B)

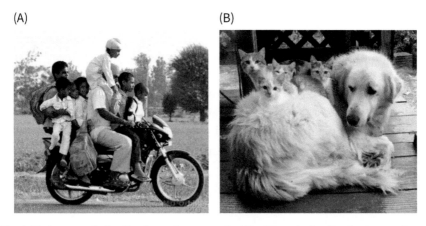

Fig. 4.11 Images of a family of people on a motorbike (**A**) and a family of cats on a dog (**B**). To understand the commonality between these scenes, you need to represent the relationship between the objects.
Images reprinted with permission.

Fig. 4.12 Perception is more than the sum of its parts. The image gives a strong impression of a sphere, even though none is shown.

the stimulus set gives the game away via the low-level statistics.[71] They are also poor at intuiting other Gestalt properties, such as symmetry, closure, and containment.[72]

AI researchers have yet to build deep networks that enjoy the explicit functionality of the dorsal stream.[73] But the idea that scene perception relies on object segmentation and relational inference has not escaped the machine learning community. One class of network explicitly tries to solve the problem of scene understanding by incorporating an architectural bias that objects are interrelated via a vocabulary of simple functions. Aptly called a Relation Network, the model first segments a scene into its constituent elements, by learning a set of filters (or weightings) over the image. Each filter earmarks a distinct object, so when attempting to make decisions (from pixels) about 3D tabletop object arrays in the CLEVR data set,[74] it might learn to separate the shiny blue square from the tall red pyramid (Figure 4.13). It then learns a set of relational functions that characterize how object pairs o_i and o_j relate. Each function $g(o_i, o_j)$ can itself be a simple feedforward neural network, and the output is the sum over relational functions. So for example, learnt functions

---

[71] For example, if objects are similarly sized and are black on a white background, then the number of black pixels will correlate with the number. If space is constrained, arrays with more elements may have different spatial frequency properties, which networks can also use as a clue. This has made this question controversial.

[72] For example, see (Fleuret et al. 2011).

[73] Although see (Mineault et al. 2021).

[74] See here (Johnson et al. 2016).

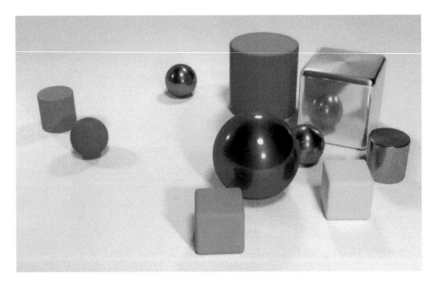

Fig. 4.13 Example image from the CLEVR data set. Example questions include: 'Are there an equal number of large things and metal spheres?' or 'There is a sphere with the same size as the metal cube. Is it made of the same material as the small red sphere?'.
Reprinted with permission from Johnson et al. 2016.

might implement a spatial vocabulary given by prepositions, such as *behind, on top of, left of,* and *next to.* This makes it easy for the network to map ground truth relations in the image onto labels or even simple phrases in natural language. When road-tested on a benchmark question answering problem set using CLEVR ('which object is behind the blue cylinder?'), the network reached 95% accuracy, trouncing the existing state of the art by 27%. It can even handle questions involving composites of multiple spatial relations in combinations it has not faced before, such as 'there is a big thing on the right side of the big rubber cylinder that is behind the large cylinder to the right of the tiny yellow rubber thing—what is its shape?'. The relation net achieved >90% accuracy on questions like these, surpassing human performance.

The foundational principle of neural network research is that intelligent agents need to be knowledgeable. They have to learn representations whose content and structure matches the way the world is organized—as Craik prescribed, their internal models should map isomorphically onto the outside world. By forming richly structured representations—abstract concepts, such as *beaver, circus, happy,* or *above*—the hope is that networks will be equipped to deal with the relentless arrival of novel sensations and experiences that are ferried towards us on Heraclitus' river. They allow us to generalize in a world where time moves ineluctably forward.

The streams of data that we access through the senses contain information about how the world is structured. However, sensory signals are variable, noisy, multidimensional, non-linear, composite, cluttered, complex, and confusing. Excavating meaning from sensory throughput is a daunting task, even for powerful networks equipped with millions of parameters and trained on millions of images. Upon arrival, useful knowledge is inextricably entangled and hopelessly undecipherable. Because training data are finite, and the problem is Herculean, machine learning researchers have turned to architectural priors—inductive biases—that build in knowledge of how the world is organized. The world has a *non-accidental structure*, that is, there are deep regularities in how sensory signals are constituted. Consider three examples: the world is *clumpy*, the world is *smooth*, and the world is *friable*.

The world being *clumpy* means that there are clusters of similar objects that physically resemble one another (such as birds) but are different from other objects (such as toasters). This means that CNNs, such as AlexNet, can use local receptivity and layerwise image transformations that are geared to disentangle shared patterns of features, and group them into distinct classes. These clumps are position- and context-invariant, so the networks can learn filters that are automatically shared across space—allowing it to intuit that a bird on a kitchen counter is still a bird, and a toaster in a tree is still a toaster.[75] The world being *smooth* means that high-dimensional sensory signals can be compactly described by a small number of latent factors. This means that generative models, such as a VAE, can extract knowledge of the axes on which faces, or trees, or cars smoothly vary, allowing the network to make predictions by interpolating or extrapolating in this latent space. Finally, the world being *friable* (or 'crumbly') means that it is divided up into discrete entities (objects) which are broken off from a larger whole (the background). A mountain is strewn with boulders; a kitchen counter is stacked with plates; a lawn is littered with leaves. Objects are numerous, spatially non-overlapping, and related in stereotyped ways. This means that Relation Networks can learn and generalize a canonical set of relational principles, such as encoding what it means for two adjacent objects to be perched on a larger object—and thus to understand the structural commonality between kittens on a labrador and a family on a motorbike.

AI researchers often strive to eliminate human assumptions about how intelligence works from the technologies they build. Luminaries such as Rich

---

[75] For the most part. Of course, the background contains important information about how to recognize objects, and networks can easily be fooled when recognizing out-of-context objects. For a nice review of context effects in biological vision, see (Bar 2004).

Sutton have argued that 'we need to build networks that discover like we can, rather than contain what we have discovered'.[76] But as we have seen in the preceding sections, deep networks have systematically incorporated computational principles which are analogous to those found in biological brains. Naively left to their own devices—to 'discover like we can'—neural networks often flounder. This is because it is simply not possible to excavate meaningful knowledge from finite volumes of unstructured sensory inputs, without a helping hand that encourages computation to focus on those parts of the structure that are relevant to intelligent behaviour. Neural networks start to succeed when researchers equip them with computational tools that are honed to account for the world's non-accidental properties. Unsurprisingly, these are the same computational tools that millions of years of evolution have provided for biological neural networks: local receptivity, convergent connectivity, divisive normalization, sparsification, predictive coding, orthogonalization, dimensionality reduction, spatial attention, and object-based relational composition.[77] In the relentless pursuit of neatness, some AI researchers forget that the world itself is not neat, and that the path to AGI, like the road taken by natural general intelligence, will inevitably be more than a little bit scruffy.

---

[76] As discussed in Chapter 2.

[77] Divisive normalization occurs when neural responses are normalized non-linearly by the average in the population. It can help accentuate contours and is a ubiquitous computational motif in biology that is frequently borrowed by machine learning researchers.

5

The problem of abstraction

5.1 Molecular metaphors

In 1876, the German chemist Hermann Kopp was having a torrid time in
the laboratory—his experiments were refusing to work. To allay his frustration, he sat down to write an unusual book.[1] Entitled *Aus der Molecular-
Welt*,[2] it describes a fantastical kingdom inhabited by atoms and molecules
with wildly varying character and physiognomy. Carbon has four arms.
Hydroxyl is arrogant, and chlorine is a real sourpuss. The chemicals—like
young children—hold hands for comfort. They pass the time dancing: partner
dances for couples or an Allemande à trois, prim quadrilles of the courtly ball
or a rambunctious Scottish jig. There is jealousy and scandal when partners
are exchanged. Six carbon atoms dance ring-a-roses, giving two hands to one
partner and one to the other, with their last hand reserved to drag a hydrogen
atom behind them—forming the famous ring structure of benzene, proposed
by August Kekulé just 20 years earlier.[3] Molecular structure is complex, and
chemical bonds are invisible to the naked eye, but Kopp brings the tiny universe of molecules to life, forging analogies with physical and social relations
in the macroscopic world. Once discovered, *Aus der Molecular-Welt* became
an instant classic.[4]

Analogies are grounded in the deep symmetries that exist in the spatial
or temporal relations between entities and their constituents. Analogies are
meta-relational, because they draw attention to how relational patterns in
data are themselves related. Chemical bonding is like children holding hands.
Chemical reactivity is like volatility of character. Atoms are like solar systems, because they involve smaller spheres orbiting larger ones. Atomic rings,
wedding bands, and the cycle of the seasons involve a steady spatiotemporal

---

[1] For a wonderful retelling of this story, see telling (Rocke 2010).
[2] *From the World of Molecules*.
[3] In a lecture in 1890, Kekulé claimed that he conceived of the structure of benzene in London in 1855,
after falling into a reverie on a horse-drawn omnibus passing through Clapham and dreaming of a snake
consuming its own tail. It is likely that Kekulé was referencing Kopp's book, or the humorous parodies it inspired, rather than recounting an actual experience.
[4] It came to light in 1882, after Kopp presented a copy to his Heidelberg colleague Robert Bunsen on the
occasion of his birthday.

Natural General Intelligence. Christopher Summerfield, Oxford University Press. © Oxford University Press 2023.
DOI: 10.1093/oso/9780192843883.003.0005

progression that gradually bends back on itself to form a circle. Military campaigns and political debates involve the strategic accumulation of territory through the deployment of opposing forces. Families, trees, and computer code can all branch recursively to form a nested hierarchy. In fact, a limited set of relational grammars, including trees, linear orders, multidimensional spaces, rings, dominance hierarchies, and cliques captures the relational patterns encountered in a variety of physical, biological, and social domains.[5]

Reasoning by analogy underpins the great flashes of insight that have impelled science forward. In the early twentieth century, in a succession of imaginative leaps, physicists conceived of subatomic interactions as a billiard table, then as a plum pudding, and finally as the solar system in miniature. But analogies are for everyone, not just quantum physicists. The way we use language is intrinsically metaphorical.[6] One analysis of TV dialogue found that we use a metaphor about every 25 words.[7] We understand that life is a journey, that writing a thesis is like climbing a mountain, that bureaucracy is a labyrinth, and that we are born into one branch of an ancestral tree. In his classic book *Metaphors We Live By*, the philosopher and cognitive scientist George Lakoff heroically attempts to catalogue the deep metaphorical structure of the English language, in which arguments are warfare and time is money, good things go up and bad things come down, and resentment is bitter and victory is sweet. Metaphors express deep patterns in the way the world works, picking out similarities across otherwise unlike domains.

Can we formalize what is meant by analogical reasoning? Consider three objects A, B, and C, each characterized by a single attribute. For example, A might be *large*, whereas B and C are both *small*. Now consider three entirely different objects D, E, and F. These new stimuli could even occur in another modality—for example, D might be *loud*, whereas E and F are both *quiet*. Thus, although A, B, C and D, E, F are entirely unrelated, the similarity in structure is analogous—both have two similar items, with a single odd one out (A and D). In fact, if you create RDMs for A, B, C and D, E, F, they will have the same form (Figure 5.1). As always, knowing how the world is structured is useful for prediction. So even if the identity of D is missing, you can assume by

---

[5] See (Kemp & Tenenbaum 2008) and (Tenenbaum et al. 2011).

[6] Metaphors, similes, and analogies all draw attention to the resemblances among relational patterns in data. They do so for slightly different reasons: a simile states that x is like y; a metaphor with poetic, rather than literal, intent states that x is y; and an analogy states the resemblance between x and y usually with a view to drawing attention to some aspect of x, which is made clearer through comparing it to y. In psychology, 'analogical reasoning' is often (but not always) non-verbal, whereas metaphors are usually (but not always) expressed in words. From a purely cognitive standpoint, however, the distinction(s) between simile, metaphor, and analogy seems irrelevant, so I will ignore them here—even if grammarians (and my grandmother) would no doubt disapprove.

[7] See (Graesser et al. 1989).

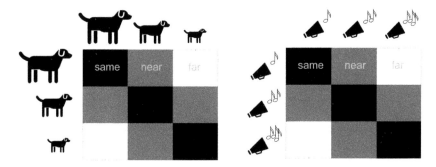

Fig. 5.1 Example relations based on size (left) and volume (right). The signals are very different, and even in different modalities (visual and auditory). However, they have the same RDMs. Each square indicates the dissimilarity between each stimulus and every other (black = most similar; white = most different).

analogy with *A*, *B*, *C* that it is *loud*, because *E* and *F* are *quiet*. This is the cognitive functionality that is needed to grasp the analogies in Kopp's book of magic molecules, where *A*, *B*, and *C* are fictional characters with human-like emotion and action, and *D*, *E*, and *F* are the building blocks of physical chemistry.

Darwin famously claimed that the difference between human and non-human intelligence is *one of degree and not kind*—that we live on an intellectual continuum with other species. Others have claimed that the ability to reason by analogy is a unique intellectual watershed that divides us from other animals, relying on as yet undiscovered cognitive mechanisms that are special to humans.[8] Whilst this view remains controversial, it is clear that many species can make judgements based on higher-order patterns of similarity and difference among stimuli. Take the simple case of deciding whether two items are the same (*A*, *A*) or different (*B*, *C*). Having learnt to select *A*, *A* over *B*, *C*, an agent should—without further training—know to choose *D*, *D* over *E*, *F*. It has been claimed that animals as diverse as honeybees, parrots, ducklings, and dolphins are able to solve this or closely related problems. Doing so relies on an ability to abstract over the specific properties of *A*, *B*, *C* and *D*, *E*, *F*. For example, in one well-known experiment, honeybees were able to match visual stimuli defined by colour after learning to match others defined by their angle of orientation.[9]

[8] For a well-known version of this argument, see (Penn et al. 2008). For a different view, see (Premack 2010).

[9] See (Giurfa et al. 2001), (Martinho & Kacelnik 2016), (Mercado et al. 2000), and (Pepperberg 1987). The parrot in question was a famous African Grey called Alex, whose extraordinary cognitive abilities are documented in the film *Life with Alex*.

This concept of *sameness* seems simple. Remarkably, however, it poses great difficulties for state-of-the-art neural networks, including both CNNs and Relation Networks. One detailed study showed that neural networks trained on vast volumes of data could learn to discriminate sameness in limited circumstances, perhaps by learning 'subtraction templates' that matched identical pixel patterns across spatial locations. However, the networks showed no propensity to generalize the concept of 'same' between different features. The networks thus failed on a task that the humble honeybee—an invertebrate with fewer than a million neurons—was able to do for orientation and colour.[10] In other work, minor cosmetic changes to the input stimuli can be shown to dramatically degrade the networks' same-difference performance, even within a single dimension, reminding us that learning in deep networks can be perilously fragile, and different from biology in often bewildering ways.

Primates are capable of sophisticated forms of reasoning in naturalistic settings, especially when their food—or position in the social hierarchy—is at stake. However, it is unclear how versatile their relational reasoning might be. In the 1940s, the primatologist Harry Harlow—better known for his controversial experiments on the effects of social deprivation on infant macaques—made an interesting discovery. In a series of experiments, monkeys learnt to choose between two visual objects, one of which was rewarded and one was not. Harlow noted with surprise that each time the task was restarted with two entirely novel objects, the monkeys learnt slightly faster. In fact, their performance continued to accelerate over hundreds of new object sets, until eventually the monkeys could respond almost perfectly from the second trial onwards. Harlow argued that over the course of repeated pairings, the monkeys had *learnt how to learn*. It seems that the monkeys learnt something abstract about the relations between the two stimuli in each pairing—that if one was rewarded, the other was not. By generalizing this knowledge to new pairings, they could learn ever faster (Figure 5.2). Human children tested in a comparable fashion showed the same ability.[11]

Human ability to reason analogically is often measured with the RPM test.[12] Each RPM problem is made up of an array of boxes, with the relations between objects and features in each box changing according to a hidden relational rule. The goal is to guess the contents of a missing box by inferring the rule. Objects exhibit lawful patterns of sameness or difference across boxes: a

---

[10] See (Kim et al. 2018).

[11] On the first trial, they had no information and were obliged to guess. The original reference for this work is (Harlow 1949).

[12] As discussed in Chapter 3. In fact, whether non-human primates can solve RPM has been controversial. There is evidence that they solve some simpler versions of RPM problems.

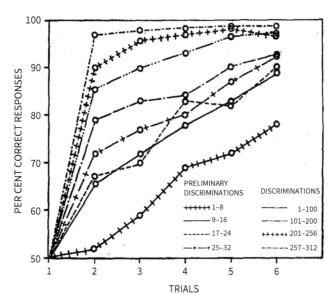

Fig. 5.2 Performance of monkeys on the Harlow task. The legend refers to the number of unique bandit tasks that had been completed.

Reprinted from Harlow (1949).

feature may vary gradually in intensity, or size, or number. Humans have to grasp the pattern from existing data (*A*, *B*, *C*) and extrapolate it to missing data (*D*, *E*, ?). The objects and features themselves are simple shapes, lines, colours, and textures, meaning that the rule cannot be inferred from the semantic properties of the stimuli. Instead, solving RPM requires the use of abstract concepts, expressing identities in the relational patterns across array elements. Most people can solve simple RPM problems, but their performance on harder examples is extremely heterogenous. In fact, the ability to solve RPM is a good predictor of outcomes in the real world, such as their lifelong levels of educational attainment or career success. This is why it has become a staple of human intelligence testing.

These observations naturally raise the question of whether deep networks can form the sorts of relational abstractions needed to solve analogical reasoning tasks like RPM. In one recent paper, researchers built a program that generated virtually unlimited numbers of RPM problems with unique visual configurations, and rules defined by exhaustive combinations of object types (shape or line), feature types (colour, size, or number), and relational primitives (AND, XOR, progression). This ability to generate huge numbers of training examples permitted the application of data-hungry deep learning methods to the problem. They then combined several Relation Network modules into a single deep network (called 'wild relation network' or WReN) that output scores for each of the eight candidate answers to the RPM puzzle. When the authors used their generator to sample RPM problems involving new, unseen combinations of all these variables, WReN performed at nearly 62.6%. Although not perfect, this was far above chance level of 1/8 or 12.5%. Thus, after training on progressions of blue squares or matches of red circles, it could solve new progressions of blue squares that had different sizes or positions, or even handle progressions of red circles. However, when more shapes, or colours, or rules were systematically omitted from the training data, WReN started to falter. For example, after training on a rule involving only red squares, it was much poorer at applying the rule to blue circles. For some strong transfer conditions, such as generalizing between shapes and lines, the network's test performance was ultimately no better than chance.

The *problem of abstraction* is to learn explicit representations of the relations that exist in data. By learning relational abstractions, we can understand that what concepts like *same*, or *more*, or *cyclic* mean in ways that go beyond the sensory inputs. For example, two horses can be the same, but so can two political views. One horse can be faster than the other, but equally one wine can be more delicious than another. A circus ring allows a performing horse to trot around and around; the hypothetical Wheel of Fortune, which raises King Lear's hopes up and then dashes them down again,[13] turns inevitably on itself in a similar fashion. An explicit representation of an abstraction occurs when a neural population displays these sorts of invariances, coding for sameness, magnitude, or cyclicity (rather than horses, political views, or circuses). If we could build machines that understand the meaning in these patterns, perhaps they would have the imaginative insight and gift for creative expressions that are currently reserved for humans.

Even the more constrained problem of analogical reasoning remains unsolved in AI research. The work above is emblematic of the challenges that researchers face. Advanced network architectures, such as relation nets, can explicitly segment object arrays into their elements and compute spatial relations between them. When the domain of the relation is similar—requiring generalization from colour to colour, or shape to shape—the network can transfer the relational functions $g(o_i, o_j)$ to new pairs of objects o_i', o_i'. But the network never learns more abstract relational concepts, that is, those that are untethered from concrete input features. Indeed, one can even imagine

---

[13] In Shakespeare's great tragic play of that title.

theoretically stronger transfer conditions—for example, if the visual lines and shapes had been replaced at test by auditory tones with different pitch and volume, or with 3D landmarks in a navigable open area, or with verbal descriptions of the problem in natural language. Here, the network would have failed catastrophically.

The reason for these failures is a familiar ghost that haunts AI research: the grounding problem. Recall Peirce's tripartite distinction: representations can reference the world by physical likeness (iconicity), by contextual congruity (indexicality), or by arbitrary convention (symbolism). For an abstract representation of an analogical relation—such as 'sameness'—to transcend a specific feature or dimension, it cannot be merely iconic. Horses and political views do not resemble one another. Nor when bees generalize the similarity of orientation to infer a similarity rule for colours, can their neural code be grounded in physical resemblance—because two blues and two vertical stimuli are not themselves similar.

For these abstract relational concepts, which go beyond physical likeness, it is the relationship in space and time that binds a stimulus and its representation together. A tricorn hat, the Holy Trinity, and Pascal's triangle are seemingly unrelated concepts with no physical correspondence, variously beloved of pirates, priests, and mathematicians. But they are linked through their tripartite structure. To understand these sorts of similarities, we need a form of neural representation that explicitly represents how items relate in space and time. Recent work in neuroscience has offered tantalizing hints about the nature of this code in biological brains, and how it is used to solve relational reasoning problems.

5.2 Playing Twenty Questions with space

If you are on a long and boring car journey, the game called Twenty Questions can be a good way to pass the time. It is played between two people: a setter and a solver. The setter chooses a secret object—which can be any object, anywhere in the world[14]—and the solver attempts to discover what it might be. The solver can pose any query, to which the setter must reply truthfully, as long as it can be answered with yes or no.

We can think of neural decoding as being a bit like Twenty Questions. The secret object is the state the animal is currently experiencing, which we

---

[14] Or out of it. Twenty Questions is particularly interesting if you allow hypothetical or fictional entities, such as the Cheshire Cat or Wonder Woman.

assume is unknown. The questions are single neurons whose activity we can read out. In this analogy, different neural coding schemes correspond to different querying strategies that might be adopted by the solver. For example, a very inefficient approach, popular among younger players of the game, is to list candidate objects one by one, asking: is it x? Is it y? Is it z? This is like attempting to read out from a neural code in which information is stored in a series of unrelated slots, in a fully localist manner. A more cunning strategy for the solver is to exploit the structure of the world to generate queries that rule out approximately half of the remaining possible options, thereby maximizing the expected information gain.[15] For example, if you ask in the first question whether the object is human-made, then irrespective of the answer, you can potentially rule out a vast set of either natural or artificial objects. You can then successively ask whether it is an animal (or not), a person (or not), a female (or not), and so on, zoning in on the secret object by halving the options each time. In fact, this strategy exploits the coding hierarchy for semantic concepts, such as *living*, *animal*, and *dog*, that is learnt by a neural network trained on image classification tasks.

Now imagine that instead of guessing a secret *object*, the solver has to guess a secret *location*. To make it simple, let's say that the set of possible locations is drawn from an open, rectangular arena, such as an empty squash court. As Tolman proposed, we can think of each location in the court as a discrete state, and the ensemble of states collectively make up a mental map. How, then, should location be encoded in a neural population?

In the late 1960s, a neuroscientist called John O'Keefe was recording from somatosensory cells in the rodent thalamus.[16] In one animal, an electrode was inadvertently inserted more laterally into the hippocampus. O'Keefe noted that the neurons he found there varied in striking ways with the animal's running speed and head movement. He found this surprising, because these variables seemed unrelated to memory formation, then thought to be the primary function of the rodent hippocampus. This serendipitous finding triggered a chain of events which led to a remarkable discovery: that when a rodent moved through an arena, neurons in the CA1 field of the hippocampus fired whenever it passed through a circumscribed location. Their activity was largely independent of the precise heading direction of the animal, and did not vary

---

[15] The best strategy is to choose a question for which the probability of yes is as close as possible to 0.5. Of course, this also depends on the setter's tendencies. If a favoured teddy bear is chosen as the object in approximately half of games, then 'is it x' might actually be worth a shot.

[16] A subcortical structure involved in relaying sensory information to the cortex, among other things. This work was being done with Jonathan Dostrovsky. See https://www.nobelprize.org/prizes/medicine/2014/okeefe/lecture/.

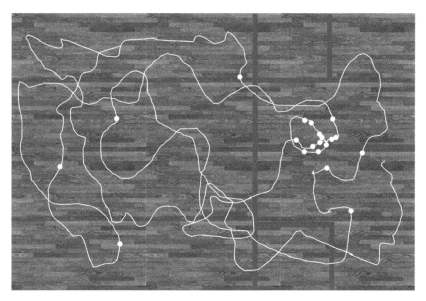

Fig. 5.3 Schematic illustration of place cells in a squash court. The white line is the trajectory of a theoretical rat. The white dots indicate action potentials from a single CA1 place cell. This neuron codes for a location in the centre rear of the court.

with relevant sensory cues such as visual landmarks or odours. In fact, they even fired in the dark. These neurons, called *place cells*, were thus representing the animal's current spatial location in allocentric (or map-like) coordinates.[17] Thus, a rodent let loose on a squash court might have hippocampal place cells that, respectively, became active when it crossed the top of the right-hand service box, paused to groom at the front left of the court near the tin, or scurried along the back wall near the door (Figure 5.3).

O'Keefe quickly realized that these cells might form an important component of the cognitive-like map of the environment that Tolman had proposed two decades earlier. His findings triggered a wave of interest in the nature of the hippocampal code and how it might act as a neural compass for the brain. Over the intervening 40 years, neuroscientists have learnt a great deal about the representation of space in the hippocampus and nearby structures that make up the medial temporal lobe (MTL) (Figure 5.4).[18] In 2014, O'Keefe was awarded a share of the 2014 Nobel Prize for Medicine for this discovery.

---

[17] Formally, allocentric space is defined in object-to-object (rather than self-to-object) coordinates. A map of the world viewed from above is thus an allocentric representation.

[18] The MTL is the name given to a constellation of mammalian brain regions that are important for both spatial cognition and memory formation, including the hippocampus, entorhinal cortex (ERC), perirhinal cortex (PRC), and dentate gyrus (DG). Figure 5.4 is taken from (Murray et al. 2007).

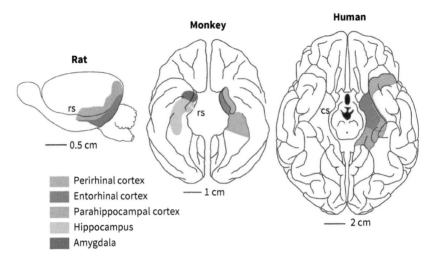

Fig. 5.4 Illustration of the medial temporal lobe, including the hippocampus in the rat, macaque monkey, and human, viewed from the underside of the brain.
Reprinted with permission from Murray et al. (2007).

A canonical place cell is active for just a single location.[19] Thus, together place cells form a localist code, carrying limited information about how space is organized. For example, the population place cell activity would be no more similar for two nearby locations in the left-hand service box than any two spots on either side of the court. Querying place cells one by one, like listing objects one by one in Twenty Questions, would thus be an ineffective strategy to infer the animal's location. Imagine that the court is tiled by ten regularly spaced place fields in each direction, or $10^2 = 100$ fields in total. Even with 20 'questions'—or opportunities to decode the location—there is only a 20% chance that the solver would actually choose a cell that allowed the animal's location to be inferred. However, the question budget could be used more wisely by capitalizing on the way space is structured. For example, the solver could first ask whether the location was at the front of the court (or not), then whether it was to the left of the court (or not), confining the possible locations to a single quadrant in just two questions. They could then narrow it down from a quadrant to a hexidecant (a 16th) with two further questions, and so on. This would

---

[19] In reality, individual place cells often have a small number of distinct fields in different parts of the environment, so it is a sparse (but not fully localist) code. Moreover, if place cells are organized hierarchically, with different neurons tuned for different scales, then they can also encode the structure of space.

be the quickest way to guess the secret location—and also the most efficient way to code the location in a neural population.[20]

This neural coding scheme entails cells that code for space with a series of quadrilateral lattices (or checkerboards) that vary from coarse (e.g. quadrants) to fine (e.g. hexidecants). It predicts the existence of neurons that respond when the animal occupies regularly spaced locations in an open arena, say every 20 cm or 2 m apart in either direction. Remarkably, neurons that fire in a regularly spaced lattice have been found in the rodent medial ERC, an MTL structure that is strongly interconnected with the hippocampus. Edvard and May-Britt Moser shared the 2014 Nobel Prize with O'Keefe for their discovery of these neurons, which are called *grid cells*. The lattice (or grid) in question is not, in fact, quadrilateral, but hexagonal (it has sixfold, rather than fourfold, symmetry), but nevertheless it seems very likely that these neurons collectively represent the animal's position in the efficient fashion implied by the Twenty Questions example.[21] Rodent grid cells have different spatial scale, with the coarser scales being found in more ventral portions of the ERC, and the finer scales more dorsally. This tells us that the MTL—and the ERC specifically—houses an efficient code for space. More recently, sophisticated analyses of BOLD data have been used to imply the existence of a similar grid code, whilst humans navigate in a virtual environment, extending beyond the ERC to the medial prefrontal and parietal regions.[22]

Unlike a localist code, a hierarchical grid code conveys how space itself is structured. Each location is coded by overlapping cells with different levels of spatial scale. This means that nearby regions will be more likely to evoke more similar patterns of population grid cell activity. Two spots near the left-hand service box will both evoke activity in neurons coding for that back left quadrant, even if they drive different firing patterns at finer scales. It seems strange to propose that we need neurons that encode the structure of space itself. Space just seems to be everywhere. It does not naturally feel like it has any structure. But this is an illusion borne of an abundance of familiarity. The Euclidean world we inhabit has lawful properties that are defined by the mathematics of vector addition and can be exploited for navigation. For example, if you are standing in the middle of a squash court, after repeating the action

---

[20] If there are n possible states, querying them in turn (akin to reading out from place cells), it would take, on average, $n/2$ questions to find the setter's state. Using this grid-like strategy will take $log_2(n)$ questions, which is fewer for any problem with $n > 8$ states.

[21] One theory is that sixfold symmetry emerges naturally under a computational constraint that neurons cannot produce negative firing rates. See (Dordek et al. 2016).

[22] See (Doeller et al. 2010).

take two steps forward, and then turn 90° clockwise exactly four times, you end up more or less where you started.

In fact, even the humble rodent can exploit the geometry of space to make a beeline for a tasty food reward. In a classic experiment, Tolman placed rats in a circular arena with multiple possible exits. All but one exit was blocked, with the open exit leading via a convoluted route to a reward. After multiple training trials, other exits were unblocked, including those that headed directly towards the food reward. According to Tolman's reports, animals chose the direct route at the first available opportunity—which they could only do if they understood how space itself is geometrically arranged.[23] This sort of behaviour would be hard to explain with a place code alone but can be explained if the animals know how space is organized.

Thus, knowing the structure of space can help you predict what will be around the next corner. If you are standing outside your favourite deli in Manhattan, you can predict that by heading a city block north, then taking the cross street west, then south down the avenue, and finally back east, you will arrive back at the same location. One recent modelling study created a virtual grid in which locations were tagged with salient landmarks, just like Manhattan street corners are recognizable by distinctive hotels, laundromats, and diners. They then trained a generative model that was loosely based on a VAE (called TEM)[24] to predict the landmark that would occur after each action. During training, the neural network formed units that behaved like place and grid cells, and others with more exotic coding properties (firing in bands or along borders) that have also been found in the rodent MTL.[25] Critically, after forming these codes, the network was able to navigate a new environment with the same grid structure, but alternative landmarks, as if it had generalized the knowledge of the structure of Manhattan to a new point in the city with unfamiliar delis, bars, and subway stations. In a different study, agents trained with deep reinforcement to navigate mazes developed grid-like coding patterns in their hidden units, and the ablation of these units was particularly detrimental for behaviours that required geometric inferences in space, such as exploiting shortcuts to reach a goal.[26] Together, these findings

[23] The original study is here (Tolman et al. 1946). Although more recent studies have failed to replicate this finding in its original form, there seems to be little doubt that rodents behave as if they understand how space is structured.

[24] Which stands for the Tolman Eichenbaum Machine. Howard Eichenbaum was a distinguished researcher who argued that the hippocampus coded for relations among objects in memory (Whittington et al. 2020).

[25] Border cells only when the agent was biased to hug the corners of the environment, like rats do. There are many other MTL cell types, including those that fire close to objects. For a great review, see (Bicanski & Burgess 2020).

[26] See (Banino et al. 2018) and also (Cueva & Wei 2018).

imply that a simple predictive principle is sufficient to learn neural codes that permit structure learning in space and might subserve remarkable geometric inferences like those displayed by Tolman's rats.

Our mental maps encompass more than physical space. Collectively, they encode a mosaic of knowledge about how everything relates to everything else. One promising idea is that the computations performed by place and grid cells might also allow inferences about non-spatial domains.[27] In fact, TEM was able to learn and generalize patterns of correlation in the value of two objects, like in Harlow's monkey experiments. It could also draw inferences by learning relationships in other canonical structures, such as family trees, and generalize them to new instances. Like humans, having learnt concepts such as *aunt* and *sibling*, TEM could infer relations between mothers, sisters, and daughters of novel families. To return to an earlier example: elements with a triangular structure (such as a tricorn hat, Pascal's triangle, and the Holy Trinity) are all composed of three elements which are equally dissimilar to one another. The tricorn hat exists in physical space, with three equidistant corners; we use our conception of space to understand the relational form for the other concepts, which are, respectively, spiritual or mathematical objects with no overt physical form.

Thus, we know that the Eiffel Tower is adjacent to the river Seine and the *Champ de Mars* in our mental map of Parisian geography. We know that it relates to a tepee, a traffic cone, and the Great Pyramid of Giza in our mental map of 3D object shapes. But it also lies in between the Washington Monument (1880–1884) and Chrysler Building (1930–1931) in the more abstract space given by a timeline of the world's tallest free-standing structures. In this space, it is closer to the Empire State Building (1931–1967) than it is to Lincoln Cathedral (1311–1549) in both rank ordering and metric time measured in years. The suggestion is that grid-like coding schemes might be one way in which we mentally organize abstract conceptual knowledge. Mental timelines lie on a single dimension, so grid-like cells would form unidimensional oscillatory codes that carve up this abstract space across different scales from coarse to fine. For example, coarse-scale neurons would fire for either ancient structures (Tower of Jericho, the Anu Ziggurat, and the Red Pyramid of Sneferu, that all held the record before 2000 BC) or those from the modern era (Notre Dame Cathedral, Empire State Building, and Burj Khalifa). These

---

[27] This idea has been developed and promoted most enthusiastically by the Oxford neuroscientist Tim Behrens. For two great reviews on this topic, see (Behrens et al. 2018) and (Bellmund et al. 2018). In the modelling study from his group, TEM was able to learn and generalize patterns of correlation and anti-correlation between two objects (like in Harlow's monkey experiments) and to draw inferences across other varieties of structures, such as family trees, by learning concepts such as 'aunt' and 'sibling'.

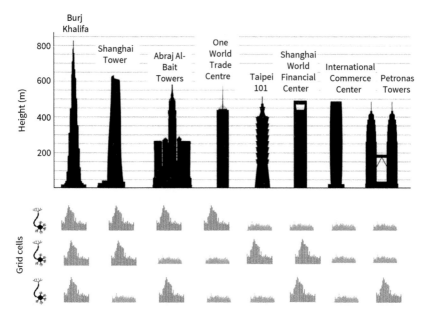

Fig. 5.5 Illustration of grid cells for coding for building size. The top illustration shows the world's eight tallest buildings in 2015. The three schematic grid cells below are shown with different scales of tuning in building height space. The grey icons denote either large or small neuronal responses.

Adapted from work by Ali Zifan; used data from Emporis.com, CC BY-SA 4.0, see https://commons. wikimedia.org/w/index.php?curid=41356641.

would be complemented by fine-scale grid neurons, with preferences for early or late halves of both the early and late eras, and so on. Together, these cells would make up a grid-like code for the abstract space of the *tallest free-standing structure timeline* (see Figure 5.5 for a similar example). In fact, a recent study in which rodents learnt to map lever responses onto variation in the pitch of auditory tones reported the existence of ERC neurons with such oscillatory patterns, exactly as predicted by this theory.[28] Neuroimaging studies have also reported evidence that non-spatial concepts, like those traced out by varying physical features of birds (neck and leg length) or concentrations of odours (pine and lemon), might be represented with 2D grid-like neural codes,[29] consistent with the idea that there exist shared coding principles for physical and abstract space.

[28] See (Nieh et al. 2021). If true, this would be a delightful finding, but the data in this paper are quite preliminary.

[29] This is a very recent line of research and remains controversial. In particular, the studies cited use fMRI, which cannot measure grid cells directly but must infer from the relationship between the BOLD

Although the idea that place and grid cells code for conceptual spaces is recent, the idea that people use spatial representations to reason about concepts
is a familiar one among cognitive scientists. Dedre Gentner has proposed that
analogies are understood via the isomorphic mappings of relational structures in mental space. Peter Gärdenfors has argued that thought is intrinsically spatial: that we understand the meaning of words, propositions, and
arguments through their relative mental geometry. Lakoff calls this the 'spa-
tialization of form hypothesis' and argues for the ontological primacy of spatiotemporal archetypes, like those shared by container and contained, centre
and periphery, part and whole, and the triad of origin, path, and goal.[30] The
idea that space and time have a special cognitive status connects the physics
of Newton and Einstein with the philosophy of Kant and Leibniz. According
to this view, spatial *position* and temporal *instant* are not mere properties of
objects, like colour and shape. Instead, space and time are the mental axes in
which thinking itself happens.

5.3 Abstractions as affordances

The last common ancestor of humans and chimpanzees lived about 7 million
years ago. But if we turn back the clock a further 50 million years, a more
significant split occurred in the primate ancestral family tree, when a group
known as *Haplorhines* broke away from the Euprimate line. Unlike their
Strepsirhine counterparts, which evolved into modern-day bushbabies and
lemurs, *Haplorhines* found a new niche foraging by day, high up in the forest
canopy. This diurnal, arboreal existence may have placed selective pressures
on brain function which were critical to the evolution of the intelligence we
recognize in their primate descendants, including old world monkeys (such as
capuchins), new world monkeys (such as macaques), and hominids (such as
gibbons, gorillas, and humans).

If you live in the trees, a major concern is to avoid tumbling accidentally
to the forest floor. Haplorhines thus developed dextrous hands and feet, an
opposable thumb, and forward-facing eyes, which allowed them to judge

---

signal in the ERC and a direction of travel in feature space, which involves some theoretical leaps of faith
(Bao et al. 2019; Constantinescu et al. 2016).

[30] Lakoff makes this point here (Lakoff 1987). René Thom, who pioneered a theory of dynamical systems
known as Catastrophe Theory, argued that the world bifurcates into just 16 basic topological types, with
relational forms such as *begin, unite, capture,* and *cut*. This is described in Gärdenfors' book *Conceptual
Spaces* (Thom 1970). Gentner's work on analogy is extensive (Gentner et al. 2001).

distance accurately using binocular vision. These innovations helped them leap agilely, but safely from branch to branch. Foraging by day makes it easier to find fruits, nuts, and seeds that are abundant in the forest canopy, but they need to be recognized and selected by their size, shape, and colour, which requires spatial and feature-based attention. Moreover, they can be hard to reach among the flimsy fine branches, which encourages risk sensitivity and judicious action selection. A diurnal existence exposes you to a greater risk of predation, so it may be sensible to band together in groups, rather than living a solitary existence. In their book *Neurobiology of the Prefrontal Cortex*, Dick Passingham and Steve Wise argued that these pressures drove the evolution of primate cognitive function, which is characterized by precise visuomotor and oculomotor control, high-acuity colour vision and shape recognition, selective visual attention, complex decision-making, and advanced social cognition.[31]

These pressures also drove the evolution of a representation of space in the PPC. The parietal cortex encodes space with a coordinate system that is centred on the self. This is the mental canvas that is lost in patients with Bálint's syndrome such as R.M. This spatial map charts the spatial positions to which we can move our eyes and limbs. Consider the view of a tabletop strewn with objects, like in the CLEVR data set: a spatial representation of this scene maps out the locations to which we can reach (to grasp an object with our hands) or saccade (to fixate an object with our eyes). The primate notion of space thus prominently reflects the objects around us, what we are holding, what we can reach, and what might attract our gaze. This is especially true for humans living in a modern, carpentered world, where almost all our actions are taken through the medium of a hand-held tool.

Primates, thus, represent space with two different frames of reference. One frame, shared with rodents and housed in the MTL, codes for location in an allocentric or object-to-object frame of reference, like a marker on a visitor map indicating that *you are here*. The other, which is more mature in primates than rodents and relies on the parietal cortex, codes for locations that can be reached or fixated with the eyes in a self-to-object format. Above, we saw that allocentric space might be recycled to represent the more abstract relational concepts which give human knowledge its semantic richness, such as relational patterns among city grids or family trees. Intriguingly, there is also good evidence that a similar principle applies to the code for egocentric space in the parietal cortex. We use our concept of egocentric space to understand

---

[31] See (Passingham & Wise 2012).

abstractions such as the magnitude of a quantity, the length of an elapsed passage of time, the number of items in a scene, or the monetary value of different choice options.

Psychologists have long known that there are mysterious interactions between the way we respond to space, time, and number.[32] For example, a behavioural phenomenon, known as the SNARC effect, occurs when participants are asked to make a numerical judgement, for example about parity or magnitude, with a button press or eye movement. Responses are faster when lower numbers occur on the left of the screen and higher numbers on the right (than vice versa), as if people intrinsically map numbers onto a mental line that increases from left to right. The passage of time seems to be projected to the same mental line: we are faster to respond to earlier events on the left and to later events on the right.[33] These findings are linked to the parietal cortex, because patients with unilateral spatial neglect following right parietal damage tend to ignore not only the left side of space, but also the left side of time (earlier, rather than later, events in a story), as well as showing biases mapping numbers onto left–right space. In an astonishing demonstration of how space and time interact cognitively, participants who viewed, explored, and imagined themselves in doll's houses of 1/6, 1/12, and 1/24 scales experienced time passing at different rates, with those playing with larger environments reporting that a 30-minute period had elapsed more slowly. A replication study also found a similar effect when participants played with model railways of different scale.[34] These findings imply that coding principles for physical space, including its organization along a horizontal axis and its linear scaling, are recycled to permit perception of time and number, such that congruency effects occur between the three domains.

If we dig deeper into the coding properties of neurons in the Posterior Parietal Cortex (PPC), we find that they do more than map spatial locations onto actions. In the macaque, the activity of PPC neurons varies with a symbolic cue whose size or colour indicates the probability or volume of a forthcoming liquid reward. When shapes or dot motion patterns predict which of two responses will be rewarded, PPC neuron firing rates scale with the level of evidence provided by the cues (with higher responses for less ambiguous shapes or motion signals). In a timing task, PPC firing rates vary with the

[32] This was pointed out very succinctly by Vincent Walsh in 2003 in what he called ATOM ('A theory of magnitude') (Walsh 2003).
[33] The original SNARC paper is (Dehaene et al. 1993). See also (Casasanto & Bottini 2014). Participants may even generate larger random numbers when their head is turned to the right than to the left (Loetscher et al. 2008).
[34] The original study is (DeLong 1981) and the follow-up is (Mitchell & Davis 1987).

duration of an interval during which a response must be withheld. Finally, some PPC neurons exhibit firing rates that vary monotonically with the number of stimuli (dots) in an array during a task in which the monkey decides whether to accept a standard juice reward or a variable amount dictated by the numerosity.[35] In each of these cases, the average neural firing rate signals that there is 'more' of something: more valuable reward, more sensory evidence, more time elapsed, more dots on the screen. This coding scheme is known to neuroscientists as a *rate code*, as the quantity that can be decoded from the neurons depends not just on whether it is active or inactive (like the yes/no answers in Twenty Questions), but also on its rate of response in impulses per second.

A single explanation helps us make sense of this thicket of data: that the PPC allows us to express abstract information on a mental line. We call this dimension *magnitude*, and it can be used to relate unidimensional concepts such as time (now vs later), space (left vs right or up vs down), number (more vs less), value (good vs bad), and belief (sure vs unsure). In fact, there is evidence for a sort of mental line, even in patterns of neural data recorded from humans. In one study, participants both learnt the reward probability associated with arbitrarily coloured animal stimuli (donkeys) and performed a numerical judgement task with Arabic digits. Computing RDMs from both data sets, they revealed that neural similarity was greatest for both nearby numbers and nearby donkeys, and that one could be predicted from the other. This implies that humans use a shared neural code for number and event probability. Another fMRI study has suggested that estimation of social, temporal, and physical distance may recruit overlapping neural patterns in the parietal cortex.[36]

In fact, even in tasks where there is no obvious sense of 'more' or 'less', the PPC seems to behave as if there is. For example, across studies in which monkeys learnt to group random shapes into two or three categories, PPC neurons started to signal that category with a global increase or decrease in firing rate, as if they mapped arbitrary categories *A*, *B*, and *C* onto points on a line expressing *more*, *some*, and *less*.[37] This occurred across different animals, but with different orderings, as if the monkeys had idiosyncratic preferences for one category over another. Humans, too, have a tendency to express a preference, even when there is no particular reason to do so, such as when a child is

---

[35] See (Gold & Shadlen 2007), (Jazayeri & Shadlen 2015), (Platt & Glimcher 1999), and (Roitman et al. 2007). Many of these results also hold in the PFC (see Chapter 7).

[36] For the donkeys study, see (Luyckx et al. 2019). For the fMRI study, see (Parkinson et al. 2014).

[37] See (Fitzgerald et al. 2013).

adamant that green or purple is his favourite colour. One is tempted to specu-late that there is a computational advantage to representing arbitrary, high-dimensional information on a mental line that we describe as preference.

It thus seems plausible to assume that our human penchant for relating space, time, and number derives, at least in part, from some sort of shared neural code with its basis in egocentric space. As Lakoff notes in *Metaphors we Live By*, in English, we use the terms *up* and *down* to distinguish not just a position on the *y*-axis of Cartesian space, but also to denote mood (on *top* of the world vs feeling *depressed*), value (*overpriced* vs bargain *basement*), level of consciousness (woke *up* vs *fell* asleep), social rank (*top* dog vs *under*dog), volume (sales are *rising* vs *falling*), and virtue (*high*-minded vs a *low* trick), and many other concepts that are not intrinsically spatial. In fact, across dif-ferent linguistic cultures (Dutch and Farsi), the way in which the words *high* and *low* are used modulates how people think about auditory pitch, another non-spatial dimension that we describe with spatial vocabulary.[38]

In fact, the macaque brain seems to code for number in the parietal cortex with both an approximately localist code and a rate code (Figure 5.6). The localist code involves neurons whose tuning is approximately bell-shaped (Gaussian) on the magnitude line itself.[39] In other words, they are like place cells in magnitude space. These cells have been observed in numerical match-to-sample studies where a monkey experiences a visual array of dots, or a vari-able number of tones, and has to match the exact number to a pair of probes that follow a delay period. A neuron might fire most strongly to an array with six dots and show weaker responses to arrays of five or seven dots, but not de-viate from baseline for arrays of three or 20. In fact, when both modalities are used in the same experiment, cells will often show overlapping tuning curves for visual and auditory stimuli, in a neat demonstration of how even the ma-caque brain learns abstractions that transcend the physical nature of the in-puts.[40] However, one outstanding puzzle is why the brain might variously use coding schemes that rely on rate, place, and grid codes. What are the relative merits of each format?

One potential answer is that the meaning of a quantity can change dramat-ically with context. If I am generous enough to offer you £30, you are happy—and if I double my gift to £60, you are probably even happier. This is similar to the experiment reporting a rate code for number, where the volume of liquid

---

[38] See (Dolscheid et al. 2013).
[39] As in the case of place cells, the code is not strictly localist because the tuning curves overlap, allowing the system to represent how magnitude (or space) is structured.
[40] For a review of these results and how they relate to behavioural effects, see (Nieder & Dehaene 2009).

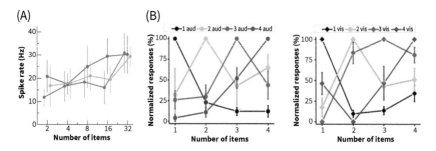

Fig. 5.6 Neurons coding for numerosity in the posterior parietal cortex (PPC).
(A) A single cell coding for numerosity with a rate code. Its firing rate increases for larger
numbers, irrespective of the value of a standard against which they are compared
(different coloured lines).
Reprinted from Roitman et al. 2007.
(B) Average tuning curves for PPC neurons tuned to numerosities 1–4 in the visual and
auditory domains. Many neurons had shared tuning in both modalities.
Reprinted with permission from Nieder 2012.

reward was proportional to the number of dots. Six dots would slake my thirst
twice as much as three dots, so here a rate code is appropriate: double the firing
is twice as good. However, now imagine that we are participating in a raffle
where you can win first prize—a £30 book token—with ticket number 30.
I have that ticket and generously pass it to you. But now if I change my mind
and instead give you ticket number 60, you are not twice as happy. In fact, you
are annoyed—because now you end up with nothing at all. That's because a
prize raffle is like a match-to-sample trial: the winning ticket must match the
prize number exactly. Similarly, if the sample array contains three dots, then
the monkey needs to choose the probe with exactly three dots to receive a liquid reward on that trial. In these cases, a place code is suitable, because six
is not twice as good as three. You need to know the exact number. This is presumably why allocentric representations use place—and grid-like—coding.
For example, on a squash court, you could, in theory, represent location with
just two rate-coded neurons, signalling your location in the x and y coordinates of Cartesian space, respectively. But this would imply that the location
at the T in the middle of the court is somehow 'worth' half of that in the far
corner, which is not very helpful for navigation and is even worse for playing
squash.

Philosophers and cognitive scientists have long proposed that our mental
representations of space and time are critical to grasping analogies, using
metaphors, and reasoning analogically. But only recently have neuroscientists
begun to unravel the neural and computational principles by which spatial

coding might be adapted for the coding of abstract concepts. These ideas draw upon a remarkably detailed picture of how neural codes for space are formed and used in rodents, monkeys, and humans. Notably, these ideas have had limited impact in machine learning research thus far. For AI researchers, building systems that understand the deep relational identities in data remains an aspiration for future work.

Questions of abstract representation are haunted by concerns over grounding. What is the sensory information that allows us to grasp the connection between a tricorn hat, the Holy Trinity, and Pascal's triangle—when the physical embodiment and semantic context of these three concepts are so radically different? This question remains unsolved, but a venerable theory in psychology, dating back to the 1930s, offers some tantalizing hints. The idea is that abstractions might be grounded in actions or, more precisely, in the *affordances* exhibited by objects and locations.

We owe the term *affordance* to husband-and-wife team J. J. and E. J. Gibson, who collectively pioneered what became known as the *ecological approach* to visual perception. J. J. Gibson defined the term as follows:[41]

> The affordances of the environment are what it offers the animal, what it provides or furnishes, either for good or ill. The verb to afford is found in the dictionary, the noun affordance is not. I have made it up. I mean by it something that refers to both the environment and the animal in a way that no existing term does. It implies the complementarity of the animal and the environment.

A chair affords sitting, a button affords pressing, and a mailbox affords posting. Affordances are the actions that an object invites by virtue of its physical form and habitual uses.

What does it mean to say that abstractions are grounded in affordances? Recall that neural codes in the dorsal stream strip away the details by which an object might be recognized or discriminated, and instead signal the spatial target of the action that it invites. In other words, they code for affordances. For a hungry diner, a knife and fork on the table afford reaching and grasping, but a similar neural code would represent the anticipated movement towards a hammer and chisel on the workbench. For a birdwatcher, a sudden flash of colour above the trees affords a saccadic eye movement and pursuit with the gaze to identify a potentially rare species, but the same neural code would be used if the sudden colours in the sky were fireworks ushering in the New Year.

---

[41] Gibson first defined the term in his 1966 book *The Senses Considered as Perceptual Systems*, but this quote is from his classic text *The Ecological Approach to Visual Perception* (1979).

By stripping away the details of the objects in question (is it a knife or a chisel? A bird or a firework?) and focussing on the action it affords, the representation carries invariant (or abstract) information about the relations between objects.

Imagine two images, one in which three kittens huddle around a bowl, and another in which three apples nestle in a juicy bunch. Apples and kittens do not look alike, but the two images share a relational property: they portray three elements in a group. This three-ness is not conveyed by the objects themselves (kittens or apples) but is carried by the actions the scene affords: three kittens to be petted (in three successive reaching movements), three apples to be picked (in three grasping movements), or in either case, three objects to be fixated in turn with the eyes. An explicit relation of the action sequence to be taken is thus simultaneously an abstract representation of the relations among elements themselves. In fact, one early study revealed cells in the parietal cortex that coded explicitly for the number of repeated actions (either pushing or turning a handle) that remained to be taken in a sequence.[42] One can imagine this principle extending to more abstract relational spaces. In the kittens and apples example, the affordance involves three successive actions (reaches or saccades), but one can imagine recycling this affordance for more metaphysical objects: a devout Christian might pray to each member of the Holy Trinity in turn, or a mathematician might perform three sequential arithmetic operations (take digit 1, take digit 2, add to get digit 3) to compute each new entry in Pascal's triangle.

These ideas remain speculative. But it is worth recalling that we only know about space in the first place because we take actions in the world. This is most evident in the case of allocentric space, where we learn about how space is organized by moving around—and experiencing the transitions that occur in space. I take a step forward: am I closer to my goal? I open a door: where does it lead? I follow the trail: do I arrive back at the lake? Formally, of course, place cells are learnt: they emerge as the animal moves through the arena. We do not know whether place cells form from grid cells, or vice versa, but grid cells could be learnt by a Hebbian process, as two orthogonal vectors x_i and x_j coding for two adjacent places i and j, become linked by association as the animal repeatedly transitions from i to j. In fact, this is one basic principle by which a mental map like that proposed by Tolman could be formed: learning the association between each state and every other state by moving through

---

[42] A long-form version of this argument is given in (Summerfield et al. 2019). The recording study is (Sawamura et al. 2002).

the environment. Such a representation has been called the *successor representation*.[43] We can think of grid cells as encoding the *principal components* of the successor representation, that is, a set of bases that allow us to encode it in compressed form.[44] The key point, however, is that only by moving around that you get a sense of how space is structured.

Similarly, if we were immobile and unable to impinge on the world in any way—like a deep network passively labelling natural images—it is unclear that we would be able to know that objects exist in space, or even to form any real sense of space at all. Presumably, this is why CNNs rely instead on low-level features, textures, and image statistics to apply labels and captions. As we have seen, this can be effective when training data are huge (e.g. more than 6 million photos on ImageNet) but leaves networks vulnerable to adversarial attacks, and brittle in the face of strong tests of generalization. It is unclear whether an agent could ever know *what objects are* without being designed in a way that computes their affordances—a form of representation that is a natural precursor to action. It seems plausible, thus, that neural networks may never know what an object is until they can pick it up. They may never understand the relational information in a scene until they can take actions towards its various elements. This, in turn, may allow humans to learn the relational abstractions that underlie analogies and metaphors, and to use basic building blocks of meaning to construct a complex reality.

5.4 Luke Skywalker neurons

When the first instalment of George Lucas' blockbuster *Star Wars* trilogy was released in the summer of 1977, it took the box office by storm, racking up record ticket sales and winning six of its 11 Oscar nominations. The *Star Wars* trilogy taps deeply into the narrative archetypes on which Western culture is built. It references the great clashes of civilization that have rent human history, from the fall of the Roman Empire to the Vietnam War.[45] The battle between Luke Skywalker and Darth Vader evokes an ancient psychic maelstrom that pits father against son. The scene where they duel with glowing blue and red lightsabres—for contemporary audiences, colours that, respectively,

---

[43] See Dayan (1993).
[44] See (Stachenfeld et al. 2017).
[45] In fact, although *Star Wars* is most often viewed as an allegory for the rise and fall of the Nazis, Lucas said in a later interview that Nixon (not Hitler) was his real inspiration for Emperor Palatine, and (perhaps bizarrely) that the Ewoks represent the Vietcong.

symbolized the United States and Soviet Union—would have brought vividly to mind the chill of the ongoing Cold War.

Humans understand the world through the stories they tell each other.[46] By creating stories, we mentally animate objects and people into causal narratives that are scaffolded by themes of hope, frustration, and denouement.[47] Our stories breathe meaning into happenstance, explain cause and effect, and help us relate recurring thematic patterns in life and art—a process known to the Greeks as *mimesis*. In his celebrated 1933 essay, Walter Benjamin writes that the *mimetic faculty*—the ability to see the similarities in real and imagined stories—is the ultimate realization of the human mind.[48] When great waves of stormtroopers rallying before Emperor Palatine evokes Leni Riefenstahl's 1935 Nazi propaganda film the *Triumph of the Will*, or when the obliteration of Princess Leia's home planet *Alderon* conjures the terrifying prospect of an imminent nuclear annihilation, Lucas is harnessing this *mimetic faculty* to imbue his great saga with portentous meaning.

If we want the artificial systems we build to be generally intelligent in ways that are intelligible to us, they will need to grasp the rich seams of meaning that permeate human culture and to make sense of the simple narratives that frame everyday discourse. To achieve this, agents will need to do more than learn the generative factors that scaffold the perception of faces, apples, or chairs. They will even need to do more than learning the shared relational patterns in scenes and abstract ideas. They will need to learn representations that refer to the world in ways that Peirce denoted *indexical* and *symbolic*—that are independent of physical resemblance altogether. They will need to grasp that Harry, Hermione, and Ron are students at Hogwarts, that lanterns, firecrackers, and red envelopes are associated with Chinese New Year, and that a plateful of spindly pasta with meat sauce is linked to the oldest university in the world via a town in north-east Italy.[49] Today, how to learn these deep conceptual patterns in human knowledge remains an unsolved problem in AI research.

In the mammalian brain, repeated co-occurrence of two stimuli leads to the formation of a conjoined neural code—a neuron (or population) that codes for them both. Above, we have encountered this idea for locations, when

---

[46] In recent years, this idea has been expressed most eloquently by the anthropologist Yuval Noah Harari in *Homo Deus: A History of Tomorrow*, his panoptical vision of human society.

[47] In his book *The Seven Basic Plots*, Christopher Booker argues that these three elements are basic to all narratives.

[48] See (Benjamin 1933).

[49] Spaghetti Bolognaise comes from the town of Bologna in the Italian region of Emilia-Romagna. The University of Bologna was founded in 1088.

repeated transitions between states coded as x_i and x_j led to the formation of a wider representation of both states x_{ij}. The same holds for objects. In a series of studies beginning in the 1990s, Yasushi Miyashita and colleagues recorded from the anterior parts of the temporal lobe (TE) and the PRC, whilst macaque monkeys performed a paired-association task, which involved grouping two distinct fractal images into the same arbitrary category. The areas TE and PRC lie at the apex of the primate ventral stream, with the PRC channelling complex visual information to the hippocampus via the ERC and DG. After training, the authors observed *pair-coding* neurons that fired in the presence of either fractal in a pair, as if the cells had learnt a concept that embraced both items. These neurons were relatively rare in area TE (5% of observed neurons), but much more common in the PRC (33%), suggesting that the latter is a good candidate for linking physically dissimilar stimuli in space and time. Human brain imaging methods, such as fMRI recordings, are far too coarse-grained to measure signals from individual neurons, but proxies for pair coding can be observed by calculating similarity between patterns of BOLD activity across voxels.[50] When humans repeatedly view temporally adjacent pairs of fractals or random objects, multivoxel representations evoked by each stimulus tend to become more similar, implying the formation of a shared neuronal code. When objects are arranged in a graph, so that the spatiotemporal distance is preserved between both adjacent and non-adjacent items, it is possible to use multivariate analysis to read out and visualize the mental map on which they lie (Figure 5.7). In humans, this has been observed primarily in MTL regions including the ERC and hippocampus proper.[51]

A handful of studies have offered privileged insight into concept formation by directly recording from neurons in the human MTL. In one landmark study from 2005, participants undergoing neurosurgical procedures[52] viewed images of celebrities and famous buildings. MTL neurons were found to respond uniquely to highly specific people or places, such as Bill Clinton, Homer Simpson, or the Sydney Opera House.[53] The remarkable specialization of these *concept neurons* in the MTL, reminiscent of grandmother coding, might be due to a computational step that takes place in the DG, where neural population codes are explicitly *sparsified*—that is, each concept is encoded by a reduced group of more specialized neurons (i.e. with a sparser code). Concept neurons also show pair coding, but with acquisition times that are

---

[50] Voxels are 3D pixels and are the smallest unit of observation in a neuroimaging study.
[51] See (Garvert et al. 2017) and (Schapiro et al. 2012).
[52] Surgery for intractable epilepsy.
[53] See (Quiroga et al. 2005).

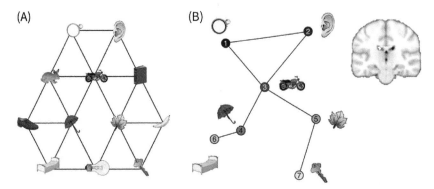

Fig. 5.7 Mental maps in the human medial temporal lobe (MTL). Humans were shown a succession of single images that were sampled by traversing the hexagonal grid shown in (**A**). Later, BOLD signals were measured for a subset of images shown in random order. The patterns of similarity in the MTL evoked by the images (when reduced to two dimensions) recapitulated the shape of the map.
Reprinted from Garvert et al. 2017.

much faster than observed in the macaque. When pictures of familiar people (such as Clint Eastwood) were juxtaposed with images of salient, but semantically unrelated, places (such as the Eiffel Tower), human MTL neurons came to code for both in a conjoined fashion.[54] This occurred after just seven instances of paired presentation, unlike in the original macaque studies, where training unfolded over many days, offering hints as to how rapid (or 'few-shot') learning occurs in humans.[55]

Another striking findings is that some human MTL neurons code for diverse objects that are united by a high-level semantic theme. For example, the authors identified a neuron that seemingly coded for *tall historical monuments*—responding to both the Leaning Tower of Pisa and the Eiffel Tower. This was not a pair-coding neuron, because these images were presented at random times in the experiment.[56] Moreover, the neuron did not simply respond to tall buildings per se, as it was silent to an image of New York's former Twin Towers. Another neuron responded to images of both Yoda and Luke Skywalker, who do not look at all alike but share the latent property of being *Jedi Knights* in the *Star Wars* saga. Yet another neuron coded for two different female characters in the TV sitcom *Friends* that was grinding through its final season just as the neural recordings were being made. Critically, the

---

[54] See (Ison et al. 2015).
[55] Discussed below.
[56] And are presumably not routinely experienced together in real life.

neuron failed to respond when one character (Jennifer Aniston) was shown alongside her then romantic partner (Brad Pitt), who was not among the cast—suggesting that the neuron might code for the entire concept of the show *Friends*, and not just the identities of the individuals in question.[57] These cells have thus been proposed to be important building blocks of human conceptual knowledge.

Pair coding in the primate MTL implies the existence of *indexical* concepts, which jointly encode objects that do not resemble one another physically, like Clint Eastwood and the Eiffel Tower, but have been experienced together. But the observation that single neurons code for broad semantic themes—Jedi Knights or characters from *Friends*—implies the existence of *symbolic concepts* or those that transcend both physical resemblance and spatiotemporal contiguity. These are neurons whose coding properties span the abstract spaces carved out by human stories—fictionalized accounts of love and friendship in Manhattan, or the noble exploits of intergalactic warriors. These neurons are great candidates for underpinning our sense of how objects and events are organized into thematically coherent narratives. From their earliest years, children start to associate people, practices, and plotlines that are linked by a common concept. For Western children, this might be knowing that Winnie the Pooh is a Bear of Very Little Brain who loves honey and is friends with Tigger, or that Christmas revolves around fir trees, and carols, and the excitement of Santa Claus coming down the chimney. It is here that Benjamin's *mimetic faculty* begins. The human brain has evolved neural machinery for grouping objects that are united by these high-level themes into a symbolic concept. In humans, a key site for this integration may be the hippocampus and surrounding MTL structures.

For AI researchers, the pressing question is what computational constraints allow the formation of abstractions such as these. How will we ever train an AI to understand the meaning of Winnie the Pooh or Christmas? Ultimately, of course, the knowledge that humans acquire about these high-level semantic concepts—that Pooh and Tigger are friends, and that Santa comes down the chimney—is acquired from experience, that is, they must be mined from the great streams of sensory data that we experience over our lifetimes. To pick out these themes—to learn the concept of *Winter Olympics* from the ground up, just like the VAE learns the concept of *age* or gender expressed in pixels of a face image—seems like a very daunting task. This is particularly so for

---

[57] Concept neurons, as they are now called, were originally named 'Jennifer Aniston neurons' in honour of this example. Coincidentally, *Friends* was filmed at Warner Bros Studios in Los Angeles, just a short drive from where these MTL recordings were being made at UCLA General Hospital.

symbolic concepts where all physical similarity and spatiotemporal contiguity are stripped away—in what could these concepts possibly be grounded if they do not benefit from patterns of correlation defined in space, time, or physical features?

One possibility is that we owe concept neurons to the extraordinary versatility of our memory systems. Consider the ensemble of physically different entities associated with the concept of *Christmas*—fir trees and carols and mince pies. If you live in a Christian-majority country, then these objects tend to materialize together during the second half of December. Thus, a sophisticated memory system might, in theory, be able to delicately extract latent factors, like *Jedi Knight*, *Winter Olympics*, or *Diwali*, from the spatiotemporal contiguity of events in feature films, sporting events, and religious festivals. Perhaps a *Jedi Knight* neuron could emerge from the spatiotemporal overlap between Luke and Yoda: they occupy the big screen at the same time, they both have green lightsabres in the later films, and they can both use the Force to lift rocks (albeit with varying degrees of mastery). Perhaps, with terabytes of daily sensory throughput, humans are able to self-supervise the learning of obscure latent variables that map onto the most abstract of symbolic concepts. This neurocognitive account of concept formation blurs Peirce's distinction between *indexical* and *symbolic* concepts. According to this view, even if Christmas is a cultural convention—cemented by stories, songs, and rituals—ultimately our concept of *Christmas* is formed by the spatial and temporal contiguity of experiences with the Yuletide theme.

However, even if our memory systems are very versatile, this account seems to stretch credulity to the limit. The MTL would need an otherworldly ability to link seemingly disparate events across time, picking out relevant details from a jumble of irrelevant inputs. The characters of Luke and Yoda also co-occur with elevators and rainforests, neither of which are particularly related to the core concept of *Star Wars*. Over the winter holiday period, you probably continue to feed to the cat and wash your socks, but these probably are not part of your canonical concept of *Christmas*. To learn the links between the objects and events that characterize Christmas, we need something else. It would be very handy if there existed a cognitive mechanism—or an additional constraint—that allowed us to extract and group sensory data into meaningful concepts, even when they are not drawn from circumscribed locales in Euclidean space, time, or the physical space of object features.

Fortunately, there is. It is called natural language, and humans use it readily to ground the most abstract of concepts. We link Luke and Yoda in our minds not just because of their coincident exploits on screen, but because we have learnt the verbal label *Jedi Knight* and heard others apply it jointly to the two *Star Wars* characters. This is not a radical claim: as humans, language is our pre-eminent symbolic system, and thus our readiest vehicle for grounding symbolic concepts.[58] In fact, another defining feature of concept neurons in the human MTL is that they respond to the identity of people and places expressed either verbally or pictorially. For example, one neuron that responded to visual images of the actor Jackie Chan also coded for his name in either written or spoken form (Figure 5.8).[59] These cells thus represent the concept of personal identity in a way that transcends the format and modality of the input data. They thus code for definitively symbolic concepts, because it is by convention that we decide which written traces or phonetic patterns denote this individual.[60]

Cognitive neuroscientists have argued that in the human brain, perceptual and semantic information is initially processed in independent streams, and then combined. The 'hub-and-spokes' model argues that concepts are assembled from a patchwork of modality-specific information (including vision, emotional valence, praxis, and speech) in a convergence zone in the anterior temporal lobe (ATL). This region, like the MTL, receives visual inputs from the ventral stream and auditory signals from more superior temporal regions—those that, when stimulated in Penfield's experiments, elicited auditory hallucinations of music and conversation. Echoing the concept neuron results in the MTL, BOLD signals in the adjacent ATL respond in an overlapping fashion to words and pictures, and cortical degeneration in this area is strongly associated with the loss of conceptual knowledge in semantic dementia.[61] However, there is also evidence that the visual signals and speech are far more intricately enmeshed in the cortex. For example, one recent study used sophisticated brain imaging analyses to reveal the existence of multiple cortical sites at the border of the visual cortex where neural tuning varied gradually from perceptual to semantic. At each site, the authors identified a gradient whereby conceptual grounding gradually morphed from video to spoken word, suggesting that the posterior cortex constitutes a mosaic of semantic hubs in which concepts are alternately more iconic and symbolic.[62]

The contrastive language–image pre-training (CLIP) network is a foundation model that can generate amazing new images from a text-based query.[63]

---

[58] In fact, studies using category names as targets for supervised learning in CNNs implicitly assume that producing labels for things is a sufficient condition for object recognition, as if names were not just ways of organizing knowledge, but ends in themselves for cognition.

[59] See (Rey et al. 2020).

[60] Whose real name is actually Datuk Fang Shilong.

[61] Reviewed in (Ralph et al. 2017).

[62] See (Popham et al. 2021).

[63] Discussed in Chapter 1. The multimodal selectivity for CLIP is described in (Goh et al. 2021).

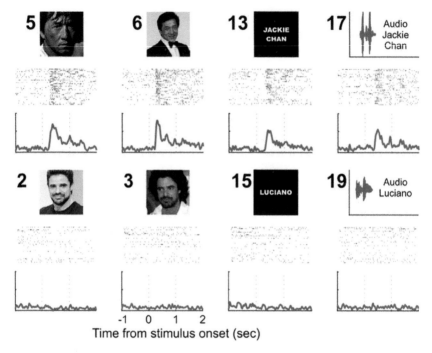

Fig. 5.8 A cell recorded from the human hippocampus that responds to images, text, or audio denoting the actor 'Jackie Chan', but not another actor known to the participant (Luciano Castro). Each red line shows the average neuronal response to multiple presentations of the image, words, or sound.
Reprinted from Rey et al. 2020.

Instead of being trained with human-annotated data (such as ImageNet), it learns from a gigantic corpus of weakly supervised data gathered from the internet. To assemble a training data set, the team at OpenAI generated 500,000 search queries (from all words that occurred at least 100 times in Wikipedia) and scraped 400 million corresponding images from the web. Firstly, they encoded the image data with a CNN and its accompanying text with a transformer, and combining them in a multimodal embedding space. They then adapted the contrastive approach in CPC by applying it to {text, image} pairs, so the network learnt a set of representations that maximally discriminated whether an image and its corresponding annotation belonged together. Not only is the network able to produce remarkable annotations for images, but when the authors explored its coding properties, they also found it had formed units that responded maximally to *Christmas*, including winter wonderland and nativity scenes, trees, lights and presents, and the words 'Merry Christmas' in the cursive fonts typical of seasonal greetings cards

Christmas   **West Africa**

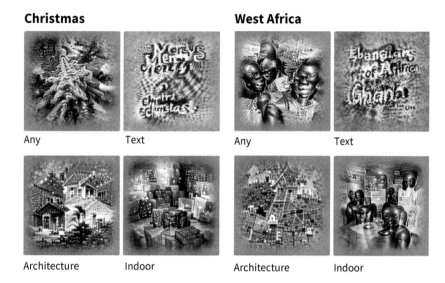

Any   Text   Any   Text

Architecture   Indoor   Architecture   Indoor

Fig. 5.9 Images generated using a feature visualization method to identify those concepts that drive a unit of CLIP most vigorously.

(Figure 5.9). Other neurons responded to concepts like Star Wars, Pokémon, or other interlinked motifs—one neuron coded jointly for rainbow flags and the acronym LGBTQ+. The network had acquired concept neurons like those in the human MTL—units responding to high-level semantic themes that are grounded in abstract symbols which humans define by cultural convention.

Language is thus the glue that holds the most abstract concepts together. By translating experiences into words, we can tag them with common semantic themes—those that will ultimately constrain what knowledge we share with one another. No doubt this is why the range of concepts we can grasp is bounded by the set of words whose meaning we understand. This echoes claims of weak linguistic relativity made by Whorf, that the nouns and verbs we learn from our linguistic communities sculpt the *relational groupings* we learn. Recall the Hopi, a Native American group, who have different concepts for water according to whether it is in a lake or in a cup—their concept of *water* is different to most other Americans.[64] By using very large generative models that meld image and text together in latent space, we can learn mental maps that begin to show the semantic richness of human memory.

---

[64] As discussed in Chapter 3.

6
The value of action

6.1 Climb every mountain

As dawn was breaking over a day in late May 1985, British climber Joe Simpson found himself stuck on a narrow ice bridge, halfway down a deep crevasse in the Peruvian Andes, many miles from help. His right leg was badly broken, robbing him of any chance of climbing out. He knew that his climbing partner Simon Yates believed he was dead and had already headed back to base camp. With all other options exhausted, Simpson decided to lower himself deeper into the unknown darkness of the crevasse. His rope was just long enough to drop him on another precarious ledge, from where, to his astonishment and delight, he saw a shaft of sunlight. It was streaming through the snow-hole from which he would eventually escape. In the book describing his adventures called *Touching the Void*, Simpson describes the effect this had on his mental state:

> The change in me was astonishing. I felt invigorated, full of energy and optimism. I could see possible dangers, very real risks that could destroy my hopes, but somehow I knew I could overcome them. It was as if I had been given this one blessed chance to get out and I was grasping it with every ounce of strength left in me. A powerful feeling of confidence and pride swept over me as I realised how right I had been to leave the [ice] bridge. I had made the right decision against the worst of my fears.

The possibility of escape inspired Simpson to new heights of bravery and endurance. He was able to haul himself out of the snow-hole and onto the glacier above, and despite dehydration, frostbite, and his shattered leg, he managed to hop and crawl his way back to camp. He arrived just hours before his companions, who had given him up for dead, were due to set out on the long trek back to civilization.[1]

---

[1] Which you can read for free here: https://booksvooks.com/touching-the-void-the-true-story-of-one-mans-miraculous-survival-pdf.html. The book was co-authored with Yates.

Natural General Intelligence. Christopher Summerfield, Oxford University Press. © Oxford University Press 2023. DOI: 10.1093/oso/9780192843883.003.0006

Simpson's story shows the extraordinary power of human motivation. Against all the odds, he found the ingenuity to hatch a plan of escape, the courage to leap blindly into the unknown, and the fortitude to carry on in the face of great adversity. But from the standpoint of both AI and neuroscience, this also poses a deep theoretical question. As biological organisms, where does our sense of purpose come from? What was it that drove Joe Simpson forward when it seemed that all was lost? For those of us who are safe and well at home—or at least not injured and stranded in the depths of the Andes—what is the ultimate cause of our behaviour? What is it that impels us to get out of bed in the morning, to sneak a second helping of cake, to give money to a stranger in need, to complete a Sudoku, to go to war for our country, to take a run in the rain? Why would anyone decide to scale a 6000-metre Peruvian mountain in the first place?

In earlier chapters, we considered the challenge of defining intelligence in both humans and machines. What qualities would a general intelligence have, and what should it be able to do? A popular answer—captured in the well-known synthesis by Legg and Hutter—is that intelligent agents are those that know how to perform many tasks and can thus meet a diverse multitude of objectives.[2] But within this seemingly sensible definition lurks a fundamental ambiguity. Is the intelligent agent one that knows how to perform many tasks *in theory*, or one that autonomously chooses to execute many tasks *in practice*? Thus far, we have focussed on agents that make inferences using the power of reason (*machines that think*), and discussed computational principles of knowledge acquisition in neural networks (*machines that know*). But are thinking and knowing about the world enough for intelligence?

Some people believe so. These tend to be philosophers or computer scientists that envisage general AI as an *oracle*. One vision of an oracle is a system that can be queried in natural language, and that provides truthful and knowledgeable answers via voice, text, or illustration. Such a tool would be immensely powerful. It would have the world's knowledge at its fingertips. Ideally, it would be able to harness powers of creativity and reason to forge new plans and develop new theories, to inject its answers with new ideas that push the frontiers of human understanding. Let's say our objective is to stem the spread of a rapidly spreading infectious disease. An oracle might explain, step by step, what public health measures should be put in place and when, how to synthesize the relevant messenger ribonucleic acid (mRNA) for a

---

[2] See (Legg & Hutter 2007).

vaccine, and how to solve the logistics of ramping production for equitable global distribution.[3]

In fact, the AI systems that we have considered thus far mostly cleave to this vision for intelligence. The early theorem provers sought to reason over hard-and-fast premises provided by the researcher, thinking around logical corners too tortuous for most human minds. Modern deep learning systems trained to map generatively from images to images (such as the β-VAE), from text to images (DALL-E), from images to text (CLIP), or from text to text (GPT-3 and Chinchilla) all open the door to new ways to digest, synthesize, and disseminate the world's knowledge. A general oracle would be the ultimate expression of *epistemic intelligence*. Its goal would be to generate knowledge and share it efficiently with humanity: to solve tasks in theory, but not in practice.

An alternative vision for general AI is an agent whose intelligence is realized by taking actions in the world. Such an agent would have *instrumental intelligence*—it would not only solve problems in theory, but also tackle them in practice. Faced with the challenge of a new virus, it does more than offer biomedical or public health advice from a lofty academic perch—it dons a virtual lab coat and, working through effectors that impact either the real world or the online world, it starts conducting research: it analyses data, adjusts beliefs, and charts a new scientific course where required. At first glance, this might seem like an unnecessary addendum to our characterization of intelligence. Surely the clever agents are those who *know*, not those who *do*—the scientist who formulates the theory, not the lab technician who mixes the reagents? The strategic brains in command and control, not the foot soldiers slogging away in the field?

However, an agent with merely epistemic intelligence has no sense of purpose. Ultimately, the goal of the giant foundation models we have met so far is just to mimic patterns in data, whether via a discriminative or a generative function. These models are not motivated to bring about any particular state of the world. They do not count the costs and benefits of different courses of action. They have no values of their own, no sense of right or wrong,[4] and no plans to make the world a better place for the programmers that created them or the wider population of planet Earth. They are strange beasts—as if Joe Simpson, alone in the crevasse, coldly calculates his chances of survival but

---

[3] It has to be said that in the Covid-19 pandemic humans actually did a pretty good job on making the actual vaccine but could definitely have done with some help on the public policy and equitable global production fronts.

[4] Of course, agents like Delphi can pass moral judgement on statements in natural language. However, it is not their moral judgement, reflecting the worth of a state of the world to the agent. It is the output of a generative model trained to predict the most likely human response.

formulates no plans for escape, and is ultimately indifferent as to how his story ends. Without the motivation to act, we squander the best part of our mental powers. Intelligence is inextricably bound up with a sense of purpose—not just a desire to consider means, but an urge to meet ends. In fact, when we talk of an artificial *agent*, this is exactly what we are referring to—an intelligence with *agency*, with the power to affect the world in order to achieve its objectives. In this chapter, thus, we will consider *machines with motives*.

In AI research, the subfield that builds machines with motives is called *reinforcement learning* or RL. In the book by Rich Sutton and Andy Barto that carries this title, which has biblical status for students in this field, RL is defined as follows:

> Reinforcement learning, like many topics whose names end with 'ing', such as machine learning and mountaineering, is simultaneously a problem, a class of solution methods that work well on the problem, and the field that studies this problem and its solution methods.

Sutton and Barto are saying that when we begin to contemplate how to motivate machines to act intelligently, we need to rethink of not just the computational space of solutions, but the nature of the problem that they face.

RL rewrites the problem for AI research by closing the reciprocal loop between agent and environment. Agents with epistemic intelligence receive queries from the world, but the answers they spit out do not directly impact the environment.[5] In the ImageNet challenge, the class labels produced by AlexNet do not influence which image is sampled next. For classical AI, the proof of one theorem has no bearing on the validity of the next. This is in sharp counterpoint to the experience of biological agents, whose actions powerfully constrain the next observations they receive. Where you move your eyes determines the visual inputs that fall upon the retina. What you grasp dictates what you hold in your hand. What you say affects how others think and feel. What you buy in the market decides what your family will eat for dinner. Whether or not you study hard for an exam in school can mould the lifelong trajectory of your career. Humans—like other biological agents—are part of the world, and our actions affect the forthcoming states that we and others will encounter in the future. By operating within a paradigm in which agents can influence their own environment, RL opens the door to machines that can behave in purposeful ways.

---

[5] At least not within their training loop.

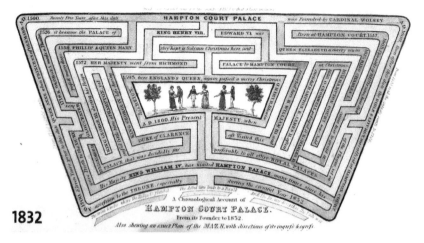

Fig. 6.1 Hampton Court maze.

To build machines with their own motivations, AI researchers have borrowed a concept from control theory known as the *Markov decision process* (or MDP).[6] An MDP is a mathematical tool for compactly specifying the dynamics that link an environment, an agent, and an objective. In the context of RL, it provides the minimum information needed to unambiguously specify how an agent could and should act, via four mathematical objects, denoted by the *states S*, *actions A*, *transition function P*, and *reward function R*. The states, actions, and transition function specify the scope of the agent's behaviour and how it affects the world. The reward function describes the agent's objective, in the form of numerical rewards received for achieving certain states. Adopting this framework allows us to cleanly specify a goal for the AI researcher: to train the agent to maximize rewards—and thus to meet the objective specified by the environment.

Hampton Court Palace is a magnificent Tudor residence, built by King Henry VIII, in the London borough of Richmond (Figure 6.1). Its gardens contain a famous trapezoidal hedge maze that has delighted and frustrated both royalty and commoners for more than 300 years. When it was planted in 1700, the maze included a radical innovation: paths that branch off confusingly towards dead ends, so that the goal is only reached by making the correct turn at each fork[7]. Solving Hampton Court maze is precisely the sort of problem that RL agents are built to tackle. Imagine that I tasked you with

---

[6] A branch of engineering that studies how machines can be configured to meet externally specified goals.
[7] Prior to this, mazes were *unicursal*, meaning they followed a single winding route to the goal.

designing an agent that could reliably find its way to the exit—one that could solve Hampton Court maze. How would you begin?

AI researchers would answer that you need to formulate the problem as an MDP, and then apply one of the many computational solutions to RL problems developed over recent decades. To specify the maze as an MDP, we need to define states, actions, transitions, and rewards. The *states* are the locations that make up the environment. We might define these as discrete positions in the maze, for example in allocentric coordinates. The *actions* constrain the scope of agent behaviour. For simplicity, we might assume that our maze-solver can move forward, backward, and turn left or right. Finally, the *transition function* determines the consequences of action. In a navigation task, these are relatively simple: if I move forward, I advance; if I move backward, I retreat. At a T-junction, a leftward move takes me down one branch, and a rightward move down the other. The transition function takes a state and action as inputs and returns the next state that will be observed.[8] Combining these elements, the MDP is a dynamic process that unfolds in discrete time. In each step, it controls the interaction between agent and environment—the agent observes a state and chooses an action; the transition function dictates its consequences, and thus the next state experienced by the agent.

To finalize the problem specification, however, we need to define the objective. In an MDP, this is the province of the *reward function*, which provides positive or negative reinforcement upon attainment of designated states. If the goal is to exit the maze as quickly as possible—like a lost tourist in desperate need of a cup of tea—then we might (for example) specify a reward of 100 for reaching the exit, and a penalty of −1 elsewhere. The goal of the agent is to learn a policy that maximizes the reward obtained from this function. It is not hard to see that for this reward function, the best policy is to minimize the number of steps (each incurring a penalty of −1) taken prior to reaching the exit (+100)—in other words, to leave the maze via the shortest path. We might say such a policy *solves* this MDP.

The basic computational object needed to solve an MDP is known as a *value function*. The value function is the subjective counterpart to the reward function. The reward function is given by the environment; the value function is computed by the agent. The reward function lives in the world; the value function lives in the brain. The reward function is part of the problem; the value function is part of the solution. The value function encodes the subjective worth of each state in the environment (or state–action pair). How good is it

---

[8] This transition function can be probabilistic, so that the same state and action might have distinct consequences on different timesteps.

to be three steps from the exit? What is the value of turning right, rather than left, at this junction? We can think of the task of RL researchers as designing agents that will learn the *optimal* value function, that is, the function which—if obeyed—will lead to maximization of reward in the environment.

Fortunately, since the 1950s, we have known how to compute the optimal value function for any given finite state MDP. The secret, which we owe to the mathematician Richard Bellman, is that the optimal value of any given state $v^*(s)$ is equal to any reward obtained in that state, plus the expected discounted value of the next state.[9] The discount is a multiplier that downweighs future value—it can be thought of as an *impatience* parameter, reflecting the heighted value of instant pleasure over delayed gratification.[10] An agent that makes choices that respect the optimal value function will also maximize objective reward on the maze. It is important to note that the optimal value function does not simply reduce to the reward function. For example, in Hampton Court maze, it is better to be two steps from the exit than 20 steps away—even if the objective reward obtained is −1 in both cases. This is because the expected discounted return from the latter—the reward you can expect in the near future—is higher in the 2-step than in 20-step case.[11] The Bellman equation thus formalizes why we savour positive experiences—such as when a child is excited on the eve of her birthday, even though presents and cake have yet to arrive.

RL dramatically ups the theoretical ante for AI research. It opens a Pandora's box that otherwise conceals the full promise and perils of powerful AI. It raises thorny philosophical questions about the meaning and purpose of existence in both animals and machines. The grand vision that animates RL researchers is that we can conceive of real-world problems in terms of an MDP—from flying a helicopter to playing the board game Diplomacy—and solve them using the computational toolkit from RL. Some have even dared to contemplate a broader ambition for the field. What if we could write down the entire natural world as an MDP? Then the problem of 'solving' intelligence is reduced to the problem of satisfying whatever reward function it entails, using scaled-up versions of the computational tools that we might deploy to solve chess, or autonomous driving, or Hampton Court Palace maze.

---

[9] We can write the Bellman equation as $q(s_t) = R(s) + \gamma q(s_{t+1})$, where $0 < \gamma < 1$.

[10] This preference is vividly illustrated by the famous Marshmallow Test, in which children wrestle with their immediate temptation to gobble up a lone treat, with the promise of a second if they can resist (Mischel et al. 1989). However, note that the discount is required, even if agents are perfectly patient. Otherwise, the value function grows without bound, because the expected reward over an infinite time horizon is infinitely large.

[11] Unless your agent's discount factor is 1, meaning it is infinitely patient.

This vision might sound outlandish, but it is the core tenet of some of the most fervent advocates of the RL paradigm. At DeepMind, Dave Silver and Rich Sutton have argued that solving intelligence reduces to the problem of maximizing reward. They boldly claim that *RL is enough*—that we will ultimately build AGI by combining the power of deep learning with the optimality guarantees that are baked into the Bellman equation. Translated to biology, this view implies that everything we do—from cleaning our teeth to swimming the channel—will be ultimately driven by a desire to maximize a reward function that is mysteriously built into our biology. According to this view, great displays of genius—from the solving of Fermat's last theorem to the composition of the legendary jazz album *Kind of Blue*—are in the end motivated by the pursuit of personal satisfaction. RL thus provides tidy answers to messy questions of motivation and purpose. It offers an explanation for what drove Joe Simpson onwards: he knew that the ultimate reward—the opportunity to live out the rest of his life—could only be attained by painfully dragging himself out of the crevasse and back across miles of boulder-strewn moraine. This claim is known as the *reward hypothesis*, and we shall give its plausibility due consideration in the sections below.

In this chapter, we will consider the intertwined history of RL in psychology, neuroscience, and AI research. We will consider the shared intellectual genesis in these fields of the computational methods that tile the solution space for RL. We shall also consider RL as a theory for biological brains. Advocates of the RL paradigm can appeal to its pleasing congruity with the natural world. Biological systems, like RL agents, take actions that determine their own future observations. This allows them to gather information by exploring the world, and to exploit that knowledge by harvesting rewards. Animal behaviour, like that of RL agents, is powerfully shaped by the rewards that follow from our actions—from a thirsty mouse pressing a lever in expectation of a drop of liquid to a habitual smoker buying cigarettes to staunch their craving for nicotine. As we shall see, the computational mechanisms that underlie reward-guided learning in animals bear a striking resemblance to the algorithms AI researchers have developed to solve RL problems.

6.2 The atoms of memory

If you have visited the coast, you might recognize a sea anemone—a brightly coloured polyp stuck fast to the rock below, whose oral disc (or mouth) is ringed with stinging tentacles (Figure 6.2). These creatures are among your most distant relatives. In fact, sea anemones, like other *cnidaria*, such as

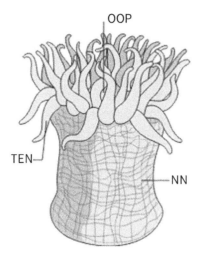

Fig. 6.2 An adult sea anemone, showing the oral opening (OOP), the tentacles (TEN), and the nerve net (NN).
Reprinted with permission from Arendt et al. 2016.

jellyfish and corals, do not even have a brain. Instead, they have nerve nets that encircle the mouth in concentric rings, controlling buccal contractions in response to stimulation, which is the basis for their predatory behaviour.[12] Humans last shared a common ancestor with these creatures some 680 million years ago, during an extended glacial period known as *Snowball Earth*. However, one phenotype that has remained conserved across the intervening aeons is the tendency to learn associations between stimuli and outcomes. This is a class of learning that psychologists call *classical conditioning*.

Classical conditioning was discovered independently on the two sides of the Atlantic at the outset of the twentieth century. In 1902, a psychologist at the University of Pennsylvania by the name of Edwin Twitmyer wrote a doctoral dissertation about elicitation of the patellar tendon reflex—the involuntary jerking of the leg that follows a sharp tap to the knee. He reported that when the tap is systematically preceded by a bell, the bell alone will come to provoke the reflex. A year later, at the 1903 International Medical Congress in Madrid, the Russian physiologist Ivan Pavlov announced his celebrated discovery that dogs learn to salivate in response to a ticking metronome that predicts the arrival of food. For reasons that are not clear, Twitmyer's work was

---

[12] For a great review on the evolution of the nervous system, see (Arendt et al. 2016).

largely ignored, whereas Pavlov bagged the 1904 Nobel Prize for physiology. Today, classical conditioning is also known as Pavlovian conditioning.[13]

When sea anemones receive low-voltage electric shocks, they fold their tentacles protectively over the oral disc. In the 1970s, a team at California State University showed that when the shock was systematically preceded by illumination of a bulb hung over the surface of their tank, the tentacles began folding pre-emptively in response to the light. The nerve nets contain cells that respond to both light and electrical stimulation. When these are activated together, their mutual connection is strengthened via Hebbian learning. Learning this association allows the sea anemones to protect their most sensitive organs from harm. Classical conditioning is a very rudimentary form of learning: two sensory representations become associated by repeated temporal co-occurrence. It does not give an agent a sense of purpose, nor does it even require a brain. However, classical conditioning is the fundamental mechanism by which *secondary reinforcers* obtain their value. It is the reason that we enjoy the smell of delicious food that we cannot yet consume, treasure a photo of a loved one who is not there, or carefully guard the money in our purse, even if it is printed on worthless scraps of paper. Viewed via the lens of the RL paradigm, classical conditioning exploits the basic computational principle by which a value function is learnt by experience.

The Bellman equation states that the optimal value of the current state is equal to the expected discounted value of future states, plus any reward obtained. In theory, its derivation unlocks the secret of reward maximization in an MDP. In practice, however, it can be difficult to solve, because it involves a tricky recursive step: to compute the value of the current state, you need to know that of the next; and for this, you need to know the value of the subsequent state, and so on. This demands tools for recursive optimization, such as dynamic programming, which in turn requires the agent to have perfect knowledge of states, actions, transitions, and rewards in the MDP, as well as great computational power. Unfortunately, agents do not always enjoy this privileged purview on a problem. For example, as animals, we are obliged to tackle life with incomplete knowledge of the states and transitions that define our environment. Stepping out of your hotel in an unfamiliar city, you won't instantly know where to find the nearest café or metro station. Venturing your ideas in a meeting, you can only guess how they will be judged by colleagues. Lost in a maze, you don't know where each branch will lead. How, then, can we

---

[13] Perhaps just as well, because 'Twitmyerian' conditioning does not have quite the same ring to it.

learn an optimal value function without knowing in advance how the world is structured?

In the 1970s and 1980s, whilst neural network researchers were working out the mathematics of backpropagation, the pioneers of RL were developing a suite of tools that allowed the Bellman equation to be solved by sheer dint of experience alone.[14] In fact, just as early neural networks were proposed as models of human semantic cognition, the first RL algorithms were advanced as computational accounts of classical conditioning in experimental animals.[15] In the early 1980s, a major breakthrough arrived in the form of temporal difference (TD) learning. TD learning capitalizes on the basic learning mechanism that underpins classical conditioning: it assumes that value is shared between temporally adjacent states. With repeated experience, value estimates gradually diffuse backwards through time and between states until the optimal value function is learnt.

To illustrate, consider an agent that is lost in Hampton Court maze. With no idea of where to go, at first it moves entirely randomly. Eventually, it stumbles by chance on the exit and, under our proposed reward function, receives a large positive reinforcer. TD learning assumes that it then travels mentally back in time to update the value of the immediately preceding state. The update $\Delta v(s)$ is proportional to the *temporal difference*—the discrepancy between the value of this preceding state $v(s_t)$ and the (discounted) value of the current state $\gamma v(s_{t+1})$, plus the reward r_{t+1} obtained by visiting it. Because this reward is 100 points, there is a large update to the preceding (next-to-exit) state. On its next random sweep through the maze, the next-to-exit state is now more valuable, so when reached, its value will flow back to the next-to-next-to-exit state.[16] Importantly, this incremental backup of value does not require either of the states to be objectively rewarded. Over many repeated samples of experience, TD learning thus allows value to diffuse from rewarded states to those that predict them. This is exactly what happens in classical conditioning: for Pavlov's dogs, the reward value of food becomes attached to the metronome, and in the sea anemones, the aversive response occasioned by the shock infuses the light flash. TD learning thus provides an elegant theory of secondary reinforcement, and its discovery fired the starting gun on several decades of fertile conversation about reward learning between neuroscientists and AI researchers.

---

[14] In fact, Paul Werbos contributed to both endeavours.
[15] See (Barto & Sutton 1982).
[16] Because $\gamma v(s_{t+1})$ is now large, thanks to learning on the previous trial.

RL thus offers both a theory of how AI should learn and a model of how animals do learn. However, before we can propose RL as a mechanistic theory for biology, there is a major conceptual hurdle to overcome. What is 'reward' in the natural world, and where does it come from? The MDP framework invites the researcher to define the reward function as a property of the external environment. If the agent is playing chess, it is rewarded for winning. Controlling a power plant, it is rewarded for increasing production and penalized for spiralling costs. Flying a glider, it is rewarded for staying aloft. But what is the reward function for natural agents going about their everyday lives, and who or what is the external entity that specifies it?

In the natural world, rewards do not arrive via a dedicated sensory input channel. In fact, they are not bequeathed by the environment at all.[17] Instead, they are the result of a subjective internal process by which we evaluate the world in the context of our need to survive and reproduce. Food, warmth, and sex are not intrinsically rewarding but instead bring us pleasure when we are hungry, cold, or aroused. Rewards are made in the mind, not given by the world. This simple intuition has far-reaching consequences for understanding motivated behaviour, as well as its disruption in psychiatric illness. However, it also poses a major inconvenience for advocates of RL as the pathway to general intelligence, because it raises the potentially intractable question of how to design a reward function for AGI with human-like purpose.

Conveniently, in biological brains, stimuli that are experienced as rewarding activate stereotyped neural circuits. In mammals, these originate in the dopaminergic midbrain and project widely to the striatum, hippocampus, and PFC, brain structures that are critical to action selection, memory, and planning. In the 1950s, two researchers working at McGill University in Montreal implanted rats with stimulating electrodes in a diverse set of brain regions and wired the stimulator up to a lever that the rats could press at will. When the stimulating electrode was placed in the thalamus, the lever was ignored. When it was placed in the hippocampus or cingulate, the rats spent between 10% and 30% of their time pressing the lever. However, when it was placed in the basal forebrain—close to a dopaminergic pathway linking the ventral tegmental area (VTA) to the nucleus accumbens—the animals went at it like crazy. One animal racked up more than 7500 presses in a 12-hour period—that is, an average of one every 4–5 seconds—before falling asleep exhausted. The researchers James Olds and Peter Milner realized that they had found the hedonic headquarters of the mammalian brain. The existence of a

---

[17] Or even by the body, which we might consider to be part of the agent's environment.

brain region that directly signals reward allows proponents of biological RL to sidestep the problem of where value comes from—by treating the dopamine system as a kind of auxiliary input channel through which hedonic experience is sensed in the world. Under this sleight of hand, the dopamine system has thus been dubbed the *retina of the reward system*.[18]

This logic has allowed neuroscientists to harness TD learning as a model of the neurobiology of reward-guided behaviour. Perhaps surprisingly, this project began with an invertebrate species—the honeybee. Instead of a fully fledged dopamine system, honeybees have a single neuron (called VUMmx1) that responds to the receipt of sweet nectar.[19] Bees will extend their proboscis to approach an odour that has been paired with electrical stimulation of VUMmx1, as expected from classical conditioning. Bees will also tailor their foraging behaviour to the concentration of sucrose in artificial yellow and blue flowers. In 1995, a team of neuroscientists working at the Salk Institute realized that TD learning could account for both of these behaviours if VUMmx1 was encoding the TD update signal—or, in neuroscientific parlance, the reward prediction error.

A few years earlier, working in Switzerland, the neurophysiologist Wolfram Schultz and colleagues had shown that dopamine neurons in the primate VTA are activated by cues that predict primary rewards, such as food and fluid, as well as by their direct receipt. In 1993, the same authors extended this finding to show that the VTA dopamine response dies away when training is established and pauses neural firing rates below baseline levels in trials where reward is unexpectedly withheld (Figure 6.3). Putting two and two together, the Salk Institute team realized that this was exactly what would be expected if the dopaminergic neurons signalled TD error: a positive response when a reward occurred unexpectedly, a neutral response when it met expectations, and a negative response when hopes of a reward went unmet. They joined forces with Schultz to write a classic paper outlining this argument, which has since become a canonical plank in our understanding of reward-guided learning.[20]

In parallel with these successes at modelling reward-guided learning in the brain, TD learning was also proving to be a powerful tool for AI research. In 1992, an IBM researcher called Gerald Tesauro used the algorithm to train a computer to play grandmaster-level backgammon. Unlike IBM's much-vaunted victory over Kasparov at chess five years later, Tesauro's program

---

[18] See http://www.scholarpedia.org/article/Reward_signals.
[19] With the release of octopamine, a transmitter that may play a similar role to dopamine in insects.
[20] The Salk Institute researchers were Read Montague, Peter Dayan, and Terry Sejnowski. Dayan and Schultz (but perplexingly, not Montague) shared the European Brain Prize in 2017 for this discovery. See (Hammer 1993), (Montague et al. 1995), and (Schultz et al. 1993, 1997).

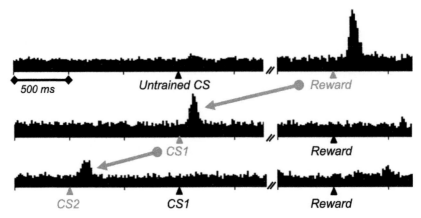

Fig. 6.3 Temporal difference (TD) learning in the monkey ventral tegmental area (VTA). The black traces show the average firing rates of putative dopamine neurons in the VTA during three phases of the experiment. Early in learning, the neurons respond to reward (a drop of liquid) alone. Subsequently, they respond to a conditioned stimulus (CS1) that predicts reward, but no longer fire to the reward itself. Finally, when another CS is introduced that predicts CS1, the neurons fire to this cue, but not to CS1 or the reward. In TD learning, this is the mechanism by which learning is 'backed up' from reward to reward-predictive stimuli.
Reprinted with permission from Schultz (2015).

(TD-Gammon) was unique in that it learnt entirely from scratch by playing against itself. In fact, the story of the development and deployment of TD-gammon reveals a striking resemblance to that of AlphaGo and AlphaZero some 25 years later. TD-Gammon used a simple connectionist model to map the board state onto a value estimate, training the model end to end with TD error. By predicting the value of forthcoming board states, it could choose whichever was most likely to result in a win. Later versions, which added a simple two- or three-ply forward search algorithm, were reckoned by experts to play at levels that equalled or bettered the strongest players in the world. Like AlphaGo's much-lauded move 37, TD-Gammon discovered new strategies which changed the way the professional game was played. For example, it showed that the then-ubiquitous strategy of 'slotting'—moving a single piece to point 6 early in the game—was suboptimal, and within a few years, it has disappeared from the standard repertoire of moves in grandmaster backgammon.

TD learning builds off the most basic memory processes—relying on the sharing of information between temporally adjacent states—what we might call the atoms of memory. It allows even the simplest organisms, like sea anemones, to learn to predict future states. However, as brains evolved, neural circuits matured to permit more complex chains of association. By the time of the early vertebrates, some 500 million years ago, a new region had emerged in the dorsal telencephalon, a brain area adjacent to the olfactory bulb, that was to become a central exchange for stimulus–outcome learning. Some 225 million years ago, this region took its place among other *allocortical* structures nestling below that signature mammalian innovation, the newly evolved neocortex. Today, we call it the hippocampus, and in humans, it is the great associative nexus that allows us to encode rich conceptual knowledge relating people, things, and places.

6.3 The basements of the brain

In 1898, a doctoral student at Columbia University decided to apply methods of psychological experimentation to study learning in animals. His name was Edward Thorndike, and his work would launch a century of behaviourist research.[21] The experiments are described in his doctoral thesis, entitled *Animal Intelligence: An Experimental Study of the Associative Processes in Animals*. Thorndike's experimental tools resembled non-spatial versions of Hampton Court maze—puzzle boxes in which hungry cats, dogs, or chicks had to pull a wire, press a lever or treadle, prise open a door, or push a bar to exit through a trap door and receive a food reward.

Thorndike's animals objected heartily to confinement, and like a frustrated tourist lost in a maze, they tried frantically to escape.[22] Here is a description of a typical study involving a cat:

> [the cat] claws and bites at the bars or wire; it thrusts its paws out through any opening and claws at everything it reaches; it continues its efforts when it strikes anything loose and shaky; it may claw at things within the box. It does not pay very much attention to the food outside but seems simply to strive instinctively to escape from confinement. The vigor with which it struggles is extraordinary. For eight or ten minutes it will claw and bite and squeeze incessantly.

---

[21] Thorndike also had some very unfortunate views about race and eugenics. In 2020, Columbia voted to rename Thorndike Hall after the prominent African-American psychologist Edmund Gordon.

[22] Or rather, like a tourist impatient for a cup of tea in the Palace café at Hampton Court. Thorndike notes that the dogs could not be food-deprived to the same degree as the cats, because otherwise they howled in the evening. See (Chance 1999).

By observing this behaviour closely, Thorndike made a remarkable discovery. Each time an animal was replaced in the box, it solved the puzzle more rapidly than the last. After several trials, the animals engaged purposefully with the apparatus, moving rapidly to open the door and secure the food reward. At this time, on the cusp of the twentieth century, most psychologists viewed learning as a process of connecting ideas to make new inferences. As we have seen, this was how Köhler interpreted the behaviour of his monkeys, who seemed to rely on dramatic moments of insight to reach an inconveniently placed banana.

Thorndike recognized that several aspects of his data were incompatible with this connect-the-dots view of learning. Firstly, his animals learnt only gradually. Performance improved incrementally, trial by trial, as if patterns of behaviour were being slowly stamped in, rather than grasped in a flash of insight. Secondly, over time, behaviour became highly automatized. A cat trained to pull a wire loop to escape would continue to claw at the air, even in its absence. The animals were learning fixed habits, not reasoning about the puzzle. Finally, the voluntary initiation of action was essential for learning to occur. Even after Thorndike had thoughtfully applied the cat's paw to a lever to permit its escape, this never prompted the animal to reproduce the same action itself.[23] These observations seemed to suggest that the animals were unaware of the consequences of their behaviour, and were blindly learning by trial and error to take the action that led to reward.

Thorndike thus proposed a new principle of learning, which he called the *Law of Effect*. Animal behaviour, he argued, is driven by the establishment of associations between stimulus and response. These links are acquired by what he called *trial and accidental success*, becoming stronger when the outcome is positive and weaker when negative (Thorndike called these 'satisfaction' and 'annoyance'). Over time, this allows a behaviour repertoire that elicits reward to be gradually acquired by experience. Today, we call this learning mechanism *instrumental conditioning*.

In the RL framework, a value function encodes what states of the world are subjectively worth. However, an intelligent agent also needs to know how to act. If the transition function is known, an agent armed with an optimal value function can peer ahead one or more steps into the future and choose the course of action that elicits the highest expected value. In fact, this was the strategy that TD-Gammon used to triumph at backgammon. However, as we can see from Thorndike's cats, the consequences of action can sometimes be

---

[23] In other words, the animals learnt by reinforcement, but not by supervision.

obscure. His puzzle boxes are an MDP in which most actions lead to the same state (still stuck in the box), and an unknown target action leads to a rewarded state (exit the box and consume the reward), but the confined animals do not know the transition function. They are unaware (and never seem to learn) that pulling a wire or tripping the latch opens the door to food—instead, they slavishly learn to perform the requisite action when appropriately stimulated. As we can see from Thorndike's account of a caged cat, this point is reached after a lot of random flailing—scratching, clawing, and biting, yeowling, hissing, growling, urinating, and rubbing their head and flanks against the box.[24] But eventually behaviour settles into a well-oiled sequence of moves from which the animal quickly obtains reward.

Thorndike's Law of Effect proposes that rewards shape the connection strengths between stimulus and response. A variant of TD learning, known as SARSA, directly implements this idea. In SARSA, the value function is expanded to encode the worth of both states and actions $q(s, a)$ and is rebranded a Q function.[25] We can think of $q(s, a)$ as encoding the connection strength between state s and action a, exactly the association that Thorndike proposed the animals learnt. The agent's policy is then simply a means of choosing each action conditional on the state. A popular choice, known as ε-greedy, is to choose the most valuable action, except on a fraction (ε) of steps when a random choice is made instead.

In the brains of mammals, dopamine neurons with cell bodies in the VTA and substantia nigra project dorsally (upwards) to synapse on neurons in a brain region known as the striatum, which is part of a core network of subcortical nuclei known as the *basal ganglia*. The basal ganglia lie deep in the midbrain, and their murky function and inaccessible location has earned them the epithet *basements of the brain* (Figure 6.4). Like the hippocampus, the basal ganglia are a phylogenetically ancient structure and were already present some 530 million years ago in the common ancestor we shared with our most distant vertebrate cousins—slimy creatures like lampreys and hagfish that live in mud at the bottom of the ocean. Almost all neocortical signals are looped via the striatum before being routed to motor cortical regions and

---

[24] In fact, a 1979 paper argues that escape from a particular class of puzzle box only occurs in the presence of human observers, because this induces the cats to engage in flank rubbing (a form of greeting familiar to cat owners), which, in turn, trips the opening on the puzzle box. The paper is entitled '*Tripping over the cat*' (Moore & Stuttard 1979).

[25] SARSA stands for "state-action-reward-state-action" because the update occurs on each non-terminal state from the quintuple of events $(s_t, a_t, r_{t+1}, s_{t+1}, a_{t+1})$. It is closely related to another member of the TD family known as Q-learning. The difference is that in Q-learning, the TD update is off-policy, meaning it is not tied to the specific move chosen, so $\Delta q(s, a) = r + \max(s', a')$ where s', a' are the next state and action, respectively.

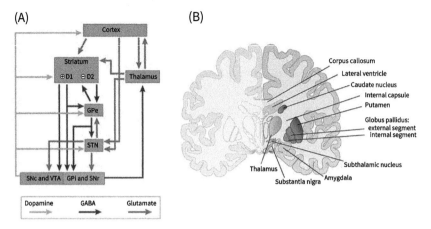

Fig. 6.4 Anatomy and connectivity of the basal ganglia. (**A**) Wiring diagram of the basal ganglia and neocortex. Arrows show dopaminergic (lightest grey), GABAergic (inhibitory; middle grey), and glutamatergic (excitatory, darkest grey) connections. GPe, external segment of the globus pallidus; GPi, internal segment of the globus pallidus. (**B**) Locations of basal ganglia and associated structures on a sagittal slice of the human brain.

Panel A reprinted with permission from Redgrave et al. (2010). Panel B reprinted with permission from Miall (2013).

down descending pathways to the peripheral nervous system to be converted into action. Striatal neurons are thus a critical waystation on the brain's all-important sensorimotor pathways.

In a classic experiment from 2001, researchers measured synapse formation in the striatum whilst rats were allowed to electrically self-stimulate their substantia nigra. Like in the VTA, the substantia nigra is a dopaminergic midbrain region where stimulation is highly reinforcing, and the rats rapidly learnt to press the lever at about 1 Hz. The researchers found that pulses of dopaminergic transmission elicited by self-stimulation potentiated synapses where the striatum received inputs from the neocortex. Across animals, the more these synapses were strengthened, the faster animals learnt to press the lever.[26] Dopamine thus acts as a gate on Hebbian plasticity that (when open) allows new links between sensory input (the sight of the lever) and motor output (depressing a paw). This triadic synaptic architecture is perfectly adapted to implement processes like SARSA, in which rewards mould the connection weights between states and actions. This finding gives

---

[26] See (Reynolds et al. 2001).

neurobiological substance to both Thorndike's psychological theory and its computational underpinnings in TD learning.

Two ancient brain structures thus govern how animals learn the value of states and actions. Precursors to the hippocampus and basal ganglia existed in our ancestors that lived half a billion years ago. The memory processes that they primarily subserve—learning of state value by association with outcome (classical conditioning) and the reward-guided linkage between stimulus and response (instrumental conditioning)—are the most basic building blocks of animal behaviour. In the parlance of the RL framework, they allow agents to learn the value of states and to connect states and actions. The rudimentary mechanisms by which we learn state values imbue the world around us with positive and negative meaning. They prefigure our learning of a rich conceptual model of the world that can be used to understand the costs and benefits of different courses of action, from the dilemma of whether to eat toast or fruit for breakfast to the great decisions that shape how our life unfolds, such as our choice of career or partner. Learning to couple states and responses is the most basic engine of behaviour, onto which all grander machinery for flexible, reasoned action selection is subsequently grafted. It is the basic process by which fruit flies learn to avoid an overheated side of their chamber, by which dogs are prompted to bound joyfully towards the door at the sight of the leash being retrieved, and by which human academics can be trained to unconsciously exaggerate an embarrassing mannerism on receiving Machiavellian smiles and nods from the students they are lecturing.[27]

Importantly, there is also evidence that these two systems team up during reward learning, especially when states and actions are continuous, rather than discrete. Where the action space is high-dimensional, state–action mappings cannot be learnt in the tabular format implied above, in which each neuron encodes the strength of a unique sensorimotor combination. Instead, a plausible alternative is the bipartite *actor–critic* architecture. The *actor* is a function that learns a potentially complex mapping from states to actions, governed by parameters θ. This function encodes the agent's *policy*, and it is often trained using an RL approach called the *policy gradient* methods. We can think of it as the instrumental learning system, with the parameters encoding the strengths of sensorimotor connections in the dorsal striatum. However, the policy is trained using TD error computed by a separate function—known as the *critic*—that encodes the value of states. A plausible substrate for this is the ventral striatum (or nucleus accumbens), which, unlike the dorsal

---

[27] This book provides a very authoritative summary (Murray et al. 2019). This is also helpful (Lynch 2009).

striatum, receives input from both the hippocampus and the dopaminergic midbrain, including the substantia nigra and VTA.[28] In fact, one brain imaging study modelled the prediction errors from both actor and critic in a bandit task, and found that they correlated with BOLD signals in the dorsal and ventral striatum, respectively.[29]

In the 1990s, Tesauro had already shown that a simple connectionist model could be used to learn a value function, with his backgammon agent TD-Gammon. By the 2010s, excitement about deep learning was setting the field alight, inviting the question of whether advanced neural networks could be harnessed for RL in yet more challenging domains. In 2013, researchers in Alberta published a paper describing the Arcade Learning Environment (ALE), a benchmark evaluation platform for RL that was based around Atari 2600 games such as Asterix, Seaquest, Boxing, and Zaxxon.[30] The challenge was straightforward: to maximize the points provided by the game emulator, just like human players might jostle for the highest score. However, it was also very daunting, because unlike other existing domains, the games were complex, naturalistic, and high-dimensional: with 210×160 spatial resolution blasting past at $60\,Hz$, the emulator generated more than 2 million unique pixel values every second, mapping onto 18 possible actions in total. Tesauro's method had worked for backgammon where perceptual inputs were much more basic—a board state could be coded with just 198 input units. But could deep networks learn a value function at scale? At first, results were not promising—it turned out deep networks trained with RL on naturalistic tasks like ALE were prone to instability and divergence.[31]

In 2014, the DeepMind team built the network known as DQN to tackle the ALE. DQN employed a deep convolutional network to map from image pixels[32] to a prediction about the value of each action, and the weights were trained with TD error. However, the network also housed a separate memory structure, which buffered reams of previous states, actions, and rewards from past episodes.[33] Throughout learning, it sampled past experiences randomly from this buffer, training from this replayed experience in tandem with active learning from the game. This mechanism, which is called *experience replay*, allowed it to overcome the challenge of learning in a dynamic environment.

---

[28] As always, the last word on brain circuitry goes to Suzanne Haber (see Haber 2016).
[29] See (O'Doherty et al. 2004).
[30] In fact, the final suite was chosen pseudo-randomly from the set of first-person games that had a Wikipedia page at the time and were not adult-themed or otherwise inappropriate. The paper is here (Bellemare et al. 2013).
[31] See (Tsitsiklis & Van Roy 1997).
[32] Downsampled to 84×84.
[33] In fact, each index in the replay buffer is the tuple $\{s, a, r, s'\}$.

DQN achieved human expert performance, or better, in 75% of the games in the ALE, surpassing previous efforts. With this result, deep RL was born.[34]

Using RL to train a deep network to play Atari at human level was a remarkable achievement. But paradoxically, it is DQN's limitations that are the most interesting. What DQN cannot do—and where it fails—has set the research agenda for the nascent field of deep RL over the intervening years. To begin with, let's glance down the list at the Atari games that DQN failed to solve. Right at the bottom of the scorecard, with a princely score of 0%—meaning that DQN performed no better than an entirely random agent—is a notorious game known as Montezuma's Revenge.[35]

6.4 The key to exploration

The greatest heist scene in cinematic history is arguably that in Jules Dassin's 1955 classic noir *Rififi*. Wearing well-cut suits and expressions of steely resolve, four seasoned jewellery thieves break into a grand apartment on Rue de Rivoli, Paris, and tie up its hapless residents. They then hammer gingerly through the floor to the exclusive jewellery shop below, collecting the falling plaster in an outstretched umbrella. Climbing through the hole in the ceiling, they disable the alarm system—which is sensitive to the slightest vibration—with fire extinguisher foam. Finally, they painstakingly drill a fist-sized hole in the back of the safe and retrieve jewels judged to be worth at least 200 million francs. Throughout the entire nail-biting 28-minute scene, not a single word of dialogue is spoken.

The ALE does not include a video game requiring players to pull off the perfect jewellery heist. But it has a good alternative. Montezuma's Revenge is a fiendishly difficult action adventure game in which players navigate a large interconnected map by opening doors with keys, dodging laser gates and fire pits, and avoiding skulls, snakes, and spiders (Figure 6.5). Like the crooks in *Rififi*, the player of Montezuma's Revenge needs to be equipped to the nines, only in this case with amulets, swords, and torches. If they make exactly the right moves in just the right order, they will eventually reach the Treasure Chamber, a central zone whose floor is temptingly strewn with priceless jewels. Unlike in *Rififi*, once snatched, this hoard is converted directly into game score, with no risk of being stolen by a rival gang of thieves.

DQN fails miserably at Montezuma's Revenge, and it is easy to see why. Like Thorndike's cats trying to escape from a puzzle box, DQN learns by trial and

---

[34] As discussed in Chapter 1. For a nice review, see (Botvinick et al. 2020).
[35] Montezuma's revenge is a slang term for traveller's diarrhoea picked up in Latin America.

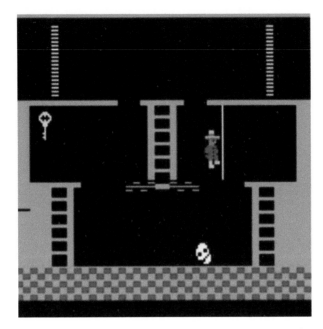

Fig. 6.5 The opening level in the Atari game Montezuma's Revenge. You have to direct the avatar (with the red coat) to collect the key and use it to unlock the yellow stripy door at the top right. Bumping into the skull, or falling off a platform, results in death.

error. This works fine for many Atari games, especially simple sensorimotor tasks in which an avatar is moved around the screen, blasting baddies and harvesting rewards. But Montezuma's revenge requires players to perform an exquisitely choreographed sequence of actions to progress from level to level. In fact, simply to advance beyond the first screen, the player has to climb down a ladder, scramble the wrong way up a conveyor belt, swing across a pole, leap with perfect precision over a rolling skull, jump to grab a key, and then perform the whole sequence in reverse to access the door that the key ultimately opens. Practically any departure from a perfectly orchestrated series of moves costs a life, and reverts the level to the start. Unsurprisingly, the probability of DQN learning to do this by chance is vanishingly small. It is a bit like expecting a toddler to pull off the perfect heist by charging randomly around a jewellery store in nappies.

How an RL agent behaves depends on its action selection policy. During learning, DQN computes the expected value of each action in each state $q(s, a)$. For example, in Pong, there are just two possible actions—the paddle can be moved up or down—for a given state, these values might be $q(s|up) = -0.2$ and $q(s|down) = 0.5$. DQN uses an ε-greedy (or epsilon-greedy) policy to select actions, which means that it chooses the best action (here, down), with a probability of 1−ε, and otherwise takes a random action. It might seem strange to deliberately bake randomness into the agent policy. However, the reciprocity between actions and observations in an MDP means that it is essential for an RL agent to be able to *explore* (gather information), as well as to *exploit* (harvest rewards). Exploration allows it to learn about different states to those it would never encounter by exploiting rewards alone. Conversely, consider a *greedy* agent that slavishly exploits the action with the highest expected return. If deterministically pursuing a greedy policy yield leaves the value function unchanged, then the agent will get stuck in an infinite loop, endlessly producing the same fixed action. To maximize reward, an RL agent needs to trade off exploration and exploitation.

In biology, proneness to exploring the environment is a ubiquitous phenotype. Even the humble bacterium—a single-celled organism—switches between two behavioural modes that resemble exploiting and exploring. Bouts of chemotaxis, during which it swims up a gradient towards preferred chemical conditions, are interspersed with phases of *tumbling*, in which their behaviour is erratic and prone to randomly changing direction—a bit like an RL agent displaying an ε-greedy policy. Similarly, in the tiny nematode worm *Caenorhabditis elegans*, the spatial scale of the random foraging is adapted optimally to the concentration of resources, so that if no food is found on a local search, the animal switches to a more global exploration strategy encompassing a wider area. Recall that in Thorndike's puzzle boxes, the cat did not sit quietly and wait for release—it flailed around with frenetic energy, satisfying a drive to explore every possible means of escape from the device. Exploration is evidently critical to organisms of many different shapes and sizes.[36]

For animals with larger brains, exploration policies can be quite sophisticated. In laboratory studies, the mechanisms by which exploration is traded off against exploitation have been extensively studied using a simple paradigm, called a *multi-armed bandit problem*, in which players choose among two or more stimuli or actions that pay out reward with an unknown probability.[37] When the payout probability is unknown, participants are obliged to trade off the reward harvesting against the gathering of information about the alternate option. Otherwise, they risk getting stuck with a policy of drawing rewards from the suboptimal alternative. This risk grows if the rewards are non-stationary, with probabilities that drift or jump over time.

---

[36] See (Calhoun et al. 2014).
[37] See (Gittins 1979).

We can think of the multi-armed bandit task as a crude version of the problem faced by animals foraging in the wild. On its nocturnal prowl, an urban fox can choose to hunt for rabbits in the local park or to scavenge for pickings among the residential dustbins, with variable probability of success or failure at either patch. In the 1960s, the Harvard psychologist R. J. Herrnstein[38] was studying instrumental conditioning in pigeons, training them to peck levers that offered variable rates of reward. He found that the pigeons consistently matched their foraging behaviour to the rate of reward provided by either lever, so if one offered a 20% change of grain and the other an 80% chance of grain, the pigeons would peck at them with a 1:4 ratio. Herrnstein called this *matching behaviour*.[39] Similarly, a common choice for exploration in RL is to choose action probabilities roughly in proportion to their respective Q-values, a policy that is sometimes called Boltzmann (or softmax-based) exploration.[40]

In policy gradient algorithms, where a parameterized function maps sensory states onto action probabilities, the rate of exploration cannot be controlled directly. Instead, a *maximum entropy* regularizer is often added to the cost function to keep the action values as entropic (or broadly distributed) as possible. This serves to promote greater diversity in behaviour, and thus a tendency to explore new states. A comparable form of regularization can be achieved by deliberately injecting neural networks with noise—adding stochasticity to the actions, observations, or model parameters. Paradoxically, although noise will disrupt learning, it has the side effect of ensuring that the network does not settle into narrow, inflexible behaviours that may be overfit to the past, but unsuited to dealing flexibly with what is to come. Adding noise to the then state-of-the art policy gradient algorithm for Atari, the asynchronous advantage actor–critic (A3C) algorithm, boosted performance by a median of nearly 20% per game.[41]

The fact that noise regularizes networks toward exploration is particularly relevant to biology, because computation in the nervous system is intrinsically variable. Neural noise is expressed at every scale, from transduction channels where ions permeate the cell membrane to drive spikes, through neurons and

---

[38] Later notorious for co-authoring the controversial book *The Bell Curve*, which advanced discredited views on race and intelligence. He died just before the book was published.

[39] Matching behaviour is not optimal if the bandits are stationary and payouts are issued with replacement, but pigeons (and monkeys and humans) seem to do it anyway. This can be explained if they assume that the bandit resources are being depleted by their actions.

[40] This policy is controlled by a free parameter, the softmax temperature. For high temperatures, this policy becomes equivalent to maximizing (always choosing the greedy option).

[41] For entropy regularization, see (Ahmed et al. 2019). For noise regularization, see (Fortunato et al. 2019) and (Plappert et al. 2018).

populations to behaviour itself.[42] In fact, there is evidence that noise—rather than a deliberate proclivity for choosing randomly, via an overt exploration policy such as ε-greedy—might best explain patterns of human behaviour in bandit tasks. A model in which noise was added to the TD update—as if prediction errors include a small amount of variability—was enough to capture the human explore–exploit trade-off, as well as explain a stickiness bias whereby humans preferred to select the same option on several trials in a row. This simple and biologically plausible innovation also explained why participants still tended to choose the less valuable option from time to time in a variant of the bandit paradigm in which the payout from both chosen and unchosen bandits were revealed on each trial, which precludes the need to overtly explore.[43]

Exploring alternative options at random—like tumbling—can prevent an agent from getting stuck with a single, suboptimal outcome. However, a yet more adroit policy is one that explicitly promotes information gathering with a view to future success. One way to do this is to endow the agent with *curiosity*—the preference to explore states that are novel or uncertain. In biology, animals are intrinsically prone to sampling novel states. Given the choice, rats will cross an electrified grid for the pleasure of exploring unfamiliar sections of a maze. Monkeys will perform a task when the only reward is a glimpse out of the window at the normal goings-on in an adjacent room. In developmental psychology, human infants will look longer and more intently at novel or surprising events, such as objects that seemingly violate the laws of physics.[44] Animals also learn faster when stimuli are new. During Pavlovian conditioning, the value of unfamiliar states is updated faster than that of familiar states, a phenomenon discovered in the 1950s, known as *latent inhibition*. There is good evidence that rapid learning about novel stimuli is dopamine-mediated. Dopamine neurons are prone to responding to novel or salient stimuli, even when they predict the absence of reward, and dopamine responses in the VTA and substantia nigra are enhanced when learning about novel stimuli. This phenomenon has been incorporated into the TD learning framework with inclusion of the *novelty bonus*, a premium that is added to the novel states as the value function is updated.[45]

---

[42] A useful review is (Faisal et al. 2008).

[43] See (Findling et al. 2019). In a follow-up paper, the same authors also showed that noise-added recurrent neural networks promote a form of generalization displayed by humans (but not non-noisy networks) (Findling & Wyart 2020).

[44] This provides a foundation for the *preferential looking paradigm*, a major tool for assessing preverbal cognition.

[45] For novelty seeking in rats, see (Dember & Earl 1957). For latent inhibition and its dopaminergic substrates, see (Lubow & Moore 1959) and (Morrens et al. 2020). For a review of dopamine responses to novelty and accompanying theory of exploration, see (Redgrave & Gurney 2006). For novelty bonuses, see (Kakade & Dayan 2002).

However, indiscriminate novelty seeking is not always a good idea. For example, you would probably find the fuzzy black-and-white patterns displayed on a malfunctioning vintage TV quite boring to watch for any length of time, yet they are the *sine qua non* of novelty—each frame is entirely unpredictable and different from all the others. This reminds us that uncertainty comes in different forms and flavours. Some sources of uncertainty are irreducible (or aleatoric), meaning that—like the noisy TV—they cannot be modelled or predicted, so exploring them is a waste of time. In other cases, however, uncertainty can be reduced by learning from experience. This is what happens as you learn a foreign language: at first, the speech sounds seem garbled and nonsensical, but with increasing proficiency, they morph into meaningful words and sentences. A sensible exploration policy is one that promotes not just novelty seeking, but also uncertainty reduction—that directs you to explore where learning is most beneficial.

In fact, this is largely what humans do. People seek out stimuli that are neither completely predictable nor completely unpredictable, but instead lie in a Goldilocks zone of intermediate novelty. One well-known observation, associated with the psychologist Daniel Berlyne, is that a piece of music is often enjoyed most when it is neither completely fresh nor repeated *ad nauseam*—so that musical appreciation has a U-shaped relationship with both familiarity and complexity. You might agree that whilst Karlheinz Stockhausen's quartet for string players and four helicopters is a trifle difficult to follow, and Beethoven's *Für Elise* is awfully hackneyed, Schubert's piano sonatas fall in that delightful middle zone.[46]

This Goldilocks zone is present from a young age. The developmental psychologist Celeste Kidd showed 7- to 8-month olds animations in which salient objects popped up from one of three distinctive gift boxes. The probability that the infants looked away (in presumed boredom) was a U-shaped function of the complexity, as measured by the negative log probability of the sequence. Similarly, adults will pay to find out the answers to trivia questions about which they have middling levels of confidence, but not those where they are totally clueless or sure of being correct. We also tend to direct our gaze to parts of a natural scene that are neither most predictable (a uniform expanse of sky) nor least predictable (the intricate textures formed by leaves on a tree), but that are somewhere in between (the prominent shape of a rock). Moving the eyes in this way can be shown to maximize a quantity called Bayesian

---

[46] See (Chmiel & Schubert 2017).

surprise (measured in units of 'wow'), a proxy for how much an observer can learn from making that eye movement.[47]

RL algorithms can also be primed to explore where learning is most beneficial. In tabular RL, a common approach is known as the upper confidence bound (or UCB) algorithm. The UCB adds a term to the action value which is inversely proportional to the number of times it has been sampled before, specified in such a way that exploration gradually gives way to exploitation.[48] Early in learning, this strongly encourages the agent to try out new actions. In domains where no two states are exactly alike, such as in Atari, proxies can be computed for how often an action has been tried in a specific situation. When exploration bonuses based on these pseudo-counts were built into DQN, it learnt a policy which was able to navigate through at least 15 rooms of Montezuma's Revenge, obtaining over 3000 points on average. However, this approach remains susceptible to the noisy TV problem—as it encourages the seeking of novelty for novelty's sake, rather than urging the agent to explore the Goldilocks zone. Thus, adopting a more sophisticated approach, the team from OpenAI used a fixed random neural network to pre-process each game frame, and trained a predictor network with supervision to mimic the output of this network. The states where the predictor fails are those where there is the most interesting information to learn in the environment, and so this loss is used as the exploration bonus. Equipped with this random network distillation (RND) bonus (and more than a few other tricks), their policy gradient agent was thus prone to exploring the most interesting parts of the world, which helped it achieve 8000 points and become the first AI system to play Montezuma's Revenge at superhuman levels.[49]

More generally, curiosity is a salient characteristic of many animals—and especially humans. It is the insatiable human drive for information that has urged us to dissect the microscopic wonders of biology, plumb the depths of the oceans, and scale the highest mountains, and even venture out into the cosmos. Currently, most RL systems are hampered by relatively primitive exploration policies that encourage randomness or endow agents with makeshift inquisitiveness. By contrast, humans have evolved sophisticated strategies for discovering the information needed to successfully implement a policy in advance of its execution. This allows them to engage in complex behaviours,

---

[47] Work by (Kidd et al. 2012). See here for work on trivia questions (Kang et al. 2009). For Bayesian surprise, see (Itti & Baldi 2009).
[48] In DQN, the value of epsilon was also gradually annealed towards zero over the first million steps.
[49] See (Burda et al. 2018).

including—among other things—the commission of devilishly sophisticated jewellery robberies.

6.5 Is reward enough?

You probably know the story of King Midas. Recounted by Ovid in his epic narrative poem *Metamorphoses*, it tells the tale of Midas of Phyrgia, who tends patiently to the hoary old Satyr Silenus after he passes out drunk in a rose garden. As a reward for his kindness, Silenus' foster father—the wine god Dionysius—grants Midas any wish of his own choosing. Foolishly, Midas asks that everything he touches turns to gold. Of course, Midas soon realizes his terrible mistake—but has turned his bed, his dinner, and his daughter to cold, hard metal before Dionysius consents to reverse the spell.

The Midas myth is a classic fable of reward function misspecification. Midas knew that gold was valuable, and thus he sought to obtain as much of it as possible. Unfortunately, however, relentlessly seeking to maximize a single, monolithic objective can have catastrophic side effects. In his book *Superintelligence*, Nick Bostrom imagines a powerful AI system that is given an innocuous-sounding objective—to make as many paperclips as possible. His worry is that a superintelligent AI given this simple objective will make paperclips at all cost—even if it involves diverting all the world's resources and eliminating all the world's population in the process.

Bostrom's thought experiment is commonly quoted to motivate research into AI safety. However, it also serves to highlight a serious translation gap for contemporary AI research. RL agents are mostly developed and road-tested in environments with universally agreed, clearly defined objectives: board games such as Go where the goal is to win, or video games such as Atari where the score provides a metric of success. However, in the messy reality of the real world, there are no points to be earned for a life well lived. What does a success at life look like? No doubt everyone from Donald Trump to the Dalai Lama has a different answer. In the natural world, nobody is keeping score (or counting paperclips).

The RL paradigm is premised on what is known as the reward hypothesis. One version of this hypothesis states that:[50]

---

[50] See (Silver et al. 2021). In an earlier blog post, Rich Sutton uses a slightly less ambitious formulation: 'that all of what we mean by goals and purposes can be well thought of as maximization of the expected value of the cumulative sum of a received scalar signal (reward)'.

the generic objective of maximising reward is enough to drive behaviour that exhibits most if not all abilities that are studied in natural and artificial intelligence.

The implication is that if AI researchers can manage to inject exactly the right constraints into the objective function, then hey presto—the resulting agent will acquire a full set of intelligent behaviours, because doing so is the optimal route to maximizing reward. The hope is that such an agent—endowed with general intelligence—will then consent to do our bidding flexibly, safely, and effectively, and in a way that is aligned with human values.[51]

The 14 quadrillion dollar question is how to specify such a reward function.[52] The Midas myth reminds us of the perils of the underspecified objective. Midas forgot to ask that his daughter and his lunch be exempted from the golden touch. But a perfect reward function for Midas would need to exhaustively list all the objects in the world, and whether (or how) they should be subject to his golden touch (cutlery—sure, why not. Toothbrush? Fine—but only the handle, not the bristles. Shirt—definitely not! But the buttons might be OK). The job of specifying such a reward function for an AGI, assuming this were even possible, would probably be even more daunting than designing the algorithm that attempts to satisfy it. In fact, the exhortation to build maximally general agents without researcher priors—expounded in the *bitter lesson*—often seems to surreptitiously offload the liberty to hand-engineer solutions into the reward function, substituting a handcrafted agent for a handcrafted objective. It is absolutely right that we cannot 'special case' our way towards intelligence by building agents with a unique capacity for every circumstance. But neither can we write down a reward function in sufficient detail that an agent behaves appropriately in every possible scenario it encounters in the natural world.

The alternative is to build agents that reward themselves. This is, of course, exactly what biological systems do. In life, there are no points gained for eating chocolate or reading a thrilling novel, nor are there leader boards for happiness or well-being. Instead, each organism is endowed with a function that maps observations onto internal (or *intrinsic*) rewards. We can thus replace the extrinsic reward function (which is specified in the world) with an intrinsic reward function (which is computed in the agent's brain). Unfortunately, the nature of this computation—the mapping from observations to intrinsic

---

[51] Whatever those might be. I am not doing justice to the complexity of the alignment problem, but fortunately two wonderful books give deep consideration to this issue (Christian 2020; Russell 2019a).

[52] That is Stuart Russell's back-of-the-envelope calculation of the value of AGI, as described in his 2021 BBC Reith Lectures.

rewards—remains an open problem in AI research. For biological intelligence, understanding the nature of the cost function for motivated behaviour is perhaps the greatest unsolved mystery of all. Knowing the true objective function for biological learning has the potential to unlock great secrets about how and why people behave the way they do.

Whilst the nature of the intrinsic reward function is unknown, there are at least three principles that might be helpful for cognitive scientists and computer scientists alike to consider.[53] Firstly, motivation can be *homeostatic* or *heterostatic*. Homeostasis is the computational principle by which a system attempts to keep some quantity in equilibrium. For example, a mechanic maintains the levels of oil, fuel, and water within a desired range in an engine, and a thermostat keeps your house at a comfortable temperature. In biology, motivation for basic needs is readily described by a homeostatic motivational system. When we are hungry, we eat until sated, and when we are thirsty, we drink until hydrated. Thus, a homeostatic intrinsic reward function will return negative values when various environmental states (e.g. our levels of food or liquid) fall below certain levels, encouraging the agent to take action to meet the relevant need. The idea that biological behaviour obeys *drives* that satisfy *needs* dates back to the theories of the psychologist Clark Hull in the 1940s.

By contrast, the extrinsic rewards provided in conventional RL studies are heterostatic. A heterostatic reward function is one in which the organism is encouraged to self-perturbate out of its equilibrium, for example by reaping extreme quantities of a given asset. In Atari, this works just fine, because attaining a superlative score is precisely the goal. But in the natural world, heterostatic reward functions invite pathological behaviours. A third, fourth, or tenth slice of chocolate cake is not going to increase your health or happiness. If Bostrom's superintelligence had been asked to make exactly as many paperclips as people need and no more, then perhaps it would have spared humanity when meeting its objective. Economists, of course, are in favour of heterostatic objectives, because their theories assume that utility is a monotonic function of monetary wealth. However, blind maximization of material assets by avaricious individuals is undoubtedly the root cause of many pathologies that afflict our society today.[54]

Secondly, an intrinsic reward function might be *fixed* or *adaptable*. We can think of a fixed reward function as one that is hardcoded into the brain,

[53] I am indebted to the thinking of Pierre-Yves Oudeyer for this summary. Oudeyer proposes the first two distinctions that I reference here in his 2009 paper (Oudeyer & Kaplan 2007).

[54] There is so much to say here. Where to start? Perhaps (Piketty & Goldhammer 2014) and (Saez & Zucman 2019).

specified either by our genes or by the hard constraints of the network architecture, whereas an adaptable intrinsic reward function can be learnt from experience. An fully adaptable intrinsic reward function is a dangerous thing. An agent with dominion over its own reward function can simply decide to reward itself *ad libitum*, a shortcut sometimes known as *wireheading* in the AI community.[55] When animals are given the opportunity to wirehead, they tend to lose all interest in everything else. This was the case for the rats in Olds and Milner's experiments, which ignored offers of chow and water and spent all day tirelessly pressing the pleasure button. Humans have invented ways of wireheading too, using drugs of abuse to directly stimulate the brain's transmitter systems. As everyone who has seen the film *Trainspotting* knows, this rarely ends well. On the other hand, a completely fixed intrinsic reward function risks being overly restrictive, unless it happens to be perfectly tailored to demands of the environment. In the natural world, it seems probable that intrinsic reward functions are prespecified, but partly malleable—leaving room for us to learn what we like. Presumably, this is why tastes, temperaments, drives, proclivities, and preferences are, at least partly, shared within socially defined groups, and why we can acquire new tastes across the lifespan, like learning in adulthood to enjoy dissonant atonal music or the bitter taste of marmalade.

Finally, intrinsic rewards might be *specific* or *generic*. For example, humans have evolved some biases towards specific intrinsic rewards that are tailored to the requirements of our evolutionary history as foraging primates: children, for example, have a strong tendency to accept sweet-tasting foods and reject bitter ones, and we tend to find hairy spiders scary and koala bears cute. Monkeys who have never seen a snake before are nevertheless terrified of wriggly animals with swarthy skin, and cats leap in terror on sudden glimpse of a roughly snake-shaped object such as a cucumber, to the amusement of millions of YouTube viewers. But the most generally useful intrinsic reward functions are those—like a thirst for knowledge, an imperative for control, or a drive to explore—which are not tied to specific sensory states.

As humans, many facets of our behaviour betray the ways in which intrinsic rewards are computed. For example, we engage enthusiastically in activities that can be tiring, taxing, or gruelling for no apparent hedonic gain. You might tussle with a cryptic crossword in the morning paper, play an explosive game of badminton with your boss, or go shopping for an elderly neighbour with no expectation that the favour will ever be returned. Some people

---

[55] See (Russell 2019b).

strive for positions of power influence or dream of being world champion, whereas others crave intimate knowledge of the personal lives of others, delight in poetic uses of language, or yearn for the vast emptiness of desolate places. Some people—the most fearless and inured to hardship—might take it upon themselves to climb a mountain in the Andes, risking life and limb just to be the first to ascend via a face that has not yet been conquered. Where do all these human desires come from?

In the previous section, we discussed one class of intrinsic reward—the satisfaction of curiosity, which may serve as an auxiliary objective for RL, for example by promoting exploration and thus reward harvesting. However, another more radical conception is that we should do away with the concept of reward altogether.[56] In many ways, this is the polar opposite to the reward hypothesis: it claims that rewards are just a convenient label for states that emerge as a by-product of *belief formation*. The claim comes in various forms, but the shared theme is that organisms are guided by a cost function that is minimized when the world is predictable, controllable, or orderly. In one version of this theory, known as *active inference*, actions are selected to make the world as predictable as possible. In another, known as *empowerment*, the consequence of maximizing this intrinsic reward is that it furnishes maximal preparedness, by maximizing the future degrees of freedom available for an agent to act in the world.

Unsurprisingly, these ideas have been controversial. However, the idea that people strive for orderliness in perception and cognition falls within a long psychological tradition dating back to Festinger's *Theory of Cognitive Dissonance* in the 1950s. Festinger argued that we always seek to minimize inconsistency in our beliefs and values. His work was partly based on interviews with people holding strange prophetic or apocalyptic beliefs, such as a Chicago-based group who believed they would be rescued from Earth by UFOs on Christmas Eve in 1954. Festinger studied the mental stresses that the group experienced and the coping mechanisms they adopted, when reality did not line up with their predictions. He concluded that people are motivated to seek psychological consistency between their expectations and their observations of the world—to minimize cognitive dissonance.

One contemporary instantiation of this idea is a framework known as the free energy principle (FEP). The FEP has attracted criticism for the grandiosity of its claims and the impenetrability of its mathematical foundations. However, broadly, it claims that in order to resist a tendency to disorder,

---

[56] See (Friston et al. 2012).

biological systems seek to control their observations to minimize *surprise* (or its proxies).[57] Surprise is a measure of how much a model of the world needs to be updated in order to account for new observations. The FEP proposes that agents use a principle of active inference to choose actions that will render sensory signals as predictable as possible. An implementational scheme based on predictive coding has been proposed, and the FEP claims to explain canonical morphological and physiological features of the primate brain, such as neural responses to prediction errors, recurrent connectivity, and gain control.[58]

Is it really plausible that our ultimate goal in life is for sensation to be as predictable as possible? Philosophers and cognitive scientists disagree sharply on this point.[59] One common critique of the FEP is that it seems to imply that people will strive to be left in peace—in a 'dark room' with minimal sensory stimulation. This seems out of kilter with our irrepressible love of rock music, carnivals, and rollercoasters. More conceptually, the FEP collapses desires (I want an apple) entirely into beliefs (I want to satisfy the prediction that I will eat an apple when hungry, and so I do), which, for all its theoretical elegance, seems rather inconsistent with the quotidian experience of munching on a piece of fruit.

For AI research, the proof of any theory of intrinsic motivation is in the empirical pudding. Is it possible to train an agent to display intelligent behaviours without extrinsic reward, and with the goal of attempting to minimize its own surprise alone? Recently, a group led by the computer scientist Sergey Levine have begun to put this question to the test, using a paradigm called self-supervised RL—where the agent is trained with intrinsic rewards alone.[60] They find that an agent that models a partially observable environment with a VAE and is optimized to minimize the belief updates on each state will not, in fact, learn to hide in a dark room, but will instead gravitate towards a 'busy' room where it can tag moving items to bring them to a halt. The same agent is successful at a 3D video game that involves rotating to shoot encroaching monsters. However, there is clearly a long way to go to demonstrate that surprise-minimizing agents can display intelligent behaviours in naturalistic environments.

A closely related idea is that an intrinsic reward function should drive agents to exert influence over their environment. In the 1950s, Harlow studied

---

[57] Formally, the quantity minimized is free energy, which is a bound on surprise, and can be computed from sensory signals and brain states, rather than requiring a perfect model of the world.

[58] See (Friston 2009) and (Gershman 2019).

[59] See (Sun & Firestone 2020).

[60] See (Rhinehart et al. 2021).

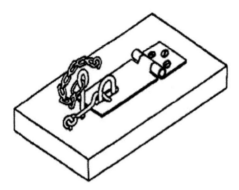

Fig. 6.6 The mechanical puzzle apparatus explored by macaque monkeys in the Harlow study (1950). It involves a hasp restrained by a hook restrained by a pin. Monkeys solved the problem more readily in the absence of an extrinsic reward.

how monkeys behaved when a puzzle apparatus (Figure 6.6) was placed in their enclosure. Like a commuter doing battle with their morning Sudoku, the monkeys enthusiastically set to work and learnt to efficiently solve the puzzle apparently just for the fun of doing so. Remarkably, Harlow reports that when the monkeys were reinforced for solving the problem (with juicy raisins), this actually hurt, rather than helped, performance.[61] Harlow's monkeys were doing something familiar to every parent: they were playing. Play serves many potential roles, but one is learning how actions influence the world. For example, Piaget famously described how his son Laurent learnt that he could provoke an interesting sound by touching a rattle and, delighted with this new knowledge, chose to do so over and over again.

This idea of environmental control as intrinsic reward comes in many guises, but the most influential modern version is probably the concept of *empowerment*, commonly associated with the computer scientist Daniel Polani. Here is his definition of empowerment:[62]

Empowerment aims to reformulate the options or degrees of freedom that an agent has as the agent's control over its environment; and not only of its control — to be reproducible, the agent needs to be aware of its control influence and sense it. Thus, empowerment is a measure of both the control an agent has over its environment, as well as its ability to sense this control.

---

[61] See (Harlow et al. 1950). We have already encountered Harlow in the context of learning to learn (see Chapter 4).
[62] From the simple primer here (Salge et al. 2013).

Cast in the language of information theory, the concept of empowerment formalizes the degree of influence that an agent has over its future environment. Those actions with the highest empowerment are those that allow the greatest variety of subsequent observations to be experienced.[63] If I am a cat locked in a cage, I will be determined to escape, to see the world beyond its bars. If I lack a corkscrew, I will search for one, so I can sample the fine wine my friend just gave me. If I am in a lowly professional role, I will seek promotion, so that I can have greater influence over the actions of my colleagues and the policies of my organization.

In AI research, empowerment can be estimated using an approach known as variational inference, and has proved to be a useful concept for skill learning in unsupervised RL. For example, empowerment has been used to discover *options* under the framework known as hierarchical RL, where the agent learns multi-step macro-actions, the completion of which is (pseudo-) rewarded, leading to improved performance in studies requiring agents to navigate environments with bottleneck states (i.e. doors) or to push blocks around to reach a goal, or to learn complex motor skills in the MuJoCo physics simulation environment.[64]

In sum, thus, biological systems are powerfully motivated to act in their own interests. If we could understand the principles that animate natural behaviour and recreate them in AI systems, then this would be an important brick in the road towards intelligence. Of course, in the natural world, organisms ultimately evolved to maximize reproductive fitness. But given the difficulty of working out which actions will increase or decrease their fitness, animals have evolved proxies—internal and external variables that they seek to maximize or minimize instead. Hedonic reward—the pleasurable sensations that are evoked by consummatory behaviours—is one such variable. The demand to explore the world, finding out what is around the next corner, over the next hill, or written on the next page, is another major impetus. The desire for order and control—to exert influence over others, to solve a puzzle, to live in a tidy house and an orderly society, and to control our sensations, health, and mood—is another. It seems likely that finding the right mix of extrinsic and intrinsic variables for RL in AI research is among the most significant outstanding challenges today.

---

[63] Formally, empowerment is the channel capacity (maximum of mutual information) computed from the *interventional* conditional probability of action on observation (e.g. using the do-operator or related causal approaches).

[64] See https://mujoco.org/. The two results cited are (Gregor et al. 2016) and (Sharma et al. 2020).

7

The control of memory

7.1 The eligibility of experience

At the denouement of Orson Welles' 1941 masterpiece, the movie *Citizen Kane*, the tycoon Charles Kane has reached the end of the road. His second marriage is over, his political career is in tatters, and his friends have been scattered to the winds by betrayal. In the last moments before death, he turns his violent temper on his ill-gotten material gains and begins ransacking his palatial mansion *Xanadu*. But when his glance falls on a snow globe that he used to own as a boy, he suddenly recollects the innocence of youth. He remembers playing in the snow with his beloved sledge *Rosebud*, before his descent into the corrupt world of money and politics. For a moment, he is mentally transported back across the decades, and his whole world turns on its axis. This recollection allows him to finally die in peace, with the word *Rosebud* on his lips.

Time moves ever forward. In the natural world, its passage is marked by the ticking of the clock and the slow rotation of the seasons. For an RL agent in a dynamic environment, time moves forward too—tirelessly meted out by the cycle of observation, action, and reward.[1] As time advances, the past recedes behind us. But evolution has endowed biological agents with a means to travel back through time and visit the past—like Citizen Kane on his deathbed, who is transported back to his youthful self frolicking in the snow. For intelligent agents, remembering what occurred in the past can be useful. The world is structured in time, so what the past reveals is often relevant to the future and can be leveraged to make better decisions.

In Chapter 6, we saw how agents learn by reinforcement. By learning the value of states and actions, agents can follow policies that maximize reward. The most primitive of these mechanisms, the *atoms of memory*, are those that psychologists call classical and instrumental conditioning. Advances in RL theory have discovered algorithms—such as TD learning—that allow an agent to learn optimal behaviours by incrementally updating the value function from moment to moment. For example, in each cycle of TD learning, value

---

[1] Albeit often on multiple threads of the CPU.

Natural General Intelligence. Christopher Summerfield, Oxford University Press. © Oxford University Press 2023.
DOI: 10.1093/oso/9780192843883.003.0007

is shared between two adjacent time points: the current and immediately preceding steps. Memory systems, however, allow agents to share information
across broader expanses of time. This is particularly helpful in naturalistic environments, where events depend on variables which were signalled in the
past but are latent and unobservable in the present. For example, on the first
level of Montezuma's Revenge, to know that you can open the door, you need
to remember that you previously retrieved the key.

A simple form of memory in the RL methods toolkit is called an eligibility
trace. In tabular RL, an eligibility trace is a scalar memory for state visitation
recency. If we return for a moment to the example of navigating Hampton
Court maze, you might recall that TD learning allows an agent to back up the
value of the exit state (+100) to the next-to-exit state. But why not back up
further? An eligibility trace tags each state as fully 'eligible' when visited and
decays the eligibility of all other states incrementally down towards zero on
every step. Thus, when stumbling across the goal for the first time, those states
that have been recently visited—in the run-up to the exit—will carry eligibility that is roughly proportional to their recency. In a class of method known
as TD(λ), an eligibility trace is used to share the backed-up value simultaneously with all eligible states, which greatly accelerates learning.[2]

In biological brains, memories are formed through the adjustment of synaptic connections. When one neuron stimulates another, their shared synapse
is strengthened in a process known as long-term potentiation (LTP). When
LTP is produced in the lab, for example through artificial tetanic stimulation
in slices of tissue, it occurs in two stages: a short-duration phase in which the
cell is tagged as having been recently active, and a sustained phase in which
new proteins are synthesized to produce lasting change. These latter plastic
changes only occur in the presence of the tag, thereby creating a mechanism
by which credit can be assigned on the basis of eligibility. In the context of
RL, this mechanism could allow dopamine to selectively strengthen tagged
synapses for the learning of associations between stimuli and actions or outcomes, allowing for neural implementation of an eligibility trace. Indeed,
humans seem to be able to back up a reward incurred by completion of a sequence of actions in a single shot, and reward prediction errors measured in
pupil dilation signals obey the predictions of a TD-learning model equipped
with eligibility traces.[3]

---

[2] The parameter λ dictates the decay rate for state eligibility.
[3] For synaptic tagging (in the hippocampus), see (Frey & Morris 1997). For a review on eligibility traces in
biology and human experiment with eligibility traces, see (Gerstner et al. 2018) and (Lehmann et al. 2019).

In this chapter, we will consider how memory systems contribute to intelligence. In biological agents, and especially in humans, memory has a complex, modular structure. As we shall see, different memory processes have evolved to solve specific computational problems that are posed by natural environments. Building on the RL paradigm, we will show how the elaboration of memory systems in deep RL agents can potentially allow them to solve the same problems. We focus on three well-known computational challenges.

The first is the problem of data efficiency. Deep RL agents are very inefficient. For example, DQN was trained with 50 million frames of each game, equivalent to 38 days of continuous play in the real world. The authors of a landmark paper discussing DQN's significance for biology point out that it is possible for a human to approximate the level achieved by the expert baseline with as little as 5- to 10-minute practice, highlighting the remarkable disparity in *sample efficiency* between humans and deep learning agents.[4] Understanding how to build agents that learn efficiently—including those that learn effectively from single experiences (one-shot learning)—remains a key outstanding problem for the field.

The second is the problem of lifelong learning. In 2015, news outlets around the world reported that a female pupil by the name of Priscilla Sitienei was attending the local school in her village in the Rift Valley, Kenya, hoping to learn to read and write. Nothing unusual about that—except that this remarkable student was 90 years of age, and six of her classmates were her great-great-grandchildren. The case of Ms Sitienei reminds us that humans are able to learn continually over the lifespan, from our earliest months right through to a venerable old age. Unfortunately, the same is not immediately true of deep neural networks. When coming across a novel task or context, deep networks learn in ways that catastrophically overwrite the knowledge they have learnt previously. It is as if when you learn to cook lasagne, you suddenly forget how to speak French, or when learning to play tennis, you forget how to dance the tango.

For this reason, although in the original paper, there was one DQN *architecture*, there was a different DQN *model* for each game.[5] The model trained on Pong was unable to play Breakout—the authors were obliged to reinitialize DQN's weights for each new game. Effectvely, thus, the agent had the luxury

---

[4] See (Lake et al. 2017) and (Tsividis et al. 2017). Of course, this comparison is not entirely fair, because humans have a lifetime of experience to bring to bear on the problem, including possibly of some other video games made by humans. The authors also admitted to preparing by watching videos of people playing on YouTube. There have been more recent attempts to compare humans and agents learning video games with appropriate priors (Tsividis et al. 2021).

[5] Where a model is an instance of the architecture trained from scratch with a unique weight initialization.

of an entirely new brain for every task it encountered. Learning a single model that can play multiple games—or, more generally, that can learn many tasks in series—is called the problem of continual learning.[6] Despite recent progress, continual learning remains an outstanding challenge for the field.

The third is the problem of task generalization. Previously, we discussed how brains and neural networks might form *abstractions*, which are complex invariances over sensory inputs (images and words) that allow us to understand the meaning of *cat, inside, politics, Asia,* and *Easter.* But humans can also abstract over tasks. After having learnt to ride a bicycle, you know some bike-specific information about handlebars and pedals. But you also acquire more general motor skills, such as how to shift your body to remain upright on two wheels, the concept of how gears control propulsion, and the rules of the road—all of which would be useful for learning to ride a scooter. Similarly, when you switch operating system from Mac to Linux, the interface is different, but concepts like *drop-down menu, window,* and *terminal* can be transferred from one domain to the other. When you visit a new city, the language and currency may be alien, but you can generalize your understanding of *greeting* and *taxi* to help negotiate it with minimal mishap.

Understanding how to build AI systems that generalize effectively to novel tasks remains a frontier topic in AI research. For example, Breakout and Pong both involve the use of a *paddle*, a tool that can be moved horizontally or vertically to prevent a ball from hitting the ground, and thus incurring a negative outcome. However, despite the near-identical game logic implied by the use of a paddle in both games, DQN had to learn a unique policy in each game. As we shall see, thinking about task abstraction revives the theme we encountered with Harlow's monkeys, which are able to transfer information about one bandit problem to another. A major area of research called meta-RL provides a suite of computational solutions that allow agents to learn how to learn, so that they can potentially solve wholly new tasks on the first encounter.

These three problems—one-shot learning, continual learning, and meta-learning—are core themes in AI research today. In this chapter, we will discuss how these challenges may be met in the human brain, and highlight machine learning research that has drawn inspiration from neurobiology to build agents that can exhibit complex behaviours in naturalistic environments.

---

[6] This term and *lifelong learning* are often used interchangeably.

7.2 The butcher on the bus

Édouard Claparède was a Swiss neurologist with a mischievous streak. In 1907, he published a report of a patient suffering from anterograde amnesia brought on by Korsakoff's syndrome. Anterograde amnesia spares most past learning but precludes the formation of new memories for facts or experiences, usually without incurring a more generalized loss of cognitive function.[7]. His patient retained learning that had occurred before the illness onset, and, for example, was able to recite the capitals of European countries and perform accurate mental arithmetic. She was also able to learn some new skills, such as finding her way to the bathroom in the hospital where she was interned. However, her amnesia left her unable to recognize the faces of medical staff that she had seen every day for five years—including Claparède, whom she met for regular appointments. Famously, on one visit, he secreted a sharp pin in his hand, which pricked her painfully when they greeted. On the next visit, the patient once again failed to recognize Claparède, but she refused to shake hands—without being able to explain why.

This turn-of-the-century report anticipates the seminal study of Henry Molaison (patient H.M.) by Brenda Milner in the 1950s, on which modern understanding of the human memory system is founded.[8] Like Claparède's unnamed patient, H.M. was able to slowly acquire new motor skills, such as drawing in a mirror, and became gradually familiar with his environment through laborious interaction. However, new facts and events systematically failed to lodge in his mind. The site of the damage to the brain of Claparède's patient is unknown, but H.M.'s lesion, which has been mapped in detail with structural MRI, encompasses the hippocampus and adjoining structures in the MTL.[9]

The study of H.M. offered an early inkling of how the brain divides labour between the neocortex and the hippocampus. Hippocampal patients are unable to encode specific instances into memory but remain familiar with previously learnt facts and events. This dissociation implies the need for a

---

[7] This is often called declarative memory (and is distinct from *procedural* memory, which are for skills like riding a bicycle). The original text is translated with commentary here (Nicolas 1996).

[8] The late Sue Corkin at MIT also made very significant contributions to the study of H.M, as described in her book *Permanent Present Tense* (Corkin 2014). Brenda Milner was born in Manchester, England but went to Canada to study for her PhD under the supervision of Donald Hebb. She was married to Peter Milner, whose work on rodent self-stimulation is discussed above. At the time of writing, she is 103, and probably the living person whose work has had the greatest impact on the field.

[9] In fact, a recent reanalysis suggests some hippocampal sparing. The implications of this finding for studies involving H.M. remain unclear.

dual-process model of memory. Accordingly, in the 1970s, the idea took root that there are two sorts of long-term store: one where memories are approximate, gist-based, generalizable, and gradually formed; and another where memories are vivid and specific and can be learnt in a single shot. The former store is said to support *familiarity*, and it depends on the neocortex. The latter is called *recollection* and it relies on the hippocampus.[10]

This distinction between recollection and familiarity is perhaps one to which you can relate. Many people report an experience known as the *butcher on the bus* phenomenon, whereby a familiar person encountered out of context cannot be placed. We owe this term to the psychologist George Mandler, who gave this example in a classic paper:[11]

> Consider seeing a man on a bus whom you are sure that you have seen before; you 'know' him in that sense. Such a recognition is usually followed by a search process asking, in effect, Where could I know him from? Who is he? The search process generates likely contexts (Do I know him from work; is he a movie star, a TV commentator, the milkman?). Eventually the search may end with the insight, That's the butcher from the supermarket!

Thus, in the healthy mind, familiarity precedes recollection—but the source of a memory ('oh! it's the butcher') can usually be identified. However, in patients with damage to the MTL, familiarity exists in a vacuum. Here is an anecdote from Claparède about the same patient.

> One day we read a story to the patient about a 64-year-old woman who took her cattle to graze and was bitten by a snake. The next day, we asked her to relate the story we had told her. She could not do so and could not even recall having seen us the day before. We urged her to answer, saying that it was about a woman and asking her how old the woman was. She then asked us: 'Wasn't the woman 64 years old?' and then she quickly added that it was merely an idea that 'crossed her mind' and that she could have just as easily said something else.

In the lab, recollection and familiarity are studied using more prosaic methods. Participants are given lists of words or pictures to learn, and then asked to judge each item as old or new, and to report whether they 'remember'

---

[10] A common framing of this distinction employs the terms 'episodic' and 'semantic' memory. I avoid these terms here because I find them misleading. The episodic vs semantic distinction mixes up the content of the memory (personal episodes vs impersonal semantic knowledge) with the nature of the retrieval (specific vs general).

[11] See (Mandler 1980).

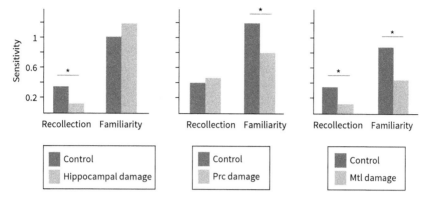

Fig. 7.1 Performance on measures of recollection and familiarity after damage to the hippocampus (left), perirhinal cortex (PRC; centre), and whole medial temporal lobe (MTL; right), relative to controls. Hippocampal damage impairs recollection; PRC damage impairs familiarity, and MTL damage impairs both. Stars show significant differences between patients and controls.

Data from Yonelinas et al. (1998) and Aggleton et al. (2005).

or 'know' that it had been presented.[12] In combination with a statistical model known as signal detection theory, this approach allows sensitivity scores for both recollection and familiarity to be computed from the same retrieval data. The plot in Figure 7.1, which is assembled from three comparable studies, illustrates how damage to the hippocampus selectively impairs recollection, whereas damage to the adjacent neocortex seems to impact familiarity. Consistent with these findings, patients with damage to both regions have a generalized impairment that encompasses both retrieval processes. Data from neuroimaging experiments support the same dissociation between a neural system for recollection in the hippocampus and a familiarity-based system in the adjacent neocortex.[13]

We can thus think of familiarity and recollection as the fruits of retrieval from neocortical and hippocampal memory stores, respectively. These two repositories retain memories in different, but complementary, ways. The neocortical familiarity system is parametric: it encodes structured patterns, summaries, or averages from big sensory data.[14] This allows it to privilege

[12] This technique requires that you explain this distinction to participants, and the simpler terminology and 'remember' and 'know' seem to make it more intuitive.

[13] The lesion data are described in this review paper (Yonelinas et al. 2010). See this earlier review, with a very authoritative historical overview (Yonelinas 2002). The imaging data are from (Wais et al. 2008). Data in the figure are from (Aggleton et al. 2005) and (Yonelinas et al. 1998).

[14] It is perhaps worth clarifying that in both epsiodes with Claparède's patient, familiarity is established in a single shot—even without recollection. However, in the more typical case, familiarity builds up gradually.

generalities over specifics, yielding an overall sense of gist ('I know that face') that is dissociated from unique instances of experience ('I saw him behind the meat counter at the supermarket'). By contrast, the hippocampus allows new memory traces to be laid down in a single shot. When the hippocampus is damaged or removed, major impairments occur. For example, removal of the entire hippocampus drastically impairs the ability of a rat to swim directly to a hidden platform in a circular pool, even after having reached it by random waterborne exploration on the immediately preceding trials.[15] Similarly, hippocampal patients cannot lay down new memory traces without pro-longed experience. H.M. was unable to recognize new acquaintances, navigate unfamiliar neighbourhoods, or recall world events that post-dated his 1953 surgery. The hippocampus and neocortex thus act together to allow agents to learn about both the many-off (averages) and the one-off (instances).[16]

As we have seen, deep networks give us a plausible computational theory for the neocortical system. Neural representations in the ventral stream, that visual highway linking V1 to the temporal lobes, closely resemble those in deep convolutional networks trained to label natural images. Indeed, connectionist models share both the strengths and shortcomings of the neocortical familiarity system. On the one hand, they learn slowly, with parameters incrementally tuned by exposure to large, diverse, well-mixed data sets. On the other hand, they encode input structure, allowing pattern recognition in held-out data. In fact, much-vaunted failures of robustness in deep networks have been ascribed to an overreliance on a general sense of familiarity. Just as you might strain to place the butcher on the bus, deep networks struggle to recognize objects in rare contexts. For example, they tend to misclassify cows on a beach but have no problem detecting them in a lush alpine pasture (Figure 7.2).[17]

One-shot learning is especially useful in the natural world because the statistics of experience can sometimes be hard to model and predict. Earlier we noted that the world is *clumpy*, that is, most stimuli belong to categories in which intrinsic variation is lower than extrinsic variation. For example, birds

---

For example, when H.M. moved house after his lesion, he gradually learnt the organization of rooms in his new residence.

[15] This environment is known as the Morris Water Maze. Here is the classic reference (Morris et al. 1982).

[16] It is worth pointing out that the status of the PRC, which is a neocortical region lying between the ventral visual stream and the hippocampus proper, has been controversial. It seems to play a role that lies midway between perception and memory—it supports perception of complex visual information and memory for simpler stimuli. In fact, CNNs trained on a range of visual discrimination tasks behave a lot like patients with PRC damage (Bonnen et al. 2021).

[17] See (Beery et al. 2018).

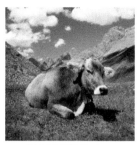 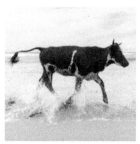 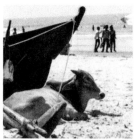

(A) **Cow: 0.99**, Pasture: 0.99, Grass: 0.99, No person: 0.98, Mammal: 0.98

(B) No Person: 0.99, Water: 0.98, Beach: 0.97, Outdoors: 0.97, Seashore: 0.97

(C) No Person: 0.97, **Mammal: 0.96**, Water: 0.94, Beach: 0.94, Two: 0.94

Fig. 7.2 Three images of cows with labels produced by a deep network. The network has no problem recognizing the cow in the Alpine pasture but does not propose 'cow' as a label for either image of the cow on a beach.
Images reprinted with permission from Beery (2018).

are warm-blooded animals with wings that can fly; toasters are not. Neural networks can learn categories by encoding their shared structure, for example inferring that sparrows, eagles, and parrots are all birds. However, our clumps of knowledge are studded with exceptions. A bat, for example, is a warm-blooded animal with wings that can fly, but it is not a bird; and penguins cannot fly, and yet they are birds. In English syntax, most regular plurals are created by adding 's', but not the nouns *sheep* or *fish*. Most calendar dates crop up annually, but 29 February only occurs in a leap year. Most heavenly bodies in the night sky are stars, but Mars and Venus are planets. We might say that the world is clumpy, but with exceptions. A system that learns summaries of the clumps alone will be prone to misassign the exceptions—for example, assuming that bats are birds—a phenomenon known as overgeneralization.

In the context of reinforced behaviour, learning from one-off, unique events helps agents assign credit for reward and punishment. For example, in the Atari game Seaquest, a submarine must be dextrously manoeuvred through a thicket of hungry sharks to rescue human divers whilst monitoring a rapidly depleting air supply. Although there are small-beer points available for shooting enemies, a major bonus occurs if you surface to collect oxygen, having picked up exactly six divers. An agent that can learn from the rare large rewards associated with that behaviour—and thus repeat it in future trajectories—will be quick to master the game. In the real world, one-shot learning can be critical to survival. Nobody would want to learn by dint of repetition that week-old shellfish are toxic or that black widow spiders pack a poisonous bite.

Exactly how the hippocampus might facilitate one-shot learning remains unknown. However, the functional neuroanatomy of the MTL gives us some powerful clues. Sensory inputs flow into the hippocampus from the ERC, from where they project via a trisynaptic pathway to the DG, CA3, and finally CA1 regions of the hippocampus.[18] One critical computational step occurs in the DG where memories are *sparsified*, being mapped from a code that is distributed across a whole neuronal population onto a representation that relies on just a handful of cells. This sparsification minimizes overlap among memories, pushing the hippocampal memory module closer to being a *non-parametric* system, where information is stored in a list or buffer, with each instance in a unique slot.[19] These sparse memories are then throughput to neurons in the CA3 region of the hippocampus, onto which they connect with unique *detonator synapses*, which can activate the post-synaptic neuron with even a single spike. Mice bred to lack a specific N-methyl-D aspartate (NMDA) receptor subunit on these cells fail on tests of one-shot learning, such as a match-to-place water maze task.[20] Eventually, memories are encoded in the CA1 region as highly individuated, *pattern-separated* units of experience, each one distinctive from the others.

AI researchers have leveraged this dual-process model as a blueprint for neural networks that can learn rapidly from limited experience. For example, *memory neural networks*[21] maintain a slot-based memory, into which snapshots of experience (such as sentences or images) are systematically written. Given any new query, the network can perform retrieval using two modules: one that produces output features by matching current inputs to one or more past outputs; and another that processes retrieved features (potentially over timesteps) to produce a response. The architecture allows similar experiences to be grouped and slotted into a long-term store, and was able to handle a range of Question Answering (QA) tasks when trained with supervision. Another architecture called the *differential neural computer* employs a recurrent neural network (RNN) to learn to both write to, and read from, a slot-based memory, which allowed it to solve complex planning problems, such

---

[18] CA stands for *Cornu Ammonis*, apparently because this region resembles the horns of a ram in Egyptian mythology. An important theory proposes that the trisynaptic pathway is accompanied by a monosynaptic pathway that projects directly from the ERC to CA1, which may explain the otherwise paradoxical involvement of the hippocampus in slow associative structure learning discussed in Chapter 5. We owe this theory to Anna Schapiro (Schapiro et al. 2017).

[19] Recalling the memory system of *Funes el Memorioso* in Chapter 4.

[20] That is, a task in which the same invisible platform must be found twice in a row (Nakazawa et al. 2003).

[21] See (Weston et al. 2015).

as charting a journey through the London Tube system after being given a start and a goal station. In fact, the network was trained end-to-end to solve variants of the classic AI puzzle game SHUDLU, responding to queries and instructions made in a symbolic language.[22]

Neural networks with external memory may be particularly useful in the RL setting. In a classic theory paper from 2007, Peter Dayan and Máté Lengyel proposed a mechanism called *episodic control*, in which samples from an instance-based memory system were used to learn a control policy. They argued that it provided a 'third way' for RL that combined the efficiency of model-free methods with the versatility of a fully planned (model-based) solution. More recently, AI researchers have road-tested this idea at scale in a deep network architecture called *neural episodic control*.[23] It uses a neurally inspired dual-process architecture, comprising complementary systems for neocortical learning and an episodic memory store which the authors call the differentiable neural dictionary (DND). Each state s (e.g. a video frame from an Atari game) is first processed by a deep CNN, mapping it onto a key h, which is used to look up the Q-values in the DND, which is an instance-based memory architecture that resembles the hippocampus (or the orbitofrontal cortex).[24] This lookup generates a linear weighting of Q-values based on similarity in the embedding of h, so that each key elicits an average of past experiences, allowing for generalization to new settings. The addition of neural episodic control allows the network to learn rapidly in more strategic games with intermittent rewards, such as Frostbite, in which players jump among ice floes in order to build in igloo, whilst avoiding a polar bear prowling on the shore.

In cognitive psychology, several theories of memory and control are based on the comparison between a current stimulus and recalled examples of experience. These are usually called *exemplar-based* models, and were originally developed to account for the effect of exceptional or outlying information on category judgements. In fact, there is evidence from experimental neuroscience that humans use episodic memory to encode state–action values, in addition to the averages of experience predicted by TD learning. In one study, participants tracked the latent value of two bandits that were intermittently paired with random, but salient, images. Presenting the images as reminders on a subsequent trial biased responses towards those choices made when they

---

[22] See (Graves et al. 2016).

[23] The third way paper is (Lengyel & Dayan 2007).

[24] The system encodes the observed return that is directly encoded after having taken several steps, so that the stored values can be reliable.

were initially viewed, suggesting that the participants had attached value to the instance-based memory and were learning via the 'third way'.[25]

7.3 The problem of a changing world

When a motion picture is being produced, individual *shots* are edited into *scenes*. Each scene is a segment of the film that takes place in continuous time in roughly the same location. In the natural world, ongoing experience is structured in a similar way. We experience life as a series of scenes (or *contexts*) which are defined by consistent sensory signals and common objectives to fulfil.[26] Imagine you are leaving the office after a long day at work. As you grab your coat and head for the door, you might leave behind the desks and computers, strip lighting, hushed tones, and the buttoned-down attire of your colleagues. If you are heading to a bar or a restaurant, the context will probably be entirely different: noisy, colourful, and crowded, full of unfamiliar people who may be eating, drinking, or dancing.[27] The way you are expected to comport yourself in these settings is quite different. If you push back your chair and crack open a beer whilst chairing a work meeting, your colleagues might look aghast. But your friends may be just as outraged if you fire up your laptop and start reply to e-mails whilst propping up the bar. We might say that the optimal policy thus varies from context to context, along with the sensory signals.

In AI research, an environment with slowly changing signals and objectives is referred to as *non-stationary*. Taken as a whole, the ALE is non-stationary, because every game is different. Some games oblige you to drive a submarine, and others to accurately roll a bowling ball to knock down ninepins. In fact, the Atari environment tends to be non-stationary even within each individual game, because developers have engineered the games so that different policies are needed for each stage or level. This is one of the key reasons why using deep learning for RL remains a significant challenge.

Take the popular game Ms. Pac-Man. For most of the time, players are tenaciously chased down by scary ghosts with whom collision costs a life. However, after munching on the power pellet, the ghosts suddenly morph from predators into prey. The optimal policy thus reverses from one moment to the next: whereas before, the ghosts were best avoided, now they should be

---

[25] The empirical study is by (Bornstein et al. 2017). For a comprehensive review, see (Gershman & Daw 2017).

[26] In fact, even if life does not have this structure objectively, we mentally experienced it as a sequence of distinct, meaningful events with discernible boundaries, akin to the scenes in a film (Kurby & Zacks 2008).

[27] This is assuming the reader has a more vibrant social life than the author.

chased to gain points. To make things even more complicated, both the visual appearance and the functionality of the game objects change systematically over time. The Ms. Pac-Man maze is pink in levels 1 and 2, but cycles through blue and brown on subsequent levels, continuing to vary deep into the game. The power pellet gradually works for shorter and shorter periods and eventually becomes wholly ineffectual. Thus, a policy that is optimal early in the game will not be advantageous later.

Deep neural networks are *parametric* learning systems, because they store memories in the model weights (or parameters), which are incrementally adjusted until convergence. Non-stationary environments pose a basic computational problem for parametric learning systems, called the *stability–plasticity dilemma*. If parameters are changed in tiny steps, the system will adapt very slowly to change (too stable). However, if parameters are changed in large jumps, the system will adjust excessively—so that weight changes provoke forgetting of past learning (too plastic). Learning systems thus need to learn in ways that admit retrieval of effective policies both now and in the unknown future.

Imagine you are headed to the beach for a week of holiday. You might pack your suitcase with swimsuit, towel, and snorkel. However, if you subsequently decide to spend an extra week in the mountains, you will have to throw your boots, binoculars, and raincoat on top of your already packed beachwear. This means that when you arrive at the beach, it will be troublesome to retrieve your swimming trunks from your luggage—because they are buried under your warm clothes. This is the basic problem that besets vanilla neural networks when they encounter tasks sequentially. When learning task A, it lays down memories in neural connection weights without due concern for what might be learnt next. On later encountering task B, new learning is layered on top of the old—potentially rendering the original policy that solves task A inaccessible and jeopardizing performance. Thus, in Ms. Pac-Man, learning to approach ghosts after swallowing the power pellet has the potential to undo learning about how to avoid the ghosts in the default case. In machine learning research, this overwriting is called *catastrophic interference*. It occurs in a parametric system when there are many distinct minima in weight space that can potentially solve either task A or task B, or both tasks A and B. If task A has been learnt and task B is being trained, the network has no incentive to learn a minimum for B that also solves A, so the original learning is overwritten. Over multiple task cycles, learning in the network oscillates from one task to the other, never mastering both—in a fruitless tug-of-war process (Figure 7.3).

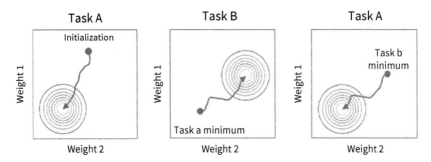

Fig. 7.3 Schematic illustration of catastrophic interference for a network with just two weights. The weights are initialized to random values. In solving task A, during the course of optimization, they move to a new setting. However, in the course of learning task B, they are moved out of this setting, and towards a new location that solves task B. There is no guarantee that this setting also solves task A, so on re-encountering task A, learning begins again from scratch.

Humans are much less prone to suffer from catastrophic forgetting than neural networks. Of course, anecdotally, we know that people can remain intellectually sprightly well into old age. But humans also seem to have evolved mechanisms that protect learning from interference. A classic demonstration of the resilience of human memory to interference dates back to the 1980s.[28] Human participants and neural networks first learnt to associate a series of pairs of words, such as apple–bicycle (task A), before learning new overlapping associations, such as apple–sofa (task B). In neural networks, performance on probed recall of task A associations (apple, _____) fell rapidly to chance during learning of task B, indicative of dramatic catastrophic interference (Figure 7.4). Interestingly, humans faced with the same task retained memory for task A associations whilst learning task B, suggesting that biological brains have evolved mechanisms that protect old learning during new learning. Perhaps this should be obvious. Learning to drive a car does not eradicate your ability to ride a bicycle. Mastering Space Invaders does not overwrite your skill at Frogger. In fact, there are numerous settings where humans seem to benefit from encountering tasks in a highly structured sequence. This is presumably why school timetables usually schedule Spanish and French classes in different slots, rather than teaching them both together in a single lesson.

---

[28] See (McCloskey & Cohen 1988).

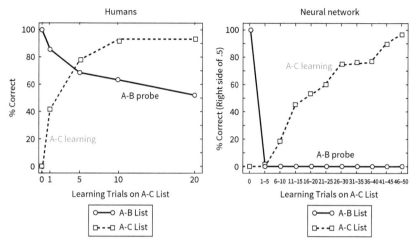

Fig. 7.4 Results of the study by McCloskey & Cohen (1989).

How then do biological systems learn continually? In the suitcase example, there is, of course, a straightforward solution. When you learn that your visit will take in both the coast and the hills, then you can reorganize your luggage to maximize access, perhaps repacking the warm weather clothes on one side of your suitcase and the cool weather clothes on the other. Similarly, a neural system that is able to consider the likely demands of task A when learning task B will be able to organize memories, such that both tasks can be retrieved in tandem—by learning a minimum in weight space that satisfies both object-ives. Understanding how to achieve this is a whole subfield within machine learning, referred to as the domain of *continual learning*. It asks how we can build agents that learn continually across their lifespan, like the admirable Ms Sitienei was able to do.

The problem of continual learning has inspired many creative solutions in AI research.[29] Some focus on how to allocate new memories to network weights in a way that minimizes catastrophic forgetting. This idea references mechanisms for lifelong learning in neurobiology, which have recently been revealed using advanced imaging methods such as two-photon microscopy. For example, in mice, new dendritic spines form in the motor cortex within two days of learning a new skill that involves balancing on a rotating rod.[30] When mice are trained to perform two distinct tasks, such as running forward

---

[29] For an excellent review, see (Hadsell et al. 2020).
[30] Dendritic spines are the post-synaptic sites of excitatory synapses. Similar results were found in the somatosensory cortex after exposure to an enriched program of whisker stimulation.

and backward, these spines form in a spatially segregated way, across different apical tuft branches. Remarkably, a sizeable fraction of these new spines is maintained stably across the entire lifespan of the animal, despite many further experiences to which the animal is exposed.[31] Moreover, the number of such persistent spines predicts how well the animals retain task memories over time. Biological systems thus seem to have evolved synaptic mechanisms that facilitate lifelong learning by explicitly protecting existing synapses from interference by new learning.

In 2017, two machine learning papers published more or less simultaneously proposed a solution to continual learning that drew heavily on these neurobiological insights. The idea was to estimate the importance of each weight in the network to past learning, and to penalize new synaptic changes in proportion to this measure. This additional penalty regularizes new learning towards the old, thus minimizing forgetting of past tasks. The method proved successful in allowing the same deep network model to learn up to ten randomly chosen Atari games, as well as navigate non-stationary problems in a supervised learning paradigm.[32]

However, many other approaches to continual learning implicitly or explicitly invoke a modular memory system. The stability–plasticity dilemma can be circumvented by a two-speed memory system, with one module that learns fast (allowing plasticity) and another that learns slowly (allowing stability).[33] Of course, the human brain has evolved a highly structured memory system that retains information over multiple intervals—from milliseconds (iconic memory) to seconds (working memory) to years (episodic, semantic, and procedural forms of long-term memory). One possibility is that two-speed learning relies on the distinction highlighted above between the neocortex and the hippocampus. There is powerful evidence that the neocortex allows slow learning of the structure of the world via a parametric model, whereas the hippocampus and adjacent structures retain information rapidly in a sparse (non-overlapping) neural code, more akin to a non-parametric model. By working together, these two systems furnish a solution to the intertwined problems of continual and one-shot learning.

Like so many core tenets of computational neuroscience today, we can trace the initial sketch of this idea back to David Marr, the visionary theorist whose career was tragically cut short by leukaemia at the age of 35. In his 1971 article

---

[31] For more than 90 months. This is about as long as a pampered pet mouse could be expected to live, and much longer than an average mouse would last in the wild.

[32] The method proposed was variously called elastic weight consolidation (Kirkpatrick et al. 2017) and synaptic intelligence (Zenke et al. 2017). There are minor differences to the two methods.

[33] See (Botvinick et al. 2019).

entitled *Simple Memory: A Theory for Archicortex*, Marr describes his bipartite vision of the neocortex and hippocampus (which he called the archicortex), arguing that:

> the neocortex […] changes the language in which incoming information is expressed by reclassifying it, as well as carrying out routine storage of associations between existing classes. […] archicortex cannot reclassify information in this way, [and instead] it performs a simple memorizing function—storing information in the language in which it is presented.

Marr proposes that the function of the neocortex, acting like a neural network, is to restructure incoming knowledge.[34] However, the hippocampus stores information in a native format (in 'the language in which it was presented'), akin to a non-parametric model, which buffers its inputs instead of summarizing them in a statistical model.

How can the two-speed systems be deployed to tackle continual learning? In 1995, researchers based at Stanford University proposed a model of biological learning called *complementary learning systems* (CLS) theory. Like Marr's model of *simple memory*, CLS theory proposes that the neocortex and hippocampus fulfil complementary roles in information encoding and storage, with the former learning slowly and the latter learning fast (Figure 7.5). Critically, however, CLS theory initially proposed that the hippocampus is wired to gradually repeat, rehearse, and replay our past experiences at quasi-random times during ongoing task performance, projecting this information back to the neocortex. This allows virtual intermixing of current and past experiences—perhaps task A and task B—so that they can be learnt conjointly. In terms of our earlier metaphor, we might think of this as the computational equivalent of repacking the suitcase for optimal access. By virtually interleaving past with current experience, this consolidation mechanism creates ensemble memories that are robust to continual learning.[35]

It was this idea that would go on to inspire DQN—and the first generation of deep learning agents to circumvent the non-stationarity problem and learn to play Atari games at superhuman levels. DQN includes a separate non-parametric memory system, perhaps akin to a primitive hippocampus, where instances of past experience are buffered. During ongoing game play, they are sampled and replayed, so that new experiences (task B) are re-encoded

---

[34] This is the idea articulated in Chapter 4.
[35] Although this depends on the level of variability in experience. For an interesting theoretical treatment of this point, see (Sun et al. 2021).

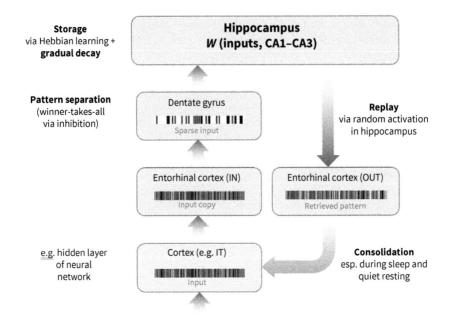

Fig. 7.5 Schematic of the complementary learning systems theory. Information is fed from the cortex to the entorhinal cortex and dentate gyrus where it is sparsified (pattern separated) before being encoded in hippocampal CA1–CA3 circuits. It is then replayed back to the cortex for consolidation.

alongside old experiences (task A) in a virtual interleaving process. This was the major innovation that allowed DQN to circumvent the instabilities of previous architectures.

In his 1971 paper on simple memory, Marr first proposed the transfer of memory from the hippocampus to the neocortex during sleep:

> [Marr] proposed that the hippocampal system stored experiences as they happened during the day and then replayed the memories stored in the hippocampal system back to the neocortex overnight to provide data for the category formation process as he envisioned it.

However, in 1995, when CLS theory was first proposed, hippocampal replay remained a conjecture. The first neurophysiological evidence had just begun to emerge, with the report that pairs of hippocampal place cells that have been coactivated during spatial learning tend to reactivate together when the rat is asleep.[36] Since then, a slew of studies painted the now classical picture

---

[36] The first demonstration of single place cell reactivation during sleep was by (Pavlides & Winson 1989), and the first demonstration of pairwise correlations was by (Wilson & McNaughton 1994). Bruce

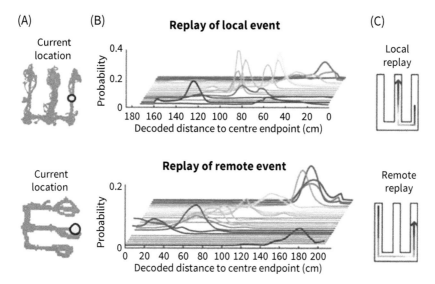

Fig. 7.6 Examples of local and remote replay recorded from multiunit activity data in the rodent hippocampus. The animal's location is shown in (**A**) (yellow dot) in each case, superimposed upon movement trajectories through the maze (grey lines). Panel (**B**) shows the activity decoded from a series of cells coding for places at variable distances from the endpoint. In (**C**), the replay trajectory starts from the location shown in darkest blue and ends at the location in darkest red. Colours correspond to those in (B). In the local case, replay is forward from the current location. In the remote case, the replay event encodes arms of the maze other than the one where the animal is currently located.
Reprinted with permission from Carr et al. (2011).

of replay as a mechanism by which sequences of experiences are rapidly re-instated offline. During bursts of irregular hippocampal activity, known as *sharp-wave ripples*, extended sequences of place cell activity are reinstated, at about 20 times the rate at which they were experienced during the waking state. Importantly, replay occurs both forward and backward, during both sleep and wakefulness, and in the latter case is related to experiences that are both remote (spatially removed from the current state) and proximal (Figure 7.6).[37] Over the past 20 years, replay has become one of the most intensively studied phenomena in systems neurobiology.

McNaughton, who led the latter paper, is a co-author on the CLS paper. There are many excellent reviews on hippocampal replay, but these may be particularly helpful (Foster 2017; Ólafsdóttir et al. 2018).

[37] The reference in the figure is (Carr et al. 2011).

The functional significance of hippocampal replay remains controversial. Because it tends to occur backward in time from a rewarded goal, replay may accelerate learning of a state value function, by mentally linking states and outcomes through offline backup.[38] When replay targets states that are successors to the current one (as has been observed in both rodents and humans) or that predict future behavioural choices, such as the taking of shortcuts, it seems reasonable to propose a role in planning. For example, in one human study, participants were asked to plan a route through a non-spatial maze composed of object images, such as navigating from the hairbrush to the kite via the watermelon. Using a neuroimaging technique that relies on measuring magnetic fields evoked by brain activity, the researchers could identify neural patterns associated with each object, and thus measure the instantiation of these patterns during planning. They found that people tended to 'replay' the objects that would be found on their intended route in reverse order, as if they were planning backward from the goal.[39]

However, there is also good evidence for its role in the consolidation of instance-based memories back into the neocortical ensemble via an interleaving process, as predicted by CLS theory. For example, disruption of replay hinders subsequent retrieval of spatial memories; and replay events seem to be propagated to the neocortex, where they are synchronized with fluctuations in activity states in several regions, including both the PFC and the visual cortex. There is thus still room for replay to play a role in solving continual learning for biological agents.

Some memories may be more useful than others. Indeed, people are prone to encoding and rehearsing events which are novel, surprising, or motivationally salient, a phenomenon known as the von Restorff effect.[40] During episodic encoding, BOLD signals in the hippocampus are particularly responsive to events which are perceptually, semantically, or emotionally salient, and these enhanced responses are predictive of successful memory formation.[41] When a rat is given uneven exposure to two spatial memory tasks, the less familiar of the two is replayed more often.[42] Privileging surprising events for replay may allow those exceptions that are most relevant for behaviour a greater weight in shaping agent policies. In fact, a later version of DQN that was biased to

---

[38] See (Mattar & Daw 2018).

[39] The imaging technique is called magnetoencephalography (MEG). The paper is (Kurth-Nelson et al. 2016).

[40] Named after the German psychologist Hedwig von Restorff, who discovered it in the 1930s (von Restorff 1933).

[41] See (Strange et al. 2000).

[42] See (Gupta et al. 2010).

replay events that led to larger TD errors, using a method called prioritized experience replay, outstripped the performance of the original DQN on the ALE suite.[43]

In previous chapters, we argued that the natural world is highly structured, and advances in AI systems should capitalize on that structure to build stronger agents. Here, the same argument is made. In this case, the structure is in time: it is given by the autocorrelation of sensory inputs and task objectives in a dynamic RL environment. Biological agents have evolved complex memory systems to handle the dependencies that exist between different moments in time. As we shall see, those relations can be idiosyncratic, which is why our memory system has a complex modular structure. To build advanced systems for RL in the real world, our agents will need to account for the temporal structure of natural experience.

7.4 Finding structure in time

Memory systems allow agents to share information with themselves across time. So far, we have highlighted a single computational principle for memory: the experience-dependent modification of synaptic weights. This is the mechanism by which feedforward deep networks like AlexNet or DQN slowly learn a function that maps image pixels onto outputs. It is how the neocortex learns stable, generalizable representations from long-term averages of experience, and is also the basis for fast plastic changes in the hippocampus that permit immediate storage of salient events. We have seen that when the world is structured in time, learning with synaptic memory alone can be challenging for deep RL agents such as DQN. Correlations in observations and rewards inflate the variance of gradients calculated during optimization, creating unstable learning dynamics, and expose the network to catastrophic forgetting.

However, this is a paradoxical claim. Structure in time should help—not hurt—learning in neural networks. Networks should be able to harness temporal structure to make predictions about the future. In the 1980s, researchers began to realize this. A paper published by the cognitive scientist Jeffrey Elman with the title *Finding Structure in Time* provided an early demonstration of how neural networks can use activation memory (or *recurrence*) to maintain information without synaptic change, with applications in sequence

---

[43] See (Schaul et al. 2016).

prediction in simple NLP tasks. Recurrence resembles the process by which biological brains share information with themselves using time-varying patterns of population activity. This innovation opened the door to the recurrent neural network, one of the most powerful tools in AI research today.[44]

Consider the Atari game of Pong. Playing in 2D, two opponents control a paddle, each trying to bounce a ball past the other. Obeying the physics of the game, the ball flies in a straight line between the sides of the screen. Imagine trying to predict where the ball will land from a short segment of game play. If the duration of the glimpse is just a single frame, the ball is frozen in time, and you can't know where it will land—or even which way it is headed. With two successive frames, you can make a rough and ready guess at where to move the paddle. However, for a precise estimate of where the ball will end up, you need to see several frames in series and to integrate across these observations to estimate its trajectory. This benefit of integration over time is even greater in the real world where sensory signals are inherently *noisy*—subject to random variation too complex to be modelled. For example, the behaviourist B. F. Skinner famously taught pigeons to play a real-world version of Pong by shaping them gradually with food rewards (Figure 7.7). In Skinner's version, the ball can move in unpredictable ways due to the unevenness of the table surface, or buffeting by a gust of light wind or spin that was invisibly applied by a devious pigeon opponent. Where a signal is noisy, it can be encoded more precisely by sampling and averaging several independent estimates.[45]

If DQN learnt to map single frames of Pong onto actions, it would probably have floundered, because each frame carries virtually no information about the direction in which the ball is headed. In practice, however, DQN was able to achieve 132% of human expert performance. This is because on each timestep, the researchers fed it the last four frames of play, so that its game experience arrived already integrated across a short temporal window. Biological brains have evolved a similar trick for visual perception. In 1960, the psychologist George Sperling asked participants to recall random letters that had been flashed briefly on the screen in a 3×3 matrix. Participants could usually name about half of the characters shown. However, Sperling realized that if cued to report just a single row or column, they could usually name all

---

[44] The Elman paper is here (Elman 1990). It builds on the earlier work of Michael Jordan in 1986. The Hopfield network, a different class of RNN, was developed in 1982 (Hopfield 1982).

[45] Assuming the noise added on each trial is independent and identically distributed (IID), then this follows from the law of large numbers, whereby the average of estimates of a noisy signal will tend towards its expectation over trials. You can try this for yourself, as my research group did at a recent lab retreat, by playing table tennis under stroboscopic conditions (it is basically impossible below about 5 Hz due to the paucity of samples).

(A)   (B)

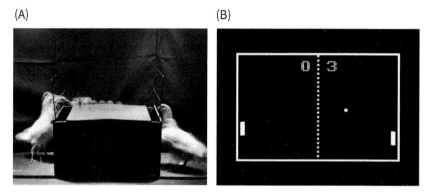

Fig. 7.7 Pong in natural and artificial intelligence.
(**A**) Skinner's pigeons playing Pong (with a ping pong ball).
Photo by Yale Joel, June 1950, © Time Inc.
(**B**) The Atari 2600 game of Pong. Players move the paddles on the left and right to hit the ball to one another.

three letters. In other words, people have capacity to remember all the items—but their memory decays very quickly. Sperling realized that he had identified a new sensory memory buffer, and he called it *iconic memory*. We might say that DQN was thus endowed with a four-frame iconic memory.[46]

Iconic memory occurs because after visual stimulation has ceased, neural activity does not shut down immediately but instead slowly relaxes back to baseline. In macaque V1, this neural decay constant predicts the retention duration for visual items in iconic memory.[47] Neural activity peters out slowly because neurons connected in a network stimulate one another, a process called recurrent excitation. The anatomical basis for recurrent excitation in a local circuit of neurons was first described by Rafael Lorente de Nó, a student of the towering Spanish neuroscientist Santiago Ramón y Cajal, whose microscopic investigation of brain circuitry won him a share of the 1906 Nobel Prize for Medicine. In 1933, Lorente de Nó wrote:[48]

> The conception of the reflex arc as a unidirectional chain of neurons has neither anatomic nor functional basis. Histologic studies with Golgi's method show the universality of the existence of plural parallel connections and of recurrent, reciprocal connections.

[46] For Sperling's classic paper, see (Sperling 1960).
[47] See (Teeuwen et al. 2021).
[48] For a historical perspective, see (Larriva-Sahd 2014).

Thus, as neuron i becomes active, it excites neuron j, which, in turn, feeds back more excitation to neuron i, and so on. Like voices that grow ever louder in a restaurant as diners strain to hear one another through the din, cells that mutually excite each other drive a self-perpetuating activity loop that serves as a primitive memory trace.

One well-studied example of recurrent excitation occurs in the parietal cortex. Neurons in the lateral intraparietal (LIP) area (part of PPC) fire just before a macaque monkey makes an eye movement to a specific location in visual space. The response properties of these cells have been explored using a popular psychophysical task in which monkeys learn to respond to the net direction of motion in a field of randomly moving dots by directing their gaze towards one of two targets. The animals are rewarded for making the correct choice, and thus learn slowly by instrumental conditioning. After training is complete, LIP signals come to code in advance for the decision that the monkey will make. The now canonical finding is that during motion stimulation, the firing rates of these LIP neurons will ramp up or down in concert with the momentary evidence that the saccade should be made to a target in their response field. This means that each neuron's instantaneous firing rate depends on both its inputs and recurrent excitation from other neurons with which it shares a response field. During decision-making, two populations with recurrent excitation—each coding for a different target—mutually inhibit each other, creating a balanced dynamic system that competes to drive the monkey's response. This model, first described by Xiao-Jing Wang in 2001, can explain the firing rate patterns of individual neurons (which tend to build up towards an attractor state, at which point a saccade is initiated), as well as the shape of psychometric and chronometric functions recorded from monkeys performing the task.[49]

In machine learning research, this model is an instance of a wider class of neural network with activation memory called an RNN. At first glance, the architecture of an RNN resembles that of a feedforward network, in that inputs x flow from the input layer via the hidden layer h to output units y, transformed at each stage by a bank of trainable weights. However, the RNN allows for an additional set of recurrent weights V that map the hidden state onto itself between timesteps, in combination with the feedforward input. For example, if weights V are set to the identity matrix, then the network will

---

[49] See (Wang 2002). The build-up in LIP was first identified by Mike Shadlen and Bill Newsome in 2001 (Shadlen & Newsome 2001). For the modelling of this problem with RL, see (Law & Gold 2009). For a more general review of this area of neuroscience research, see (Hanks & Summerfield 2017).

simply add up x over successive timesteps.[50] However, other weight settings will allow information to be dynamically transformed over time in potentially complex ways. For example, the model described by Wang requires both focal excitation and broad inhibition from a pool of theoretical interneurons. Of course, RNN weights do not have to be set by hand. Using an elaboration of backpropagation in which gradients flow back in time, they can be trained to meet a supervised or RL objective. In fact, many classical neural and behavioural motifs are also exhibited by a model that is trained to solve the dot motion task using a recurrent neural network trained with RL, via a variant of the actor–critic approach.[51]

RNNs are now a ubiquitous tool for processing time series data in AI research. One major use case is in natural language processing. RNNs were the basis for the first NLP models, known as sequence-to-sequence (seq2seq) neural networks because they learnt to predict the next word, phrase, or sentence in a text corpus. For example, consider the following quasi-Shakespearean excerpt:

QUEENE:
I had thought thou hadst a Roman; for the oracle,
Thus by All bids the man against the word,
Which are so weak of care, by old care done;
Your children were in your holy love,
And the precipitation through the bleeding throne.

This was generated by training a simple recurrent neural network to predict sequences from the Bard's complete works. The text has a vague aura of Jacobean plausibility until you attempt to seriously fathom its meaning, at which point it is revealed to be entirely gibberish.[52] As we have seen, modern NLP models that rely on transformers tend to perform a lot better.

The recurrent weights in an RNN learn to map activity patterns flexibly across time, allowing for flexible memory dynamics. Similarly, in biological brains, neural circuits are capable of maintaining complex, self-sustaining activity patterns, with dynamics that depend on network morphology and biophysics: membrane properties, connectivity patterns, transmission velocities,

---

[50] On timestep t, the hidden layer activity $h_t = tanh[Wx_t + Vh_{t-1}]$, where W denotes the first layer weights and the bias term is omitted. The identity matrix has ones on the diagonal and zeros elsewhere. Any matrix multiplied by the identity matrix is itself. Thus, if V is the identity matrix, then $\Delta h_t = tanh[Wx_t]$.

[51] In fact, the authors show that it is possible to capture a number of key neural observations that depend on recurrent dynamics using the same model (Song et al. 2017).

[52] You can try for yourself here, with instructions from Andrej Karpathy's blog (Karpathy 2015).

and the relative strength and timing of excitatory and inhibitory signals. The complex patterns of recurrent neural activity that unfold in time allow information to be maintained or manipulated in sophisticated ways, making activation memory a powerful tool for sensorimotor behaviour and more complex decision-making.[53]

In the late 1960s, a neurophysiologist by the name of Joaquin Fuster moved to California from his native Spain to take up a position at UCLA. He brought with him a research agenda that pioneered the use of newly available extracellular recording methods to study the PFC of the macaque monkey. At the time, the functional organization of memory in the neocortex remained a mystery. In 1950, Karl Lashley had published a report documenting his search for the *engram*—the elusive trace of memory in the brain—by lesioning increasingly larger portions of rat neocortex. However, Lashley's findings implied that lesion location mattered less than lesion volume—larger lesions invariably provoking greater impairment. He concluded that memory was distributed widely across the brain, a principle he called *mass action*.[54]

Fuster was inspired by experiments conducted at Yale University in the 1930s. In a series of studies, Carlyle Jacobsen measured the effect of lesions in the vicinity of the *sulcus principalis*, the major fissure that divides the dorsolateral from the ventrolateral PFC, in the macaque monkey. In one test, food was hidden under one of two cups in full view of the monkey, but the animal was only allowed to retrieve a morsel after a delay period lasting up to a few minutes. Jacobsen describes the results as follows:

> The tests of delayed response, however, revealed a profound deficit in what may be termed the recent or 'immediate memory'. Before operation the animal scored a high percentage of correct responses after delays of fifteen, thirty and forty-five seconds. As the delays increased beyond one minute, however, the accuracy of performance decreased rapidly until after delays of one hundred and twenty seconds, the percentage of correct choices had no greater than a chance value.

Jacobsen's work had thus suggested that the PFC plays a role in maintaining information over the short term. Using invasive electrodes, Fuster set out to identify the neurons mediating this effect, recording from the PFC whilst monkeys performed a similar delayed memory task. He succeeded in dramatic

---

[53] Recurrent processing may be due to either local circuit dynamics or long-range interactions between the cortex and subcortical structures such as the thalamus.

[54] See work by the late, great Howard Eichenbaum, who put Lashley's work in a modern context (Eichenbaum 2016).

form. His experiments revealed the existence of PFC neurons which fired persistently over the delay period, spanning delays of as long as a minute.[55] If their chain of persistence was broken, the baited side was more likely to slip the monkey's mind, resulting in an error. Fuster conjectured that these cells were retaining information about which side was baited, and thus dubbed them 'memory cells'. In the 1980s, Patricia Goldman-Rakic built on his findings, showing that individual PFC cells are tuned for short-term memories of locations and objects that are maintained over the delay. Today, it is widely accepted that these cells in the PFC form a neural substrate for short-term memory.[56]

Like sensorimotor integration in area LIP, the maintenance of information in short-term memory relies on recurrent excitation, and persistent activity in the dorsolateral portion of PFC (known as the DLPFC) can be modelled with an RNN.[57] As a model of memory processes, the RNN has proved a valuable tool in understanding the computational solutions that the brain may have evolved for maintaining information over time, and a means to explain their normative properties. One central claim has been that memories are maintained in a neural *attractor state*, which is a stable pattern of reverberatory activity into which a network settles over time. For example, in a mouse premotor area that is a likely homologue to the primate DLPFC, it can be shown that persistent delay-period activity in single cells is resistant to perturbation, confirming that it depends on the dynamics of the whole network, rather than on the biophysics of a single cell. It is likely that in the case of short-term memory, recurrent activation is sustained by interactions among cortical and subcortical regions (such as the thalamus), as well as within the local network.

However, the nature of the dynamic code for short-term memory remains a major open question in systems neuroscience. Attractor states remain a major candidate, and indeed, the stable delay-period activity reported by Fuster and Goldman-Rakic seems to signify an attractor state. However, neural activity is overwhelmingly heterogenous both across time and across neurons. Even where just a few, simple experimental variables are manipulated during sensorimotor control, relatively few neurons form readily interpretable activity

---

[55] Conducted with his postdoc Garrett Alexander

[56] Fuster and Alexander's 1971 paper is (Fuster & Alexander 1971) and Jacobsen's earlier work is (Jacobsen 1935). In fact, as so often happens, another group (in Kyoto, Japan) independently reported the same finding at the same time as Fuster (Kubota & Niki 1971). There is also an excellent review on lesion work in the PFC here (Szczepanski & Knight 2014) and on the computational processes underlying short-term memory here (Wang 2021). Patricia Goldman-Rakic was tragically killed in a road accident in 2003. Her thoughts about working memory are summarized in this review from 1995 (Goldman-Rakic 1995).

[57] Computational models of working memory that build heavily on Goldman-Rakic's work are described here (Durstewitz et al. 2000).

patterns. For example, during the discrimination of random dot motion stimuli, a veritable zoo of different responses accompany the canonical target-evoked and stable ramping patterns that have been consistently reported for over 20 years. One possibility is that short-term memory relies on non-stationary attractor states, such as oscillations or more complex chaotic patterns. Another possibility is that stable patterns ride upon a background of more idiosyncratic activity that is evoked by activities that are unrelated to task performance.[58]

Alternatively, a different theory suggests that memories may be encoded in a sequence of transiently encoded neuronal states, each different from the next. One study used an RNN as a normative tool for understanding when activation memory should be stable and when it should be sequential with no one single attractor state, finding that different factors shaped the short-term memory code. For example, if delay periods are of variable duration, then the RNN learns a more persistent memory code, presumably so that the network is in a common state whenever the probe arrives. By contrast, tasks with higher temporal complexity and networks with stronger intrinsic coupling tended to give rise to sequential dynamic codes for short-term memory. RNNs can thus fruitfully be used to make predictions about the neural activity underlying memory processes that can be tested in future experiments.[59]

Another school of thought rejects the idea that activity should be interpretable at the level of single neurons. We have encountered this argument before, in the context of supervised CNN models of the visual cortex, where neural codes for objects are proposed to be fundamentally entangled, high-dimensional, and uninterpretable. Transposed to the parietal cortex, the same argument is made to explain the indecipherable patterns of neural activity that unfold as monkeys decide whether two successive dot motion patterns belong in the same category. An RNN trained to perform the task shows the same heterogeneity of neural coding patterns is observed in single recurrent units. However, when neural activity is plotted at the level of the population, rather than of single cells, for example by reducing the dimensionality of the population code and projecting onto the axes, of stimulus, context, or task, the data suddenly become easy to interpret in both the RNN and the neural circuit (Figure 7.8). Similar to the results of fitting CNN models to the ventral

---

[58] For examples of the zoo of activity in area LIP, see (Park et al. 2014). For evidence that the attractor state lives in a subspace of neural activity, see (Murray et al. 2017).

[59] See (Orhan & Ma 2019).

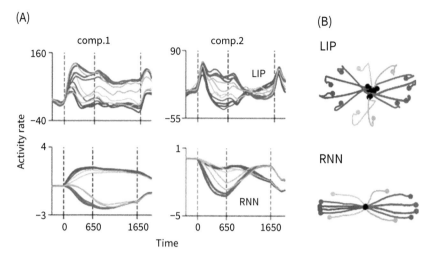

Fig. 7.8 (**A**) Upper panels: the principal components 1 and 2 of multineuron activity from macaque lateral intraparietal area (LIP) as a function of dot direction (colour) and motion strength (light/dark lines). Lower panels: the same for the hidden units of a recurrent neural network (RNN) trained to perform the same task. Both monkey and network activity are idiosyncratic. (**B**) Projection of average activity into 2D. Both RNN and LIP neurons form a similar, highly structured representation of the stimulus.

visual stream, this had led to the suggestion that neural coding is only meaningful at the level of populations, and not of individual cells.[60]

Above, we detail three examples of activation memory in the primate brain: those subserving iconic memory in the visual cortex; sensorimotor integration in the LIP area; and short-term memory in the PFC. In each, information is maintained over time through the recurrent activity of a neural circuit, whereby neurons mutually drive one another within a network. Notably, however, the three examples involve very different time courses of memory. In the early visual cortex, recurrent dynamics fade away over tens of milliseconds, allowing flashes of visual information to loiter just long enough for immediate recall (as in the Sperling task), but no more. In the parietal cortex, LIP neurons can integrate motion signals over a few seconds up to a saccadic response. This is enough to allow a weak momentary signal to be aggregated over time into a reliable estimate for fast and accurate sensorimotor control. By contrast, in

---

[60] Neural activity is heterogenous during dot motion discrimination (Park et al. 2014) and categorization (Chaisangmongkon et al. 2017). See also (Mante et al. 2013). For papers advocating for population over neuron doctrine, see (Saxena & Cunningham 2019) and (Yuste 2015).

the PFC—as we saw from Fuster's original experiments—short-term memory maintenance can persist for up to a minute or more.

This trichotomy also coheres with a general organizing principle for brain circuits, which is that windows of temporal integration grow as one moves anteriorly across the neocortex. This principle was originally proposed by Fuster, who argued that the basic function of the brain is to bridge the gap between perception and action at multiple different levels of temporal scale.[61] In 2008, a clever experiment mapped this temporal hierarchy onto different regions of the human brain by showing participants in the fMRI scanner excerpts of classic silent movies directed by Buster Keaton and Charlie Chaplin. Movies were scrambled at different timescales, so that at the longest scale, long segments of narrative (of more than half a minute, such as when the drunken millionaire is saved from suicide in *City Lights*) remained intact, whereas at shorter scales (scrambled segments of 4 seconds or less) the event sequence of individual scenes became nonsensical. The authors measured the correlation in BOLD signals across two presentations of a scrambled film.

The logic of this experiment was that brain regions with short time constants of integration should be relatively immune to scrambling, as their neural dynamics carry no memory beyond a few seconds, and thus should correlate across presentations even at shorter scales. However, correlations for brain regions that integrated information over longer time periods should only resist when scrambling occurred for prolonged segments. The authors observed hierarchy temporal receptive fields that unfolded along the posterior–anterior axis, from the earliest visual cortical regions with rapid decay constants to the PFC in which longer narrative segments were integrated and understood.

This finding echoes the detailed study of intrinsic timescales (autocorrelations in neuronal fluctuation) across data from several research groups (26 monkeys in total). Intrinsic timescales for different regions were remarkably conserved across different groups and studies, ranging from about 50 ms in the visual cortex to 200 ms in the PFC, with even longer integration windows in the orbitofrontal cortex, at the anterior pole of the frontal cortex. Building a hierarchical RNN model that is constrained to respect these time constants, one report simulated a response to a pulsed visual input, finding that it recreated the idiosyncratic patterns of dynamic activity across 29 different brain areas.[62]

---

[61] See (Fuster 2001).
[62] See (Murray et al. 2014) and (Chaudhuri et al. 2015).

7.5 Mental gymnastics

With 19 gold medals in world championship competitions, Simone Biles is the most decorated gymnast of all time. She took a historic four gold medals in the 2016 Summer Olympic Games in Rio de Janeiro, including the individual all-round artistic event, which requires athletes to excel at the vault, uneven bars, balance beam, and floor exercise. Each of these four exercises demands a finely choreographed routine with several elements. For example, on the balance beam, gymnasts mount a thin 5 metre-long beam of wood that is suspended more than a metre off the ground, and perform a sequence of dance moves, twirls, jumps, and handstands, before leaping acrobatically to the ground. In the women's final, Biles was awarded the highest scores on all four exercises. Each component of each exercise is itself minutely scripted and practised to perfection. For example, Biles' dismount from the balance beam began with a back handspring, launching her high into the air from the edge of the beam, allowing time for a somersault with full lateral rotation and a second somersault on the descent, culminating in a flawless landing (Figure 7.9). She was the only female competitor to score over 15 points on this exercise at the 2016 games.

Intelligence is often defined as the ability to perform a diversity of tasks. In English, the word *task* refers to a unit of purposive behaviour: a task is defined by an objective that we wish to satisfy in a given context, and the rules that constrain how it might be achieved. Thus, in the modern, developed world, we might find ourselves tackling tasks such as assembling a flat-pack chest of drawers, booking a city break in Prague, solving a long division problem alongside a confused child, or preparing a baked Alaska for a special dessert. For Simone Biles, there was a more daunting task to be solved in summer of 2016—to come home with a gold medal. It is instructive to consider the nature of this challenge and how it was met, as it gives us a window into how tasks are represented in the brain, and how control processes can be deployed to allow the execution of complex behaviours.

Tasks can be represented hierarchically. Most tasks contain subtasks, which may themselves be composed of smaller units of purpose.[63] For Biles and her fellow gymnasts, the task of winning gold in the all-round event can be

---

[63] In cognitive science, the term 'schema' is often used to describe a subcomponent of a task, although, as we have seen in Chapter 4, the term is sometimes used interchangeably with 'representation' or 'mental category'.

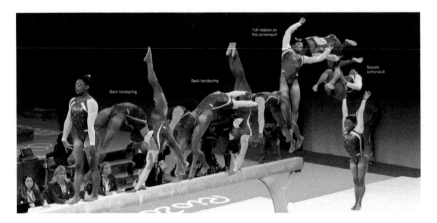

Fig. 7.9 Simone Biles on the balance beam.
From https://www.nytimes.com/interactive/2016/08/11/sports/olympics/simone-biles-winning-moves.html.

decomposed into the subtasks of gaining high scores on each of the four individual exercises. Each exercise score, in turn, depends on the quality of execution of individual components or moves, such as the complexity of the jump when leaping over the vault. Ultimately, the execution of individual moves requires the sequential activation of patterns of muscles which move the body. We can thus see tasks—from tying your shoelaces to delivering a parcel—as *behavioural objects*, much as shoes, shoelaces, and packages are basic entities that make up our visual world. The perceptual hierarchy of scenes, objects, and features is mirrored by a hierarchy of control for action. As we shall see, there are also shared principles by which these hierarchies are implemented in the brain.

Mentally organizing tasks as hierarchies confers two benefits, which we call *abstraction* and *composition*. As we have seen, in the context of perception, an abstract representation is one that is invariant over certain properties of an entity, for example, the concept of cat abstracts over whether the animal being referenced is Siamese, Abyssinian, or Moggy. In a similar vein, tasks are abstract when they are not tied to specific stimuli or context. For example, the abstract task of *assembling flat-pack furniture* can be applied to a chest of drawers or a bunk bed, and the abstract task of *booking a city break* can be deployed for Barcelona as easily as for Prague. At the Rio Olympics, each gymnast set out to tackle the task of winning in a different way. Each floor exercise had a distinct set of acrobatic tumble lines, a unique aesthetic style, choreographed dance moves, and a special musical playlist. An important principle is that abstraction increases as you ascend the task hierarchy. There are many routes to a place in the history books, but only a handful of ways to perform the perfect backflip.

The second property of hierarchical task representations is their potential for composition. Composition means that tasks are composed of subtasks that can be completed independently, and often in any order. For example, when arranging a short break in a foreign city, you can book transport before searching for a hotel, or vice versa. When making a baked Alaska, you can prepare the ice cream and sponge cake in any order, as long as they are both ready in time to coat with stiffly whipped meringue before popping your masterpiece in the freezer. Composition is important because it allows new tasks to be solved on the basis of existing skills. For example, if I know how to ride a bicycle with no hands and I also know how to play the trumpet, then I might be able to do both at once—even if I have never practised. It is our ability to compose new actions from existing building blocks that allows us to generate entirely new sentences every time we open our mouth. In the words of the linguist Wilhelm von Humboldt, composition allows us to *make infinite use of finite means.*[64]

Previously, we saw that successful task execution depends on the integrity of the PFC (and especially the DLPFC). In the classic studies of Burgess and Shallice, patients with PFC damage caused chaos when asked to perform errands in an unfamiliar high street. The behaviour of patients with PFC damage is particularly disrupted in novel contexts, where well-worn habits and routines cannot be recruited to scaffold action selection. Exactly how the PFC contributes to task performance, however, remains one of the great unsolved questions in neuroscience.

In the 1980s, on the basis of the extant neuropsychological findings, Tim Shallice developed an influential model in which the PFC exerted a *supervisory* role over perception and action. This model helped carve out one of the major distinctions in modern cognitive science: that actions could be selected using *automatic* or *controlled* brain processes. Automatic processes are those that relied on familiar links between stimulus and action, such as those that have been extensively practised or reinforced during instrumental learning. If I am approaching a set of traffic lights, and they turn red, my automatic, overlearnt response might be to press the brake pedal. However, *cognitive control* is needed when the situation is novel or unexpected. Imagine that instead

---

[64] Despite Chomsky's popularization of this pithy phrase, von Humboldt was actually pretty lukewarm about notions of a generative grammar or linguistic universals. See https://plato.stanford.edu/entries/wilhelm-humboldt/.

the traffic lights simply switch off as I approach. What should I do? Stop or go? This, Shallice argues, is where the PFC takes charge, bypassing the automatic stimulus–response pathway and using a more deliberative strategy that anticipates the future consequences of action. Perhaps it reasons that there has been a citywide power cut and that the other lights at the junction are off—so barrelling through the lights at speed is probably a bad idea.[65]

In the early 2000s, on the basis of emerging fMRI results, the psychologist Jonathan Cohen and his group elaborated this theory to argue that an adjacent medial frontal structure, the dorsal anterior cingulate cortex (dACC), is responsible for detecting the need for control, whereas the DLPFC is engaged to implementing cognitive control processes. This theory was built on studies showing that when the brain first detects conflict—a clash of different possible responses (Stop? Go?)—then BOLD signals increase in the dACC, whereas DLPFC BOLD is highest whenever conflict needs resolved. They describedree an influential computational model, in the form of a (handcrafted) connectionist model, in a classic paper by Miller and Cohen from 2001.[66]

How does the lateral PFC implement cognitive control to guide behaviour in novel situations? Shallice, Miller, and Cohen conceive of the lateral PFC as a supervisory system that regulates activity in the sensory and motor cortices using top-down attentional regulation. However, whilst this theory specifies a putative control mechanism, it is silent about how tasks are learnt and represented in the PFC. Nor does it specify how the frontal lobe is organized to allow task abstraction and composition. Over the intervening 20 years, we have learnt much about neural coding and macroscopic organization in the primate PFC. There is now good evidence that PFC neurons represent relevant stimuli, the context provided by a task, and the interaction between these two variables.

One important early finding was the identification of neurons that represent abstract properties of tasks. In a classic study, the neuroscientist Joni Wallis trained macaques to match novel images across a delay. On each trial, monkeys saw an initial image (A) delivered alongside a cue, followed by a

---

[65] For the classic Shallice theory, with Don Norman, see (Norman & Shallice 1986). The original distinction between automatic and controlled processing goes back to (Shiffrin & Schneider 1977). Note that use of the word 'control' as used here is potentially confusing because in machine learning, 'control' usually means 'computation of optimal actions in an MDP'. By contrast, cognitive neuroscientists tend to distinguish motor control (selecting actions) from cognitive control (deploying special mechanisms for dealing with unfamiliar or conflicting choices).

[66] For the integrated theory, written with Earl Miller, see (Miller & Cohen 2001). My favourite evidence for the conflict detection/resolution story comes from an ingenious study by Tobias Egner, in which participants judged whether conflicting words/faces referred to actors or politicians (Egner & Hirsch 2005).

probe image (A or B). For some cues, the monkey had to release a lever if the probe matched the initial image (match subtask), whereas for others, releasing the lever was only rewarded if the initial and probe images did not match (non-match subtask). After monkeys had learnt to perform the task, neurons in the DLPFC exhibited delay-period activity that depended on whether the monkey was performing the match or non-match task. Critically, this activity did not depend on the precise nature of the cue or response and was observed even when the images were entirely novel. In other words, these PFC neurons were signalling the abstract concept of 'match' or 'non-match', rather than an instruction about how to respond to specific images. Since then, many other studies have reported comparable results. Cells coding for abstract rules have also been isolated in the endbrain of crows, a corvid species known to have remarkable problem-solving abilities.[67]

Another macaque paper from 2007 offers a striking window into the computations performed by PFC neurons.[68] The group of Jun Tanji trained monkeys to make sequences of four actions using a manipulandum that could be turned, pushed, or pulled. Each sequence comprised two sorts of actions (e.g. push [A] and turn [B]), and they cued monkeys to perform sequences involving *pairs* (AABB), *alternation* (ABAB), and *repetition* (AAAA). Critically, cells in the DLPFC became active after the cue (but before action initiation) in a way that predicted the sequence type. For example, Figure 7.10 shows a cell that responded on alternation trials, those that had an ABAB structure, irrespective of whether the actions A and B were turn–push, turn–pull, or pull–turn. Like in the Wallis study, the DLPFC neurons are coding for the task in an abstract fashion. In both cases, we can think of PFC neurons as encoding a set of mental operations, like the steps implementing a program or function, but being invariant to the specific inputs received by that program (particular images or lever movements). Findings like these begin to put computational meat on the bone for the theories dating back to Craik and Tolman, which argue that intelligence requires the conduct of operations on mental representations.

In the late twentieth century, neuroscientists studying the PFC tended to fall into one of two rival camps. The first camp saw the PFC as controlling action selection for complex behaviour, whereas the second, continuing the tradition of Fuster and Goldman-Rakic, highlighted its contribution to

[67] See (Wallis et al. 2001). For a review detailing related findings, see (Freedman & Miller 2008). For the study on crows, see (Veit & Nieder 2013). The precise region of the endbrain is called the nidopallium caudolaterale, and it is a putative homologue of the primate PFC.

[68] For the original paper, see (Shima et al. 2007). For a helpful review, see (Tanji et al. 2007).

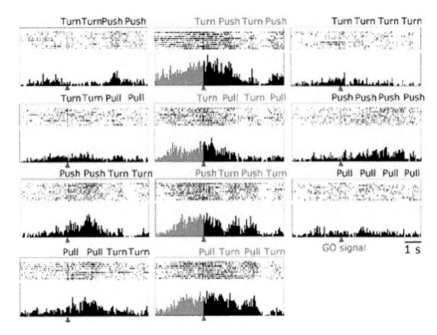

Fig. 7.10 Cells coding for abstract movement patterns in macaque prefrontal cortex (PFC). The cell illustrated responded in advance of, and during, a cued movement sequence of the form ABAB, irrespective of whether A and B were push, pull, or turn. It did not respond to other sequences, like AABB.
Reprinted with permission from Shima et al. (2007).

short-term memory maintenance. Fortunately, in the intervening period, the field has coalesced around a view that reconciles these two theories. The key is that short-term memory tasks themselves demand abstract mental operations, for example to encode and maintain a sensory stimulus before mapping the memory trace onto a matching or recall response. In most paradigms, the same operations are required for a varying stimulus set, comprising a diverse set of pictures or locations. Thus, we can think of the neurons in Fuster's study as performing the (abstract) operation of maintaining information until a response is required. In other words, putative short-term memory neurons are not maintaining specific stimulus content, but instead contributing to the overall operational demands of the task.

The neural division of labour across the surface of the lateral PFC has also been a long-standing puzzle. However, a 2003 brain imaging study led by Etienne Koechlin revealed an organizing principle for how mental operations are assigned to frontal cortical sites, called the *cascade model*, which has now become widely accepted. Closing the circle with studies showing delay-period activity, the claim is that the principal axis on which PFC processing is organized is *time*. The posterior-to-anterior (or caudal-to-rostral)[69] axis of the PFC is structured, so that more caudal regions perform more immediate or punctate task operations, whereas more rostral regions coordinate action over longer periods of time. Returning to Simone Biles, who is midway through her floor exercise routine—how does she select which action comes next? Her next move can be partly inferred from immediate contextual signals, such as her position on the mat. But given that she will visit the same spot multiple times, she needs a mental representation of which segment from the full task (her routine) is currently being executed. Koechlin and colleagues argued that selecting actions on the basis of cues that spanned longer temporal periods was the province of more anterior regions of the PFC. This idea neatly unites the two themes that reoccur in theorizing about the PFC: Fuster's notion of hierarchically ordered memory processes for bridging perception and action, and the idea that the PFC generates control signals that transcend the immediacy of stimulus and response, a view that we owe to Shallice, Miller, and Cohen, among others.[70]

To test this theory, Koechlin and colleagues designed an imaging experiment in which human participants selected responses to three different types of cue, organized according to a hierarchy of temporal abstraction. The first level involved simple mappings between stimulus and response; the second required conditional action selection, with an immediately prior context signal that changed the S–R mapping, as in the broken traffic lights example; and the third level displaced the cue to an earlier time, with or without yet another layer of selection demand.[71] Given this task, it was possible to use the information theory to compute the *demand for control* associated with decisions made under each type of cue.

The authors found that response selection inevitably led to increases in BOLD signal in the premotor cortex, the most posterior aspect of the

---

[69] The terms 'rostral' and 'caudal' refer to positions along the axis of the neocortex. In the frontal lobes, the caudal areas are nearest to the middle (sulcus of Roland) where the motor cortex lies. The most rostral portions lie at the front, near the frontal pole.

[70] For the original paper, see (Koechlin et al. 2003). For a summary and review, see (Koechlin & Summerfield 2007). For related hierarchical theories of the PFC, see (Badre & D'Esposito 2009) and (Fine & Hayden 2022).

[71] As if, for example, I told you in advance that the traffic lights were broken, and so you should wait for a roadworker to signal when to proceed, and you maintained this instruction up to the point where you reached the lights. In the original paper, this type of control signal that is maintained across time was referred to as 'episodic', but this is potentially confusing because 'episodic memory' typically refers to long-term memory for past episodes.

254 The control of memory

frontal lobe, adjacent to the primary motor cortex. This is consistent with the well-known deficit that premotor lesions provoke deficits in movement and simple action selection, both in monkey lesion studies and in human neuropsychological patients.[72] However, when a response was selected on the basis of a contextual cue, there was *additional* BOLD activity in the caudal DLPFC (Brodmann's area 8). Only when the contextual cue was displaced back in time was there also activity in the rostral portion, or Brodmann's area 46, the human equivalent to the sulcus principalis region that had shown delay-period activity in the recording studies by Fuster, Goldman-Rakic, and Wallis (Figure 7.11).

This finding betrays a key principle for PFC organization, called *subsidiarity*. The most posterior regions were always active during task performance, even for simple action selection. Thus, Simone Biles needs a premotor cortex to execute a handstand. But the more anterior regions were additionally recruited only as required. Thus, to know where she has reached in her floor exercise routine, without mat position as a guide, the DLPFC is additionally active. At the most abstract level, to strategize about her overall approach to the competition, over the full time course of the games, the most anterior PFC regions come online. One speculation is that evolution has furnished primates with the ability to extend tasks over longer intervals through the successive addition of more anterior cortical real estate.

Time is fundamental to cognitive control because tasks are temporally structured, usually involving extended sequences of actions and events. Short-term memory is the glue that holds tasks together in time, so that information from early in the task is maintained to impact later choices. Thus, if you discover low prices at your favourite Prague hotel on a certain date, in the next subtask, you can choose your train tickets accordingly. Knowing that you have tightened the bolts on the bedframe, in the next subtask, you can then add the slats and mattress to your new bunk bed. The finding that increasingly anterior PFC regions integrate information over longer and longer spans to solve more and more complex tasks is, of course, compatible with the idea that the brain is wired as a series of recurrent loops with an increasing time constant. As proposed by these theories, information cascades across time to allow for behavioural control over multiple temporal scales.[73]

---

[72] See (Passingham & Wise 2012).
[73] For example, see (Murray et al. 2014).

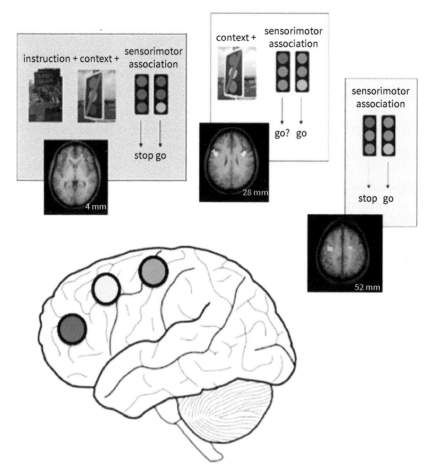

Fig. 7.11 Schematic illustration of the results from Koechlin (2003). The authors reported a rostro-caudal axis of control in the prefrontal cortex (PFC). Most caudally, the premotor cortex (green) codes for the demand for simple action selection, such as choosing stop vs go at a traffic light. More anteriorly, in the dorsolateral PFC (yellow), BOLD signals scale with the demand of context-mediated action selection, such as choosing to go through a red light when a sign indicates that the traffic lights are broken. Control that extends over longer time periods is associated with yet more rostral regions (red).

7.6 Banishing the homunculus

In the 2015 Pixar animated movie *Inside Out*, a young girl called Riley is going through turbulent times after her family move from rural Minnesota to the big city. The conceit of the film is that Riley's emotions are personified as characters inside her head, and that her behaviour depends on their choices about which levers to pull or buttons to press on a giant internal control panel. When the emotions make some dubious choices early in the film, things go haywire for Riley, and the rest of the story describes how the crisis first unravels and then is finally resolved.

Inside Out is a whimsical film, but it raises a serious question: who controls the controller? The characters inside Riley's head experience their own emotions and make their own voluntary choices, so according to the film's logic, they also have controllers in their head, who, in turn, need controllers—leading to an infinite regress. Similarly, theories of PFC function that appeal to control processes have long been critiqued for succumbing to the *homuncular fallacy*—a theoretical sleight of hand whereby complex decision-making is ascribed to 'little person' (or homunculus) who enjoys executive powers, without providing a concrete, mechanistic account of how decisions are made.[74] In the words of Tom Hazy, Michael Frank, and Randy O'Reilly in a seminal article from 2005, we need to *banish the homunculus*—and describe how memory and cognitive control actually work at the computational level.[75]

Consider a popular assay of frontal lobe function called the 1-2-AX task.[76] Participants view a sequence of numbers and letters, and the rules for responding to sequential letter pairs are modified by the occurrence of numbers. For example, following a 1, participants must respond to any X preceded by an A; whereas following a 2, a response is required to any Y preceded by a B. Thus, like in the Koechlin paradigm, actions must be selected after combining information from an (shorter) inner loop (was the last letter A or B?) and a (longer) outer loop (was the last digit 1 or 2?). This paradigm matches our conception of a task as a hierarchical action selection problem that unfolds in time.

A natural choice of computational tool for solving this type of problem is the recurrent neural network. In fact, although an RNN can learn to solve the 1-2-AX task by multiplexing information about the last letter and the last number in the recurrent weights, training it can be slow and unreliable. A more effective solution would associate each state not just with an action (via the readout weights), but also with internal operations that allow it to be *written to* (encoded), or *read from* (retrieved), a separate memory store. In

---

[74] Perhaps the best known of these is the nebulous concept of a 'central executive' in the classic model of working memory (Baddeley & Hitch 1974).

[75] Key papers from this group include these: (Hazy et al. 2006) and (O'Reilly & Frank 2006).

[76] This is an extension of the AX-CPT task, which was used in one of the very first papers showing that human BOLD signals in the PFC vary with short-term memory load (Cohen et al. 1997).

this way, some signals (e.g. the digit) could be cached over the longer term and only retrieved when needed, whereas other information could be constantly maintained in active memory using recurrent dynamics.

The architecture that embodies this principle was first described in 1997 and is among the most enduring tools in machine learning research.[77] It is called (somewhat oxymoronically) the long short-term memory (LSTM) architecture and was originally designed by the Swiss computer scientists Jürgen Schmidhuber and Seth Hochreiter to deal with the problem of vanishing gradients.[78] The LSTM rises to the challenge posed by environments—such as the 1-2-AX task—that exhibit dependencies over two or more timescales. In an LSTM cell, the hidden state units h are complemented by a second, parallel activation memory called the cell state c. The network learns to control gates which dynamically swap information between h and c on each timestep or erase (forget) information that is irrelevant to performing the task. This endows the LSTM with two memory states that can share information with each other across time, allowing control signals to be passed forward on two different timescales for task performance.

A common metaphor for the functioning of the PFC is that it behaves like a computer program. A program transforms input variables through a sequence of operations, often using recursion (maintaining and/or incrementing variables across cycles) or branching (switching variables in or out of different states according to contextual signals). One striking demonstration of the power of LSTM takes this metaphor literally. The researchers trained an LSTM to predict the latent state of variables from raw computer code written in the Python programming language. For example, if the input consists of:

```
j=8584
for x in range(8):
    j+=920 b=(1500+j)
print((b+7567))
```

then the target value should be 25011. The network did remarkably well, especially when combined with a curriculum that, like a class in coding school,

---

[77] As of 2022, the original publication has been cited more than 60,000 times—making it one of the most influential papers in the field.

[78] Schmidhuber has become a somewhat controversial figure in machine learning, due to his relentless self-publicization and strident claims of intellectual priority for many of the field's major advances. LSTMs are, however, truly one of the most historically significant contributions to AI research. Vanishing gradients occur during backpropagation when partial derivatives become numerically negligible when many small values are multiplied together during repeated application of the chain rule, as is necessary when training RNNs across multiple past timesteps.

begins with simple scripts and gradually ramps up in complexity.[79] As might be expected, the LSTM and related tools similarly have no trouble with the 1-2-AX task.

The LSTM was not built to model biology. Nevertheless, the gating function it proposes has inspired a number of computational theories of task learning in the PFC.[80] Perhaps the most elaborate and plausible is the 'Prefrontal Basal Ganglia Working Memory' (PBWM) model that was proposed by Michael Frank and colleagues.[81] As we have seen, PFC neurons maintain information via recurrent excitation, probably mediated both by thalamocortical loops and by intrinsic cortical connectivity. However, PFC neurons are prone to complex dynamics—seemingly allowing them to fulfil different roles at different times. For example, when a neuron is persistently coding for a stimulus in short-term memory, an irrelevant distracter can transiently activate the cell with a signal that fails to hijack its tonic firing. In other words, the cell switches from coding the relevant to the irrelevant stimulus, and back again. Relatedly, when a monkey is asked to report a stimulus identity and position in successive portions of the trial, the same PFC neurons represent both variables, changing their coding properties midway through the trial.[82] These observations are hard to reconcile with straightforward recurrent excitation alone. Instead, they imply that PFC neurons show *switching dynamics*, whereby they can switch between different coding schemes according to a latent contextual variables. These switching dynamics either could rely on intracellular mechanisms that modulate whether the cell is a strongly or weakly responsive mode or may be mediated by fast plastic mechanisms that occur at the synapse.

In the PBWM model, the PFC and basal ganglia work together to learn these switching dynamics. In the standard neurobiological portrait of learning by reinforcement, sensorimotor loops passing through the striatum are strengthened in the presence of dopamine-mediated reward prediction errors via three-factor learning rules, as discussed in Chapter 6. Here, however, dopamine acts to strengthen or weaken striatal signals that instead toggle information flow in the PFC, by enabling or disabling recurrent dynamics. PFC neurons are organized into a patchy topographic map in which nearby neurons have similar coding properties, referred to as stripes, and striatal

---

[79] See (Zaremba & Sutskever 2014). In fact, the curriculum that works best is one that sprinkles hard examples among the easy ones early in training. One of the authors of this paper Ilya Sutskever went on to be head of research at OpenAI.

[80] Including (Alexander & Brown 2018) and (Lloyd et al. 2012), as well as the Frank and O'Reilly model (O'Reilly & Frank 2006).

[81] Originally described here (Frank et al. 2001).

[82] See (Rao et al. 1997) and (Watanabe & Funahashi 2014).

signals may occur at the level of PFC stripes.[83] Thus, the striatum can act to set the switches in the PFC, so that information can be maintained, overwritten, or forgotten at appropriate times. The entire model can be trained using an actor–critic approach, with the striatal system taking actions and being critiqued by dopamine signals. Thus, in this model, the PFC gating mechanism is learnt in the striatum, rather than directly in the PFC.

Learning gating signals in this way can confer robustness on memories, especially for longer-term maintenance—which was the original motivation for Schmidhuber's LSTM. But another major benefit is the circumvention of a catch-22 that occurs when assigning credit to recurrent dynamics in short-term memory tasks. For persistent dynamics to be reinforced, they need to occur in the first place—but if they have not been reinforced, they will not occur. A standard RNN thus learns to bridge the perception–action cycle only very gradually. However, learning to open and close gates that enable or disable recurrence sidesteps this problem entirely. A simpler architecture that learns to gate in and out of memory using SARSA captures the way in which rats reverse between match and non-match rules in a maze task.[84]

One possible mechanism for gating relies on short-term synaptic plasticity. In one influential model of this process, a synaptic resource (such as a transmitter availability) can build up and deplete across the delay period, acting as an independent memory repository that does not require spiking activity. In fact, the resource goes through a cycle of depletion (by spike generation) and replenishment (in the refractory period) which keeps memories in an oscillating latent state during delay, and with biologically realistic parameters, the frequency of this rhythm is about 4–8 Hz, precisely matching the (theta) frequency of oscillatory activity that has been observed during the delay period of short-term memory studies. The model is more robust to noise than variants based on attractor states. It could thus be that the maintenance processes underlying memory and control processes rely on 'activity-silent' states forged with fast synaptic plasticity.[85]

This theory is tricky to test empirically, but one line of support has come from human brain imaging studies. The neuroscientist Mark Stokes and

---

[83] See the work from Jennifer Lund's group at UCL, using staining methods to track patterns of intrinsic connectivity (Levitt et al. 1993). These are reminiscent of the *hypercolumns* observed in the early visual cortex, whereby neurons with similar orientation selectivity are found in close proximity, that were originally discovered by Hubel and Wiesel.

[84] See (Lloyd et al. 2012).

[85] For this model, see (Mongillo et al. 2008). For a review, see (Barak & Tsodyks 2014). For a comprehensive introduction to 'activity-silent' activity, see (Stokes 2015).

his team cued human participants to remember one of two gratings across a delay period and used multivariate methods to assess the moment-by-moment stimulus representation of both cued and uncued gratings in electroencephalographic (EEG) signals. The cued stimulus representation died away over the delay period but could be revived with a 'pinging' stimulus—a blast of energy provided by a random visual event which occurred unexpectedly during the delay period. This is consistent with the idea that synapses, not spikes, were responsible for maintaining the memory, and thus with a gating account. A similar reawakening of latent working memories in BOLD has been reported when transcranial magnetic stimulation is applied during the delay period.[86]

Gating thus is almost certainly part of the brain's computational repertoire and may be critical to cognitive processes involving memory and control. Simultaneously, it is a major algorithmic innovation that has allowed AI systems to share information effectively over longer time periods and to train faster and more stably. LSTMs were, until very recently, the tool of choice for all complex machine learning applications, from sentence prediction in NLP and variable prediction in computer code to complex strategic control in dynamic games such as StarCraft. However, in 2017, AI researchers discovered a more sophisticated algorithmic component, known as the transformer, that tends to outperform the LSTM in almost every domain.

On a first reading, the sentence 'the old man the boat' does not make grammatical sense—it seems to be lacking a verb. But on a second glance, it is, in fact, legitimate, because in English, 'man' can be a verb as well as a noun (as in 'to crew the boat'). Misleadingly, sentences beginning with 'the old man' usually have an elderly male human as their subject. This type of sentence is called a garden path sentence, because it initially leads you astray,[87] and to grasp the meaning of a garden path sentence, you have to mentally restructure it after the event, revising your interpretation of individual words.

The LSTM allows information to be gated in and out of its cell state, affording sophisticated control over memory. But it has an important limitation: it processes sequences of data (words, music, or images) item by item, and so it cannot revise its past activation states on the basis of new information. Thus,

---

[86] See (Rose et al. 2016) and (Wolff et al. 2017).
[87] Or up the garden path.

if it has discarded some part of its memory—using the *forget* gate—then it cannot later go back and retrieve it. However, as seen with garden path sentences, even sophisticated agents (like humans) can be initially misled, and thus benefit from being able to retrospectively revise and reweigh information they have been given in the past.

This is exactly what a transformer permits. The transformer buffers its inputs and dynamically reweighs them using a process called self-attention, which allows outputs to depend on the unfolding context. Thus, in the clause 'the child ate the cake because it …', an LSTM will always process the word 'it' in the same way. However, a transformer can retrospectively, and on-the-fly, change its encoding of 'it' according to whether the sentence continues '… was hungry' (meaning 'it' refers to the child) or '… was delicious' ('it' refers to the cake). The transformer thus has a significant advantage in predicting the next chunk of text, because it can revise the weight given to 'child' and 'cake' according to the subsequently revealed context. Interestingly, to achieve this, the transformer explicitly learns separate mapping functions for each item (e.g. cake) and position (e.g. fifth word in the input phrase). By explicitly encoding both position and item, transformers can effectively learn to factorize 'what' the input is and 'where' it is in the input stream, allowing it to explicitly encode the relations between words. One possibility is that it is this encoding of item and position—or objects and space—that gives transformers their remarkable ability to seemingly compose new meaning in text and image.

The transformer is the reason for the startling success of foundation models such as GPT-3 and Gopher, and has widespread application beyond NLP. Currently, for example, state-of-the-art performance on ImageNet is dominated by approaches that use *vision transformers* to model the relations between pixels in an image, and Tesla is currently using transformers for processing image data in their driverless cars.[88] Transformers will probably continue to shape progress in AI research for some time, but it remains to be seen whether the computations they perform have a plausible counterpart in biology.[89]

---

[88] The original transformer paper is this one (Vaswani et al. 2017). The first vision transformer model, released in late 2020, is this one (Dosovitskiy et al. 2021). For some reflections on transformers and biology, see (Mumford 2020).
[89] Although see (Whittington et al. 2021).

7.7 Learning simple programs

The celebrated anthropologist Jared Diamond trained as a medical student before gravitating to the field of ornithology. It was the study of birds that first took him to Papua New Guinea, where he met people whose culture was radically different to his own—and yet strangely familiar too. As he recounts in his bestselling book *The World Until Yesterday*, many of the New Guinea Highlander practices that initially seem unfathomable—their taboos about relationships, feasting rituals, marriage practices, or trade systems—have recognizable counterparts in the Western world. For example, if one native hurts another in an accident, a formalized ceremony involving the affected parties allowed for compensation to be paid and relationships to be re-established. This practice can help forestall a costly blood feud between indignant parties, much as the Western courtroom trial is an act of theatre geared at providing the aggrieved with justice and bringing closure to an event.[90]

Thus, whilst many situations Diamond encountered were alien to him, they involved familiar concepts such as bartering, greeting, feasting, and warfare. Even if the native people behaved in unexpected ways, their activities shared a common structure and purpose with those in the West. Diamond was thus able to reuse task knowledge obtained on the streets of his native downtown Los Angeles to adapt to life in the highlands of Papua New Guinea. This ability to perform tasks in novel environments by recycling knowledge about how to achieve goals is a critical component for any general AI system. And yet, it is an area where AI research has so far made only limited progress.

As we have seen, recurrence and gating in memory systems allow agents to learn sophisticated control policies. How, then, do intertwined memory and control processes allow agents to adapt rapidly to new tasks? In recent years, machine learning researchers have tackled this challenge by building deep networks that are able to *learn how to learn*.

Recall that Harlow's monkeys were able to learn each new bandit task faster than the last, even though they involved entirely novel objects.[91] The rapid progress that monkeys made on each new bandit problem—with performance eventually plateauing after just a single trial—is in sharp contrast to that of deep networks, which are bedevilled by sluggish learning and a hunger for data. Harlow conjectured that with repeated exposure to many tasks with similar structure, the monkeys had learnt how to learn.[92] Recent work has

---

[90] See (Diamond 2012).
[91] See Chapter 4.
[92] Harlow called it *learning set*.

suggested that learning to learn may be a ubiquitous feature of natural intelligence, exhibited even in the mouse, a small mammal with a rudimental
neocortex. For example, when confronted with successive tasks in which new
odours predict rewards with a shared temporal sequence, or when performing
different reversal learning problems encountered in novel spatial layouts,
neural populations in the mouse frontal cortex encoded abstract components
(or schemas) that were shared across tasks, such as the need to alternate responses on a certain schedule, irrespective of odour or position.[93]

In machine learning, 2016 brought a sudden flurry of interest in meta-
learning—the training of deep networks to learn how to learn.[94] One simple,
but effective, approach is to first learn a good initialization for the network, so
that learning a new task reduces to fine tuning from weights set to propitious
values. This is perhaps similar to how evolution sculpts the innate connections
in biological brains, so that neonates can quickly form useful representations
like place cells and face representations, preparing them for inevitable real-
world challenges like navigation and social interaction.[95] An alternative, and
arguably more sophisticated, approach is to meta-learn a control policy for
memory, so that a network can rapidly adapt to new problems on the fly using
the activation dynamics in its recurrent units.[96] Married with an RL objective,
this method is known as meta-RL, and it holds great promise for AI research.
One algorithm, proposed in a paper led by Jane Wang from DeepMind, was
directly inspired by theories of learning in biological brains, and especially the
neurophysiology of the PFC.

To understand how meta-RL works, it is helpful to formalize our definition
of *task* in the context of a typical laboratory study where stimuli elicit actions
leading to rewards over a sequence of discrete trials. Here, we can think of a
task as fully described by how stimuli and actions (and their interactions) map
to outcomes over successive trials. For example, in a 2-back memory task, the
outcome on trial t depends on whether the agent faithfully responds that the
current stimulus matches that on trial $t - 2$ or not. Absent explicit instruction,
and provided with sufficient examples of stimulus, action, and outcome his-
tories, an agent should eventually be able to learn the rule and successfully
perform the task. The principle of meta-learning is that an RNN exposed to
many such task examples (during *meta-training*) will eventually learn to use
the evolving history of actions and outcomes (held in recurrent memory) for

---

[93] See (Samborska et al. 2021) and (Zhou et al. 2021).
[94] This interest was built on earlier work (Hochreiter et al. 2001).
[95] See (Finn et al. 2017).
[96] See (Duan et al. 2016) and (Wang et al. 2017).

a similar *new* task, to begin to respond correctly as the trials progress. Thus, having performed a myriad of tasks that require matching one step back (1-back) and three steps back (3-back), the agent can use the history of outcomes incurred by its actions over successive trials to infer that this time it is supposed to be performing a 2-back task. During its training, the agent is not learning to perform any single task or even a fixed distribution of tasks. It is learning how to learn new tasks that it has never seen before.

Typically, at the core of the meta-RL agent is an LSTM that receives as inputs both the current stimulus and the history of actions and rewards, and is trained using policy gradient methods to predict the state and action values. Interestingly, when monkeys perform a bandit task, PFC neurons code for the history of actions, rewards, and their interaction—the very information that is needed for meta-learning. Like monkeys performing the bandit task, the meta-RL agent can use this history to construct a choice signal that allows it to optimally trade off exploration with exploitation, by tailoring response frequencies to the probability of reward (matching) and adjusting the rate at which it learns to match the volatility in the environment.[97] It was also able to perform reward-guided learning tasks where the value of some stimuli could only be inferred from the correlation structure of the task. For example, in a task by Bromberg-Martin and colleagues, monkeys inferred that because saccade to one location was rewarded, the other was not, or vice versa.[98] Meta-RL displayed the same pattern of behaviour and even exhibited reward prediction errors that resembled those in the monkeys. Learning that the value of one object can be learnt from another is, of course, the essence of the Harlow task, and meta-RL was able to faithfully recreate the accelerating learning over many novel tasks that is the central feature of Harlow's data.

Consistent with the definition provided by Legg and Hutter, the meta-learning approach commits to a picture of intelligence as solving a succession of tasks. During meta-training, the network is optimized to find a sample-efficient adaptive strategy for a broad distribution of problems. Harnessing the power of function approximation that is intrinsic to deep learning, it then generalizes this strategy to new tasks that are sampled from the same distribution. In fact, we know that for a wide range of circumstances, meta-trained agents discover Bayes optimal solutions, in which the prior for a new task is a weighted mixture of past experience. For example, after training on a succession of bandit tasks, the meta-learner acquires a policy that optimally trades off exploration and exploitation, selecting actions according to the highest

---

[97] See (Tsutsui et al. 2016) and (Behrens et al. 2007).
[98] See (Bromberg-Martin et al. 2010).

Gittins index per timestep.[99] In a different setting, meta-trained agents can learn to represent a distribution over a family of functions, so that they can adapt rapidly to fit new data, mimicking the flexibility and data efficiency of probabilistic approaches such as Gaussian processes.[100]

In Chapter 3, we discussed a tradition for AI research that relies on symbol manipulation and compositional cognition, including the use of probabilistic computation to infer the structure of a generative process for tasks (i.e. the grammar that generates data produced by a formal language). In parallel, machine learning researchers have asked whether deep learning can be trained to compose and interpret structured programs for complex behaviours. One interesting example of this is training deep networks to perform mathematical operations, including arithmetic, algebra, and numerical sorting. Because maths is a tightly structured systems requiring a high degree of precision ($17 + 17 = 3.4$ is not 'nearly right'), it is challenging to learn with unrestricted gradient descent. This means that even sophisticated architectures, such as transformers, often give plausible-sounding, but incorrect, answers.[101] In humans, mathematical cognition relies on the implementation of a series of structured operations that require storing and retrieving exact numerical values in working memory, rather than learning to guesstimate a quantity by summarizing a long history of examples.[102]

Over recent years, a method known as *neural program induction* (NPI) has been developed to tackle this class of problem. In NPI, a neural controller (usually an LSTM) learns to issue instructions conditional on the current execution state of a program. These instructions have predetermined semantics that can transform the program state, allowing the network to learn to perform a structured sequence of operations on data. The system can thus learn either via supervised learning to imitate a teacher executing a program or with RL to maximize metrics for accuracy and efficiency. NPI has been applied to domains such as sorting numbers, searching lists, or combinatorial optimization problems such as the knapsack problem.[103]

A familiar feature of NPI systems is the ability to read and write to an external (often content-addressable) memory, storing information in

---

[99] See (Mikulik et al. 2020).

[100] See (Garnelo et al. 2018).

[101] For example, factorizing 235232673 as 3, 11, 13, 19, 23, 1487 (the correct answer is 3, 13, 19, 317453). See (Saxton et al. 2019). Although transformer-based foundation models are getting much better at maths, including maths word problems (Cobbe et al. 2021).

[102] See (Menon 2016).

[103] A resource allocation problem such as that faced by an air traveller in which a set of items with different weights and values are chosen to maximize utility whilst not exceeding a weight limit placed on their luggage.

dedicated slots where required, much like the hard disk of a computer with von Neumann's architecture. This choice is naturally inspired by Turing's proposal for a universal computer that writes to, and reads from, a ticker tape of infinite length. One such system, called the differentiable neural computer (DNC), learnt to control *read* and *write* heads to store information in structured ways in addressable memory. It was able to solve intricate sequential control problems, such as planning a route through the London Tube system after viewing a single instance of the map in symbolic form (along with a start and destination station). The DNC was even able to learn end-to-end to solve a version of SHRDLU, a paradigmatic challenge for classic AI in which blocks are manipulated according to verbal instructions.[104]

As we saw with Bayesian program learning, the central question for NPI is what the primitive program elements should be. For example, one report showed that many architectures fail to meet the challenge of generalizing from simple problems (such as $2 + 4 = 6$ and $3 \times 5 = 15$) to more complex ones ($4 + 3 + 5 \times 7 = 42$), and proposes that recursion should itself be a building block for program induction.[105] Another approach scaffolds computation by endowing the program with function calls, but without specifying the contents of each function. This allows the program to 'divide and conquer' a task, breaking it down into subroutines in a way that encourages reusability and composition, and led to stronger forms of generalization.[106]

A traditional conception of memory is as a storage system, in which useful information can be deposited for future use. Across this chapter, however, we have encountered a different view, in which memory is a sophisticated adaptation to the control system that releases action selection from the immediacy of the current senses. Memory processes serve up information from the past to control processes, and reward learning shapes the way in which information is encoded, maintained, and retrieved over time. This allows agents to solve theoretical computational challenges, such as grounding behaviour on a single event (one-shot learning), partitioning knowledge between different temporal contexts without catastrophic interference (continual learning), and reusing past knowledge to adapt to new tasks (meta-learning).

In earlier chapters, we encountered a theoretical distinction that has powerfully impacted how neuroscientists think about learning and decision-making: that between model-free and model-based processes. A model-free

---

[104] The DNC was adapted from an architecture called the Neural Turing Machine. See (Graves et al. 2016).

[105] See (Cai et al. 2017).

[106] See (Li et al. 2020).

agent learns a value function from experience, by taking repeated actions and sharing value estimates between states that were experienced in close proximity. A model-based agent uses knowledge of the transition structure of the environment (a 'model of the world') to mentally simulate possible courses of action and their outcomes, leveraging these offline calculations to decide how to act. It is interesting to note that this distinction becomes blurred once agents are equipped with sophisticated forms of memory, such as those we have met in this chapter. This is because in conjunction with RL methods, memory processes allow agents to share value estimates between current and past states in flexible ways. For example, one-shot learning and continual learning allow credit to be assigned to specific instances in the past or to temporal episodes defined by a contextual variable. Meta-learning agents—even with wholly model-free training—are able to learn an adaptable control policy that generalizes to new tasks, behaving as if they were forging new plans on the fly.

This is vividly revealed by the patterns of behaviour that meta-trained agents display when confronted with standard assays of model-based inference from the psychology literature.[107] A well-known probe for model-based decision-making is known as the two-step task. The two-step task is a modified bandit paradigm in which rewards are only reached after choosing two successive actions that move the participant through a miniature non-spatial maze. Making the first transition probabilistic allows researchers to distinguish between model-based and model-free accounts of behaviour following expected and unexpected transitions. A purely model-free participant, who ignores the transition structure, should repeat successful actions, irrespective of whether the first transition was expected or unexpected. A model-based agent should learn that if a positive outcome occurs from an unexpected (low-probability) transition, then reward will most likely be maximized by choosing an alternate action on the next trial. In practice, human participants show a mixture of model-free and model-based behaviours, with various factors shifting the balance between these strategies, including age, stress, dopaminergic medication, and the cover story used to explain the task.[108] Extensive use of this task has cemented the distinction between model-free and model-based learning in the neuroscience literature.

However, meta-RL agents trained in a fully model-free fashion solve the two-step task, displaying a pattern of behaviour that closely resembles that of

---

[107] See (Daw et al. 2005) and (Dolan & Dayan 2013).
[108] For the original task, see (Daw et al. 2011). Dopamine makes you more model-based (Wunderlich et al. 2012). Stress makes you less so (Otto & Gershman 2013). Children become more model-based as they mature (Decker et al. 2016). People become much more model-based if you provide a comprehensible cover story (Feher da Silva & Hare 2020).

humans. They are able to do this because they have learnt a control policy that maximizes, contingent on the history of actions and observations from comparable games. The meta-RL agent also captured human behaviours on other tasks that cannot be solved with vanilla TD learning, such as a bandit paradigm in which the volatility (rate of change of the latent bandit values) was itself a stochastic variable.[109] One interesting future question for neuroscientists is whether purported signatures of model-based inference are, in fact, just a product of sophisticated memory and control processes that depend on the primate PFC.[110]

---

[109] See (Behrens et al. 2007). These results are reported in (Wang et al. 2018a).
[110] (Botvinick et al. 2019).

8

A picture of the mind

8.1 Where is my mind?

One of A. A. Milne's much-loved stories about Winnie the Pooh begins with Christopher Robin announcing that the friends are going on an 'expotition' to find the North Pole. They round up the other animals and set off, and after some distance has been travelled, their provisions have been eaten, and a nasty thistle narrowly avoided (except by the morose donkey Eeyore), the story continues:

> Rabbit and Christopher Robin have wandered a little way up the stream to have a private conversation, because Christopher Robin is not entirely sure what a North Pole would look like if you were standing right in front of one, and he wants to ask Rabbit's advice. They both say that they used to know, although now they've forgotten, but then they decide that it must be just a pole stuck in the ground, and hence the name.

The problem that the animals face is a familiar one. When setting out to find something, it is important to know what you are looking for.

AI researchers hope to discover how to build AGI. The problem is that nobody really knows exactly what an AGI would look like. What would it be able to do? What purpose would it have? What form would it take, and under what constraints would it operate? Is the goal to build something that lives on your phone and doles out advice in natural language? Is it an embodied robot that is able to do your laundry and walk the dog? Or is it an algorithm embedded in our societal infrastructure to solve complex optimization problems, such as coordinating a fleet of autonomous vehicles, running a scientific research laboratory, or stabilizing the economy by holding the reins of macroeconomic policy? Should we aim to build a single agent that can do all of these things, or a suite of more narrow technologies, each tailored for a single problem?

Lacking a singular vision for the Singularity, AI researchers have instead turned to human generality as a blueprint. Humans are not constrained to perform a single, narrow task. A human could give sensible advice to her sister

Natural General Intelligence. Christopher Summerfield, Oxford University Press. © Oxford University Press 2023.
DOI: 10.1093/oso/9780192843883.003.0008

on the phone whilst commuting back from her job at the World Bank, and then take the dog for a walk before bed. In fact, for some people, these would be perfectly routine daily activities, a far cry from the mind-bending feats of strategy or abstraction that grandmasters display when competing for world titles in StarCraft or Go. This is the bewildering paradox at the heart of AI research: that many activities that humans find impossibly hard turn out to be relatively simple to solve with enough computation, whereas the basics—performing mundane chores and dispensing common sense advice—are way beyond the reach of even our most sophisticated current AI systems.

Since the 1950s, the vision for general AI has ebbed and flowed. In each era, the animating force was an implicit theory of the computational process that makes people smart. In the age of classical AI, research was framed by the vestiges of positivist philosophy, in which the critical human faculty was the ability to use formal systems to work out what was true. The earliest pioneers fashioned AI in the image of early twentieth-century luminaries like Russell and Frege, who sought to rebuild our systems of thought in the language of logic. However, by the 1970s, it began to dawn that most humans are, in fact, quite unreliable logicians.[1] Instead, the focus shifted to our privileged ability to communicate in natural language: a highly structured, generative, open-ended system for sharing ideas. Over the next decades, many AI researchers instead tried to ground intelligence in the human capacity for drawing inferences using semantic knowledge. Serious attempts were made to build systems that could solve general problems by reasoning from means to end, using hand-coded fact bases and inference engines, or clever heuristics that make planning tractable in very large search spaces. This led to the advent of expert systems and the genesis of algorithms such alpha-beta search, which drove the success of Deep Blue at Chess at the end of the twentieth century.

In the modern era, deep learning has come to the fore. Deep neural networks learn complex discriminative or generative functions from training data and transfer performance to novel settings. With the rise of deep learning, the focus has again shifted. Deep learning models meld computation and memory, so that the power of their inference is enmeshed with their knowledge of the world. To handle novel settings, neural networks need to grasp information in the most general way possible, which means representing maximally invariant concepts. Thus, the prevailing vision of human intelligence has turned again on its axis, and now it seems that the signature human mental ability is to learn and generalize abstractions. People know that

---

[1] See the discussion of heuristics and biases below.

keys open doors, that snakes bite, and that gold is valuable; they thus still hold their own against deep RL systems playing Montezuma's Revenge. Humans know that objects can be grasped, that people feel pain, and that yesterday is gone forever. They grasp that *equality* is relevant both when paying taxes and when dividing cakes, that *tsunami* can refer to a terrifying wave of water or a burdensome torrent of e-mails, and that *higher* can refer to a relationship in space, or quality, or society. People can even compose new understanding from existing building blocks of semantic knowledge—without ever having thought about it before, we can infer that there are no elephants on Jupiter, that vampires do not like pesto, and that Aristotle never owned a laptop.

In parallel with the advance of neural networks, researchers have devised RL methods that motivate agents to learn to solve problems for themselves. This subfield has drawn inspiration from a long tradition in psychology and animal learning that has envisaged behaviour as an attempt to reap rewards, satisfy needs, and obey drives. It places front and central our powerful motivation to meet the demands of both our bodies and the local environment. These signals drive us to seek out hedonic signals from primary reinforcers such as food, sex, and warmth. But we also create sophisticated goals for ourselves—to reach that destination, beat that personal best, or finish writing that book—generating internal motivational signals that urge us onwards towards these milestones. The RL framework for intelligence is more ambitious than its rivals. It seeks to explain the breadth of motivated animal behaviour, from the circumscribed habits of simple animals like flies and worms to the intricate policies by which humans try to realize their basest desires and loftiest dreams in the spheres of family, friends, work, and leisure.

Thus, the twin projects of understanding the mind and building a brain have historically gone hand in hand. We see in natural intelligence a vision for what AI could be: its potential for versatility, robustness, and creativity. And yet, opinion is divided. Is studying natural general intelligence a pathway towards building AGI? Will simple algorithmic solutions suffice, if they are scaled to the proportions of biological computation, with billions of neurons and trillions of connections? Or is there a special ingredient or combination of ingredients that natural intelligence enjoys, but that AI is currently missing? Do we need to build agents that form richer abstractions for strong generalization, that learn rapidly from minimal experience, or that can infer causation, exhibit curiosity, plan deeper, or display metacognition? Are there algorithms, architectures, or cognitive functions that give humans their generality, but that current AI systems lack?

8.2 Inductive biases

AI researchers and cognitive scientists continue to be divided by the question of whether knowledge obtained from the study of natural intelligence is relevant for building AGI. This issue and the clash of views it provokes have been discussed across this book.[2] Should the computations in our AI systems be hand-engineered by the researcher or learnt from experience? Should we populate the minds of our agents with dedicated constraints (or *inductive biases*) that are tailored to solve the problems that the agent is likely to encounter? Alternatively, should we take simplicity as our mantra and search for a single, undifferentiated principle or algorithm that can be scaled to massive proportions with galaxies of parameters and gallons of computation? In the modern era, the neurosymbolic architectures that IBM has used to compete at college debating championships and TV quiz shows are most emblematic of the former approach. The giant foundation models for natural language and image processing—in which a single computational tool, the transformer, is replicated millions of times—are the epitome of the latter.

As we saw, AI research was conceived in the former tradition but, in maturity, has gravitated towards the latter. Over for the past 10 years, the theoretical winds have blown powerfully towards systems, with minimal inductive biases. We want AI systems that learn about verbs and about faces, but the prevailing view is that we should not build modules that are wired to process the structure of sentences or arrangements of anatomical features. Instead, it is claimed, we need maximally generic algorithms that allow agents to acquire computation for themselves by learning from data. Knowledge about faces and verbs may *emerge* during training, but so could knowledge about tools and adjectives or about buildings and declensions. These unstructured systems thus offer not only the virtue of simplicity, but also the promise of maximally general solutions. This promise has paid off in practice. For example, after eye-popping successes in the domain of NLP, the transformer was rapidly generalized to multimodal data (mapping from text to image, and back again). By contrast, IBM's DeepQA system will never do more than answer questions—because it is tailored exclusively to that task. This motivates the pursuit of maximally neat, simple, and general solutions espoused by Sutton's *bitter lesson*.

---

[2] Especially in Chapter 2.

In psychology, exactly the same debate between advocates of *nativist* and *empiricist* theories of the mind has played out across the history of the discipline. These opposing views have risen and fallen from vogue in predictable alternation. The empiricist tradition, which dates back to Locke, sees the neonatal brain as a blank slate, ready to take its shape from the impress of the world. It found its first radical expression in the behaviourist movement of the early twentieth century, when psychologists conceived of behaviour as driven entirely by learning from reward. The later rise of cognitivism, in the era of Chomsky, Marr, and Fodor, unseated this view with a nativist rallying cry that emphasized the inevitability of language development, the hardwired structure of information processing, and the modularity of the mind. However, empiricism resurged in the 1980s, when connectionist modellers argued that the brain is initialized *tabula rasa*, allowing a maximally general set of skills and knowledge to be acquired over the training provided by the lifespan. The turn towards Bayesian models of perception and cognition in the early 2000s cut a path back to nativism, by focussing on rational inference without large-scale parameter estimation. Thus, for a century or more, psychology has danced a theoretical jig from one pole to the other of the nativist-empiricist debate.

Today, the nativist–empiricist wheel of fortune is turning again in psychology and neuroscience. The renaissance of connectionism in the form of powerful deep learning has piqued biologists' interest in undifferentiated processing systems. Biological brains are themselves multibillion parameter neural networks, which display simple, endlessly reduplicated computational motifs, such as the canonical microcircuit in the mammalian neocortex. Should we also see biological brains as monolithic processing architectures? Has evolution itself cleaved to the warning of the bitter lesson?

A resurgent idea is that our neurobiological theories are convenient fictions that serve to bend massive, messy parallel processing into recognizable form. This argument takes its cue from observations that weakly structured deep networks are currently our best model for explaining neural representation in the ventral stream of primates and humans. In the sensory neocortex, like in deep networks, computation seems to be messy and hard to interpret at the level of single neurons or local circuits. Thus, the idea has begun to circulate that hard-fought theories of brain organization and function—founded on a trove of evidence that neurons code for faces, or task rules, or spatial locations—might, in fact, be 'just-so' stories. Neuroscientists may be prone to reading complex, high-dimensional neural signals like tea leaves—optimistically finding structured coding patterns that do not actually exist. As the Princeton neuroscientist Uri Hasson has put it:

> Both [artificial and biological neural networks] produce solutions that are mistakenly interpreted in terms of elegant design principles but in fact reflect the interdigitation of 'mindless' optimization processes and the structure of the world.

This is quite a claim. We have heard the case for 'mindless' optimization in machine learning, and here it is repeated in neurobiology. Put simply, Hasson's argument is that neural computation is itself largely unstructured. However, signals from the natural world are highly organized, and so the illusion of structured computation occurs as they refract through biological networks and are read out in neural recording experiments.[3]

Neuroscientists are undoubtedly prone to see their experimental results through an optimistic lens. It is also true that the six-layer neocortex—a brain structure found only in mammals—has a repeating local circuit motif. But as we have seen, this idea that the brain is simple and undifferentiated is hard to defend. Biological brains are made up of a mosaic of functionally distinct regions, populated by an army of different cell types that exchange signals using a rainbow of different transmitters and peptides. All animals— irrespective of their bodies, habitat, or niche—exhibit brains with an intricate neurofunctional design that is strikingly conserved across healthy individuals of that species. Humans differ in many ways—we may have darker or lighter skin, speak Japanese or Portuguese, and live in the Arctic tundra or the Namibian desert. But all healthy people have a hippocampus, a cerebellum, and a thalamus. Even within the neocortex, neuroimaging studies have shown that patterns of regional specialization are striking conserved across individuals. Evolution has thus placed remarkably strict constraints on how the brain is organized. In natural intelligence, computation does not emerge blindly from the imprint of data alone. It is shaped by fundamental design principles that have been sculpted by natural selection playing out in deep evolutionary time.

Across previous chapters, we have traversed the contours of this diversity. It is seeded from the basal ganglia and hippocampus, core neural structures that have been conserved for half a billion years, phenotypes that allowed the first vertebrates to learn associations between stimuli, actions, and outcomes. In mammals, these regions share stereotyped patterns of connectivity with

---

[3] See (Richards et al. 2019), (McClelland et al. 2010), and (Hasson et al. 2020).

the neocortex, forming a dynamic partnership that allows animals to learn habitual actions, engage in sequential motor behaviours, form memories over multiple timescales, process objects in space, and represent the world in meaningful ways.

From this heterogenous brain structure springs our unique cognitive fingerprint, combining perception, attention, memory, language, and control. In the 1950s, Karl Lashley proposed the principle of mass action—the view that the brain is an undifferentiated processing device, with each zone contributing monolithically to intelligence. However, Lashley was wrong. Decades of neuropsychological evidence have since shone a light on the modular nature of the brain, with localized patterns of damage provoking extremely specialized patterns of impairment. For example, circumscribed lesions can cause an inability to recognize faces, animals, or inanimate objects;[4] failure to assume ownership of one's own body parts; generation of semantically incoherent sentences; specific impairments of gait and balance; an inability to lay down memories for autobiographical events; difficulties with planning or dealing with novelty; and unwillingness to voluntarily take any actions at all, despite no physical barriers to doing so.[5] This vivid patchwork of regional specialization implies that the brain has evolved solutions that are tailored to the stereotyped problems that the natural world produces.

Today only pockets of renegades cling to the fully fledged vision of symbolic AI that was articulated by Newell and Simon in their 1975 Turing Lecture. However, critics of deep learning—those who are quickest to highlight its unreliable image labelling, nonsensical dialogue, and failures of basic common sense—often appeal loosely to something that sounds like classical AI as an alternative. In the closing chapters of *Rebooting AI*, for example, Gary Marcus finds himself proposing that:

> Common sense needs to start with [...] either formal logic or some alternative that does similar work, which is to say a way of clearly and unambiguously representing all the stuff that ordinary people know.

Marcus' argument is that evolution has tailored the brain for the world, and that AI researchers should embrace the nativist tradition and do likewise. Drawing on the work of developmental psychologists, such as Elizabeth

---

[4] Whilst most prosopagnosic patients have difficulty recognizing people (such as their spouse), but not animals (such as their pets), for at least one patient, the converse was true (Bornstein et al. 1969).

[5] Respectively: somatoparaphrenia, Wernicke's aphasia, bradykinesia, anterograde amnesia, executive dysfunction, and akinetic mutism.

Spelke, Alison Gopnik, and Susan Carey, he argues that human children are born with *cognitive start-up tools* that allow core functions to develop with dogged inevitability. These include strong prior assumptions about how time, space, and objects interact, and powerful tendencies to pay attention to biologically and socially relevant stimuli, and a predilection for language, casual inference, and theory of mind. His claim is that the shortcomings of current AI systems—their narrowness, brittleness, and sample inefficiency—can be mitigated by building in better inductive biases. Marcus has been criticized for failure to propose plausible alternatives to the current cult of simplicity.[6] However, he is not alone in harbouring a sense of unease with the tidy vision that one generic master algorithm (or simple cost function) will ultimately rule them all. Depending on your viewpoint, this nativist vision offers either a refreshing counterweight to a monochrome empiricist view in current AI research or a naive throwback to the failed methods of a century past.

Thus, we have a conundrum. Natural intelligence, our existence of proof for generality, relies on inborn computation implemented in highly stereotyped neural circuits. However, AI researchers claim that the field has consistently advanced by shedding inductive biases and allowing big data and computation to work their magic. So what gives? Unfortunately, this debate between AI nativists and empiricists has morphed from a sober academic debate into something of a heated culture war, in which protagonists on either side talk past each other in mutual incomprehension. However, if we take a closer look, there may be more agreement than is commonly realized.

Firstly, it is unclear whether the algorithmic purity that epitomises the empiricist view is, in fact, a real driver of progress, as the *bitter lesson* proposes. Strident empiricists argue that inbuilt inductive biases hold back research, drawing their lesson from the history of AI. One popular refrain is a quote attributed to Fred Jelinek, a pioneer of NLP at IBM: 'Every time I fire a linguist, the performance of the speech recognizer goes up'. As the field embraced deep learning and rejected the baggage of hand-engineered computation, AI's most sacred milestones began to tumble. However, these coincidences of these two variables need not imply that they are causally related. Instead, they could both be driven by a third confounding factor. A plausible culprit is that over the same time period, computational power has increased a trillionfold and massive sources of digital data have become available from the internet. Thus, the fact that empiricism has stolen the zeitgeist in AI research need not be the cause of the field's progress—perhaps yet stronger inductive biases really do

---

[6] He has also not helped his own case by combining a combative style with a certain naivety about what neural networks can and cannot be expected to do.

help AI progress, but they are masked by the historical trend that as AI philosophy has tended towards empiricism, it has been powered by digital technologies that have advanced beyond measure. If this is the case, then stern warnings about not repeating the errors of symbolic AI are, in fact, simply exhortations to not revisit a bygone era of punch cards and vacuum tubes. This is a view that presumably everyone can get behind.

The main issue, however, seems as always to be a basic disagreement about the nature of the problem itself. Nativists like Marcus argue that progress in AI research is held back by a reluctance to build in strong inductive biases. But in fact, machine learning researchers are constantly developing new inductive biases, and this creativity is undoubtedly the critical engine of progress in the field.

One reason that we cannot avoid inductive bias is that the yardstick of performance in machine learning research is always the ability to generalize from training to test. By focussing on held-out evaluation conditions, AI researchers sensibly prime their agents for deployment in a world where all experiences are novel and all challenges unfamiliar. Once released in the wild, agents will not perform a single, narrow task that has been written down by the researcher but face the unknown 'meta-task' that is set by the demands of an uncertain future. However, there is a basic principle, familiar to all AI researchers, that sometimes goes unvoiced in this debate. There are an infinite number of equally viable ways to solve an optimization problem, and thus a limitless number of routes to meeting the objective provided by the training data. This means that it is impossible to assert that any algorithmic approach—from the scruffiest to the neatest—is better or worse unless you consider the nature of the generalization problem that the network will ultimately tackle.[7]

This intuition was neatly exposed in a paper from 2016, in which the authors showed that it is perfectly possible to train deep convolutional networks to convergence on ImageNet, even after randomly shuffling the object labels. The network simply learns an extremely convoluted discriminant function that maps pixels onto the nonsensical supervision, effectively memorizing the training set in its entirety. In doing so, it learns nothing about flamingos, shirts, or ambulances, and thus totally fails to generalize to new objects—so its performance on the test set is at chance.[8] The wider lesson is that the problem of how to optimize an agent for generalization is inherently underspecified. The right way to learn depends on information to which an agent has no

---

[7] This is related to the *no free lunch* theorem, and it states that any two optimization algorithms are equivalent when their performance is averaged across all possible problems.
[8] See (Zhang et al. 2017).

access—the tasks or problems that it will face in the future. In practice, it is the AI researcher who knows (or guesses) what the validation conditions will be. Thus, out of all the possible ways in which the network could learn, the researcher is obliged to bias it towards that which is best suited for the expected test set—that which allows it to generalize as effectively as possible.

Thus, inductive biases are not algorithmic gremlins that cognitive scientists foist upon AI researchers to the detriment of progress. They are the bread and butter of everyday machine learning research. The familiar algorithms to which we owe the success of deep learning—such as the convolutional filter, the LSTM, and now the transformer—are inductive biases. Each of these innovations tailors the network to a class of problem that it can expect to meet in the generalization set. As we have seen, convolutions adapt the network for a world in which objects are translation invariant, LSTMs prepare the network for environments in which decision-relevant information is available over multiple timescales, and transformers equip it to dynamically reweigh past information as new context comes to light. Each of these algorithms has supercharged progress in AI research. But each is an inductive bias, and implicitly a microtheory about the nature of the problem that AI is destined to solve.

One corollary of this observation is that it is perfectly possible for both the apparently irreconcilable views of both nativists and empiricists to be correct. The optimal strength of an inductive bias for AI depends on the breadth of the generalization conditions that an agent can reasonably expect to encounter in the future. We have seen repeatedly that the computations observed in biology are helpfully adapted to the true structure of the natural world. For humans, this means the existence of cognitive functions are tailored to account for the nature of space, time, objects, words, bodily actions, and rewards—the fundamental building blocks of our existence. But there are limits to our generality: it is bounded by what is needed, given the structure of the world. Our brain expects the world to be smooth and coherent, so we cannot cope with randomly permuted sensory signals. It expects the distant past to have diminishing relevance, so we cannot remember everything. It expects us to learn to speak a single language, so there is an early critical period for language acquisition (and many people struggle to learn a second tongue). It expects the world to be Euclidean and three-dimensional, so we cannot readily navigate in four dimensions or readily reason about high-dimensional nonlinear systems.

This means that if we imagine that AGI will experience the natural world in which we live, it will need at least the same level of generality that we enjoy. It will not need to cope with a world in which objects pop randomly in and out of existence, where gravity is inverted or time runs backwards, or where all people look exactly the same. But if the inductive biases are too strong, the system will show limited generalization. For example, if we handcraft language according to the principles handed down from psycholinguistics, an agent may be unable to capitalize on its knowledge of syntax to program in Python, read Braille, or signal in semaphore. The battle between nativists and empiricists is cast as being about whether inductive biases are a good idea. But it is ultimately a debate about what AI is for.

AI researchers are thus architects of inductive biases. But the question remains of whether it is to the human brain that we should look for inspiration when designing algorithms. Is the human brain up to the job? Do we really want AI systems that mimic natural intelligence, or might something better be possible?

8.3 The best of all possible brains?

In the opening lines of his recent book *What Makes Us Smart*, the psychologist Sam Gershman asks a simple question: how can we apparently be so stupid and smart at the same time?

He goes on to explain this paradox:

> On the one hand, the catalogue of human error is vast: we perceive things that aren't there and fail to perceive things right in front of us, we forget things that happened and remember things that didn't, we say things we don't mean and mean things we don't say [...] and yet there is an equally vast catalogue of findings in support of human rationality: we come close to optimal performance on domains ranging from motor control and sensory perception to prediction, communication, decision-making and logical reasoning.

We do indeed like to think of ourselves as rational beings. In fact, vast swathes of theory in psychology and neuroscience have been hewn from this optimistic vision of our mental powers. The idea was forged in a rationalist tradition dating back to Descartes. It was nurtured by experiments that explored our ability to think strategically in chess or infer the validity of syllogisms. Its most recent incarnation is a focus on our propensity to reason like intuitive Bayesians.[9] Even without formal training in statistics, people can often accurately guesstimate quantities and likelihoods, from the outcomes of sporting

---

[9] In Chapter 3.

events to elections to the probable length of a poem or a monarch's reign. Thus, a long tradition argues that we make credible decisions based on the information available to hand.

Others attribute credit for the trajectory of our success as a species to our ineffable powers of reason. One popular perspective is that humans occupy a *cognitive niche*—that we have eked out a special place for ourselves in the hierarchy of species by evolving dedicated cognitive abilities for solving problems.[10] This view goes hand in hand with the idea that life is a race for survival, in which all animals must run just to stand still, because in the competition for resources, one organism's predator is another's prey.[11] The niche we have found is to outwit other species through both dedicated and general-purpose systems for goal-directed thought. Our superlative brains allow us to reason in sophisticated ways about physical and social systems, and thus to fashion tools from the objects around us, formulate plans of entrapment, use plants as medicines, and coordinate with social others, allowing mutualism, conditional cooperation, and the emergence of cumulative culture. Evolution, it is argued, has selected directly for clear-sightedness and a penchant for reality over falsehood.[12] In the words of Steven Pinker:

> a hominid that soothed itself by believing that a lion was a turtle, or that eating sand would nourish its body would be out-reproduced by its reality-based rivals.

It is certainly comforting to believe that we earned our role as apex predator through brains, rather than through brawn. But are people actually as rational as this view implies? What about those shortcomings which induce even healthy, educated adult humans to fall cognitively flat on our faces? What about our tendency to make diabolical life choices, to get involved in crime or substance abuse and end up behind bars? To remain trapped for decades in a hopeless marriage or a thankless career? What about our ability to dupe ourselves with infeasible stories, and to fall prey to the tall tales of fraudsters or the fantasies of cultists and conspiracy theorists? For example, one study from the 1980s showed that 99% of US college students believed in some form of supernatural phenomenon, such as telepathy, levitation, or ghosts, and 65% reported having personally experienced these phenomena. More recently, during the 2019 coronavirus (Covid-19) pandemic, false beliefs about

---

[10] Discussed in Chapter 2.

[11] This is known as the Red Queen hypothesis, from the character in Lewis Carroll's magical fable *Through the Looking Glass*, who explains to Alice: 'Now, here, you see, it takes all the running you can do, to keep in the same place. If you want to get somewhere else, you must run at least twice as fast as that!'

[12] For a contrary view, see (Prakash et al. 2021).

quack remedies spread like wildfire, and many people believed the illness was a hoax. It is hard to reconcile Pinker's rational hominid with these distinctly irrational beliefs.[13]

Thus, as Gershman noted, there is a flipside to this story: a tirade of work suggesting that people, in fact, reason poorly about both validity and probability. This idea began with a trickle of evidence in the 1960s and 1970s, a time when most psychologists were still enthusing about human rationality. Two psychologists—Daniel Kahneman and Amos Tversky—began to quietly dissent. Over the intervening decades, the trickle has become a roar.

Kahneman and Tversky noted that in many contexts, humans seemed to ignore or abuse the laws of probability, leading to biased and suboptimal decisions. For example, the basic tenet of the Bayesian decision theory is that priors and likelihoods should carry equal weight when computing posterior beliefs. However, in their experiments, people were unduly prone to overlooking base rate (or prior) probabilities when new evidence came along. For example, when a medical test is good, but not perfect (e.g. 99% accurate), and the prevalence of the condition for which it is testing in the population was very low (say one in a million), an affirmative result has a very high probability of being a false positive. However, participants—including trained medical staff—often failed to appreciate this, seemingly placing too much faith in the likelihood (test result) over the prior (base rate).

Similarly, people often failed to grasp the basic statistical principle that larger sample sizes imply more reliable results. For example, participants did not understand that if 55% of a sample of 10,000 people said they would vote Republican in the next elections, this is better news for the Grand Old Party than if 55% of only 100 people reported the same.[14] When making economic choices, for example when choosing between gambles described by a sum of money and a probability of receipt, people often seemed to behave as if there was a premium on certainty—so whilst a sure bet of £100 should be worth just £1 more than a 99% chance of £100, people would pay a higher premium to move from uncertainty to certainty—a result on which the multibillion-dollar insurance industry is founded. People can even accept or reject the very same option, depending on how the choice is framed. In a classic experiment, the psychologist Eldar Shafir asked participants to choose between multi-attribute alternatives, such as vacation packages, that differed in price and glamour. For example, they might have been asked to choose between a cheap, but relatively unexciting, trip to Baltimore, and a costly, but exotic, holiday in

---

[13] See (Messer & Griggs 1989).
[14] See (Kahneman et al. 1982).

Bali. When asked which one they preferred, they chose Bali—presumably because it was exciting. But when asked which they dispreferred, they also chose Bali—presumably because it was expensive.[15]

These findings jumpstarted an industrious academic subdiscipline aimed at cataloguing the frailty and fallibility of human reason. We are unduly optimistic—we overestimate how much we will enjoy our next summer holiday. We are overconfident—we are sure that the capital of Australia is Sydney (it is Canberra). We seek to blindly confirm, rather than question, our theories about the world—attributing information that is inconvenient for our beliefs to error, chance, or malfeasant intervention. We show an unreasonable preference for the status quo—we will pay more to hang onto our possessions than what they are actually worth, and neglect to make self-interested financial choices unless they are presented as a default. We can prefer or disprefer a choice option, depending on whether it is pitched as a gain or an avoidance of loss. We see patterns in randomness and form superstitious beliefs about coincident events, believing that misfortune comes in streaks, or convincing ourselves that a chance meeting with an old friend is destiny and not serendipity. Our preferences and beliefs change from day to day like the weather, and we can find ourselves supporting diametrically opposing arguments in short succession.[16] It seems that despite flashes of apparent rationality, we are not always so smart.

Thus, is human rationality a self-serving fiction? If so, this casts doubt on the nativist argument. What if, in the attempt to build in human virtues, we inadvertently build in human vices?

Infants arrive in the world with strong constraints on time courses and pathways for learning, and their brains are highly structured in ways that are consistent across individuals. Thus, nativists argue that because natural intelligence does not start with a blank slate, neither should AI. However, this critique only makes sense if one sees the trajectory of learning in a neural network as recapitulating the development of an individual (ontogeny), but not the evolution of the species (phylogeny). In the natural world, computation *did* ultimately emerge from scratch and *was* entirely sculpted by experience—only this happened over evolutionary time, rather than during a single lifetime. Thus, whilst at first glance, it looks like natural intelligence owes its success to the invisible sway of our genes, acting like a researcher that adeptly

---

[15] See (Shafir 1993).

[16] Optimism bias (Sharot 2011), overconfidence (Yates et al. 1997), status quo bias (Samuelson & Zeckhauser 1988), and numerous other fallacies of judgement and decision-making (Kahneman et al. 1982).

builds in face perception or sentence comprehension, ultimately these abilities were acquired from a learning algorithm that acted upon either our synapses or our DNA.

If we see the training of a deep learning agent as recapitulating the whole trajectory of evolution, then the question arises of whether the general intelligence that we happened to have evolved—the human flavour—is the best possible solution. As far as we know, the tree of life has a single set of roots—evolution only happened once. In fact, we have already seen that diverse intelligences can emerge across animal species that occupy distinct environmental niches. Some empiricists might argue that there is a sort of naive exceptionalism to the view that we should try to build in the particular intelligence that we humans happen to have evolved. The philosopher Gottfried Leibniz famously proposed that we live in the best of all possible worlds, a view that is pilloried in Voltaire's satirical tale *Candide*. It is possible that nativist advocates of enhancing AI with human-like cognition have simply fallen prey to the Panglossian fallacy that we happen to have evolved the *best of all possible brains*.[17] If untried computational pathways are more effective, might we be stymying our AI systems by building in natural intelligence?

Gershman's answer to this question seeks to rescue us from unreason. He argues that human intelligence is uniquely adapted to make the best possible decisions under the natural constraints of limited data, computation, and time. To negotiate the real world, we harness two principles: we rely on our prior beliefs when sensory evidence is noisy, and on frugal approximations when computation is costly. The first principle entails that perception, cognition, and action are inevitably shaped by inductive biases that are just strong enough to compensate for the paucity of data that the senses are able to collect and process. These biases instantiate ways we tend to see and understand the world. They are moulded in an intertwined way by experience and hardwired developmental pathways, which carefully steer our world model towards stereotyped intuitive beliefs about physical things (how objects interact in space) and social others (how people interact in social settings). Thus, when sensory evidence is weak, noisy, or ambiguous, we can fall back on these prior biases, using the probability calculus laid out by Bayes' rule to factor them optimally into our inferences about the world.

Thus, we might say that there are good and bad news for biological agents. The bad news is that the world is an uncertain place. Sensory signals are noisy and ambiguous, information is only partially observable, and biologically

---

[17] I am indebted to Sam Gershman for this metaphor (albeit in a different context).

relevant variables are volatile, stochastic, or chaotic. We have limited time and resources to make sense of it all. The good news is that we know a lot of stuff. Our generously endowed brains allow for richly structured inductive biases—prior tendencies and knowledge that help us make judicious choices in the face of the unknown. We know how sentences work, so we can guess what is being said in a noisy bar. We know how scenes work, so we interpret a blurry oblong on the sidewalk as a pedestrian.[18] These priors are our model of the world. This model encodes our understanding of things, processes, and their interactions: our common-sense beliefs about how the world works.

However, under this view, we sink or swim, based on the quality of our priors. Where our model of the world is accurate, we appear smart—seemingly miraculous reasoners who make finely honed judgements on the scantiest of evidence. When it is fallacious, we appear dumb—we fall prey to perceptual illusions, cognitive misjudgement, and economic irrationality—leaving us at risk of gambling away our life savings or forming delusional beliefs about aliens or the dangers of vaccination. Rationality and irrationality are two sides of the same coin; they are both a hallmark of neural machinery adapted to deal with the natural world where time, information, and computation are scarce—a world where the brain runs on the power of a lightbulb, the slowest organism starves or gets eaten, billions of neurons are packed into the limited confines of the skull, and the evidence of our senses is forever uncertain.

This answer to the question thus is unfailingly optimistic. Human brains are not perfect, but they are just as good as they should be. Echoing the argument above, the claim is that the mind is exactly as structured as it needs to be, given the regularities of the natural world and the inevitable constraints of biology. Even where we fail—where our beliefs are delusional or our policies self-defeating—we do so whilst employing a computational logic that is as good as it can be, given what the world is like.

What does this mean for AI research? This picture of the mind agrees that the constraints we should impose on, or inculcate in, an AI system depends on the nature of the problem that it will be deployed to solve. If our computational budget is constrained, or agents will be obliged to make rapid, high-stakes decisions in a noisy environment, then copying human inductive biases is probably a good idea. However, if we can draw upon limitless computational resources, or permit our agents to ponder indefinitely, then other pathways to success may be more fruitful.

---

[18] See (Bar 2004) and (Oliva & Torralba 2007).

8.4 Is the mind flat?

In Douglas Adams' comedy *Hitchhiker's Guide to the Galaxy*, a hapless Englishman called Arthur Dent narrowly escapes the destruction of planet Earth and is forced against his will into an intergalactic adventure, clad only in a shabby dressing gown. As the story unfolds, Dent is, in turn, befuddled, daunted, and exasperated by a series of alien concepts: that a towel is essential for space travel, that Vogon poetry is a form of torture, that the Earth was a supercomputer run by mice, and that to understand foreign languages, you need to insert a small fish in your ear.[19] Adrift in the far reaches of the universe, Dent never really grasps the basic tenets of extraterrestrial culture and technology. He finds it all very illogical, and spends most of the story wishing he could head back home and put the kettle on for a nice cup of tea.

When we imagine AGI, we think of a system that can deal judiciously with the unexpected. Perhaps we imagine an agent that (despite an earthbound past) can grasp the idiosyncrasies of the galaxy with similar adroitness to Arthur's friend Ford Prefect, a seasoned space traveller whose relentless savvy helps extricate them from every calamity. Back home on planet Earth, we hope that AGI will be versatile, creative, and resourceful. A generally intelligent agent can adapt rapidly to an unfamiliar social situation, master the strategy demanded by a new game, or grasp the structure of a foreign language. Over the past chapters, we discussed pictures of the mind that revolve around thinking and knowing or that emphasize the learning of abstractions, or a value function, or complex memory systems. So what is it that makes general intelligence possible?

A recurring theme of this book is that humans owe their intellectual powers to an unusually lavish model of the world. We heard this argument in the immediately preceding section, with the proposal that people form powerful causal models that can be used to make sense of an inherently uncertain world. Earlier, we discussed the knowledge structures and concepts that people harness to join the dots between objects, events, and words. Abstractions allow people to express their experiences using analogies, metaphors, and stories. We saw that the human hippocampus is a nexus for high-level abstractions, housing *concept cells* that encode semantic knowledge in ways that transcend the physical properties of the referenced item.[20] Subsequently, we argued that the PFC may be important for reuse of past task knowledge, by encoding

---

[19] Vogons are green slug-like aliens with a love of bureaucracy and 'as much sex appeal as a road accident'.
[20] In Chapter 5.

action sequences and plans in ways that were divorced from their immediate targets of action, allowing Jared Diamond to make sense of the rituals of New Guinea Highlanders that were initially as alien to him as Vogon culture was to Arthur Dent.[21]

By harnessing a world model, agents can bring existing knowledge to bear on new problems. When you meet a new acquaintance, you know nothing about them, but you understand the niceties of social introductions. When you encounter a new board game, you don't know the rules, but you understand the concepts of turn-taking, meeples, and winners and losers. When you hear a new language, you don't know the vocabulary, but you understand that there will probably be nouns, verbs, and adjectives. This knowledge—our model of the world—is our toolkit for dealing with the future. Like the *Hitchhiker's Guide* itself, it equips us to make sense of forthcoming events, even if they are exotic, astonishing, or alien.

However, there is a caveat to this story. Unfortunately, there is good evidence that human mental models are much less reliable and versatile than we might hope. This invites a view that *the mind is flat*—that a tendency towards mental shallowness, rather than depth, is our most distinctive human trait.

In 2002, Frank Keil and Leonid Rozenblit published a seminal paper arguing that people suffer from a powerful *illusion of explanatory depth* that is distinctive to theory-like knowledge. People are marvellous storytellers, capable of finding a thousand inventive ways to reason about cause and effect. If I ask you why water looks blue, you might confidently tell me that it is because it reflects the sky. However, when subject to scrutiny, our stories turn out to be flimsy and self-contradictory. For example, when graduate students at Yale University were asked to assess their own knowledge of how the heart pumps blood, or how a sewing machine works, they initially reported high levels of confidence. However, when asked to provide explanations, they stuttered and stumbled. Keil and Rozenbilt found that after this botched attempt to explain, participants' faith in their own understanding plummeted. Thus, their mental models were shallower and more fragile than they realized (in fact, water appears blue because it absorbs more long-wavelength light, removing red, yellow, and green from the light it reflects back).

Adopting a similar position, the psychologist Nick Chater has argued convincingly that our mental models are flimsy and improvised.[22] He suggests that the human mind cobbles percepts and ideas together on the fly, makes up stories and fills in gaps, and fabricates our beliefs and preferences in an ad

---

[21] In Chapter 7.
[22] In his book called *The Mind is Flat*.

hoc fashion. We do not, he argues, really know what we want, or understand, or believe—or even grasp the detail of what we are actually seeing or hearing. In fact, psychologists have long puzzled over the confused or downright bizarre responses that people often give when debriefed about the experiments in which they have just participated, or the elaborate, but implausible, justifications that they give for life decisions, political views, or preferences for consumer products.[23] Contrary to the hopes of both economists and RL researchers, who wish us to have a stable, consistent, and well-defined internal value function, people seem to be remarkably suggestible—even where their own subjective preferences are concerned.

One fascinating instance of this is the phenomenon known as *choice blindness*. In a study conducted in Sweden, people were asked to fill out questionnaires about their political views. After submitting their answers, they received them back and were asked to verbally explain their views. Unbeknownst to participants, researchers switched the answer sheets, so that left-leaning people received right-leaning answers back, and vice versa. Of the 75% who failed to notice, many were happy to provide elaborate justifications for political positions opposing their own, apparently blind to the choices they had just made. Similar effects have been described with preferences about facial attractiveness and the taste of tea or jam.[24]

Choice blindness is an instance of post hoc rationalization, the tendency to invent motives in the light of actions, rather than choosing actions to satisfy motives. We have already encountered the post hoc rationalizations of disappointed millenarians who woke up to find that the world has not ended as prophesied.[25] But rationalization is ubiquitous in more mundane settings. For example, rationalization can satisfy a bias for optimism when a punter believes that the horse they have just bet on is more likely to win. It can give our decisions a sheen of morality, as when a partygoer explains to themselves that eating the last slice of cake spared the other guests from feeling awkward. Nick Chater proposes that our beliefs and preferences are invented on the fly by retrieving and interpreting memories of actions we have taken in the past. For example, I know that I like apples more than oranges because I remember that I ate a Granny Smith for lunch every day last week. Instability of preference can thus arise when we randomly sample different memories (e.g. on one random occasion, I recall eating a delicious satsuma, and thus briefly assume I have a preference for oranges over apples).[26]

---

[23] See (Nisbett & Wilson 1977).
[24] See (Hall et al. 2010), (Johansson et al. 2005), and (Strandberg et al. 2020).
[25] In the discussion of cognitive dissonance in Chapter 6.
[26] See (Stewart et al. 2006).

Of course, our beliefs, preferences, and values are not entirely stochastic, so they cannot be driven entirely by what we happened to do in the past. Otherwise, people would be equally likely to be scared of kittens as of snakes, because that subset of people who initially (randomly) ran from a kitten would interpret this as meaning that kittens are dangerous, prompting them to flee in the future and further reinforcing the belief. A softer version of this theory limits its application to our declarative knowledge, allowing preferences to be ultimately grounded in implicit behaviours, such as innate reflexes or overlearnt habits. If I am innately afraid of snakes, or implicitly desirious of cake, then my rationalized beliefs (that cake is the right way to celebrate a birthday, and that snakes are dangerous venomous animals) are ways by which I explain these implicit tendencies to myself. The psychologist Fiery Cushman has argued that rationalization may, in fact, be adaptive, because it allows us to distil our implicit habits into causal models, shoring them up more firmly within an integrated web of explicit knowledge.[27]

If our mental models (and even value functions) are unreliable and make-shift, then this places limits on our ability to generalize between old and new settings. This is important, because in both neuroscience and AI research, the idea has taken root that the special magic of the human intellect—not shared by current AI systems—is our ability to transfer. This is betrayed by the opening lines of many of the most influential research papers cited in the preceding chapters, which fondly assert that the human ability to form abstractions and generalize from a single learning example is the key to our superlative intelligence.[28] However, these claims should be placed in the context of a voluminous literature that—for more than a hundred years—has tried to assess the efficacy of human transfer learning. The answers have not always been clear-cut.

Across the twentieth century, there were numerous reports of seemingly impressive human transfer—that after tackling one problem, humans were faster at solving other problems that were related, but different. In one classic study from 1980, conducted by Mary Gick and Keith Holyoak, participants were presented with a challenging puzzle in which rays of variable strength had to be deployed to destroy a tumour without damaging the overlying healthy tissue. The counterintuitive solution is to angle several weak rays, so that their beams converge at the tumour, giving it their cumulative force, but

---

[27] See (Cushman 2020).

[28] 'Humans have a remarkable capacity for generalizing experiences to novel circumstances,' reads one. 'People learning new concepts often generalise successfully from just a single example,' reads at least one other. Or more pithily: 'Abstract reasoning is a hallmark of human intelligence.' These assertions are unreferenced, presumably because it is hard to know what to cite.

sparing the tissue through which they pass. Participants were found to solve this more readily if they had previously encountered an apparently different reasoning problem with a similar structure that involved commanding troops to storm a castle through multiple entrances at once.[29] This is, of course, an attempt to study in the laboratory the sorts of analogical processes evoked earlier, where scientists conceived of atoms as planets, or gases as billiard balls, or chemical bonds as ballroom dancers.[30]

However, others are more sceptical. Thorndike, for example, had serious doubts about whether people were able to transfer learning between domains. In an early experiment, he asked human participants to estimate the area of differently sized shapes. After training for a few thousand trials on rectangles, participants improved on estimating the area of rectangles, but not of other shapes such a circles and triangles.[31] In 1901, he wrote:

> Improvements in any single mental function rarely brings about equal improvement in any other function, no matter how similar, for the working of every mental function-group is conditioned by the nature of the data in each particular case.

Almost a century later, in a comprehensive survey of human transfer learning, Douglas Detterman sums up with a similarly pessimistic view:[32]

> First, significant transfer is probably rare and accounts for very little human behaviour. Studies that claim transfer often tell subjects to transfer or use a 'trick' to call the subject's attention to the similarity of the two problems. Such studies cannot be taken as evidence for transfer. We generally do what we have learned to do and no more. The lesson learned from studies of transfer is that, if you want people to learn something, teach it to them. Don't teach them something else and expect them to figure out what you really want them to do.

Detterman notes that in many studies purporting to show transfer, like Gick and Holyoak, participants may not spontaneously redeploy knowledge from one domain to another. Rather, there are typically two tasks, and participants receive strong hints or verbal encouragement to use knowledge obtained from one to solve the other. Transfer thus may be less of an experimental result and

---

[29] Known as the Dunker radiation problem and the Attack–Dispersion story, respectively (Gick & Holyoak 1980).

[30] In Chapter 5.

[31] See (Woodworth & Thorndike 1901).

[32] See (Detterman 1993).

more of a demand characteristic of the study.[33] Like other fleeting and spontaneous effects, transfer is hard to capture in the lab, raising doubts about its ubiquity in the wider world.

How can we understand the generality of human intelligence in the light of these failures of generalization? One answer is to note that not all generalization conditions are created equal. When studying humans, cognitive scientists have helpfully distinguished between *near* and *far* transfer.[34] Near transfer is the routine recycling of past knowledge to deal with similar, but non-identical, experiences. For example, if I know how to ride a bicycle, I might reuse those skills when learning to ride a scooter. Skills are readily shared between domains because bikes and scooters look alike—they both have two wheels, brakes, and a saddle—and thus afford a similar set of actions. Humans and other animals are good at near transfer, as are some deep RL agents.[35] For example, after training on rectangles, Thorndike's participants were able to estimate the area of new rectangles that they had not seen before. Near transfer allows us to cope with a natural world that is infinitely variable, but highly structured, so that we encounter similar streets, chores, and conversations from one day to the next.

By contrast, *far transfer* requires inference to transcend the physical properties of a stimulus and focus on relational properties, such as how the parts relate to one another. This is the sort of process that Gick and Holyoak set out to interrogate in the lab. For example, having learnt that a firebreak can be used to contain a forest fire, I might infer that social distancing can be used to stem the spread of a disease through the human population. Here, any knowledge being transferred is not about trees or people. Instead, it is about the relational property that is shared between domains. But here, the evidence that humans can spontaneously transfer relational abstractions is mixed or dubious. We may have learnt the concept of 'firebreak' in the context of geography, and we may understand its use in the context of medicine, but we cannot reliably use this abstraction to spontaneously generate solutions to reasoning problems involving the spread of one entity through the medium of another.

It is plausible that we struggle to deploy abstractions to solve far transfer problems because—as Chater argues—our mental models are much more shallow or fragmentary than they appear. We know a lot of facts. We can recount information about people, places, and events. We can tell stories about

---

[33] A demand characteristic is a feature of the task that strongly cues participants to behave in the way that the experimenter wishes them to.

[34] See (Haskell 2001).

[35] See (Kirk et al. 2022).

past occurrences and dream up plausible-sounding explanations for observed phenomena. But our mental theories lack depth. Even educated people struggle to explain basic facts about the world. How does oxygen keep you alive? How is electricity produced? To whom government debt is owed? For the most part, our understanding of even basic processes is quite patchy. Thus, our human repertoire of abstractions and our ability to use them for transfer may be more limited than we would hope.

If our mental models can be unreliable and far transfer is elusive, then where does our generality come from? What makes us quotidian polymaths? How is it that we can readily navigate the streets of a new town, conduct transactions in an unfamiliar currency, or rapidly learn the niceties of a formal social occasion? How is it that after learning five languages, we are quick on the uptake with the sixth? What makes a chess player be faster to master three-way chess, or hexagonal chess, or the Indian variant called chaturanga?

8.5 Concepts and programs

Eratosthenes of Cyrene was the John von Neumann of the third century BC. Many of his contributions to mathematics, astronomy, and geography have been handed down to the modern era. He is credited with computing the circumference of the Earth with less than 2% error, a remarkable feat for an era when intercity distances were still measured by professional pacers with constant stride length.[36] He also famously invented the *Sieve of Eratosthenes*, a tool for discovering prime numbers. It works by gradually eliminating multiples of successive integers starting from 2, each forming a sort of numerical colander that catches the composites and allows the primes to fall through. His algorithm is used to this day in number theory.

We marvel at the creative mind that solved these problems more than two millennia ago. But there are at least two lenses through which to view Eratosthenes' feat. Through one, we see a triumph of reasoning. Primes are not composites; composites are multiple integers; thus, successively remove these multiples and primes remain. Through the other, we see a masterful feat of abstraction. The sieve, a basic tool which may be as old as agriculture itself, sifts the fine grains from coarse; Eratosthenes transfers this knowledge to invent a mathematical sieve, which separates desired from undesired numbers. Thus,

---

[36] To achieve this, he used visionary flights of reasoning: he measured the distance between two cities on the same meridian, and the angles of the shadows cast at noon on the solstice, and combed them using the newly discovered trigonometric theory about how to combine the arc and chord of a circle.

Eratosthenes might be using Hebb's intelligence A, by thinking logically about sequences of integers; or he could be drawing on Hebb's intelligence B, by generalizing his world knowledge from the kitchen cupboard to the number theory. These are the two routes to intelligence—thinking and knowing—that have been weaved together across the pages of this book to tell a story about natural intelligence.

The natural world is infinitely restless, and each experience is at least partly novel. This means that intelligent agents are obliged to generalize. The problem that agents face—the meta-task for natural intelligence—is thus to learn about the environment in a way that prepares for an unspecified transfer problem in an uncertain world. The most general forms of understanding, and the strongest forms of generalization, occur when agents can acquire abstract concepts. Thus, in psychology and neuroscience, a great deal of research has been directed to studying how humans acquire the knowledge that populates their mental landscape—including semantic knowledge about people and places, and even more abstract relational knowledge such as the fact that family trees and biological taxa share a common hierarchical structure. As we have seen, the world has a stereotyped structure, so agents that learn and develop in ways that prepare for that structure will be maximally adapted to solve the meta-task.

We typically think of generalization as relying on neural codes for perceptual, semantic, or relational information in memory. For a vanilla deep learning system, such as a convolutional neural network trained to recognize natural scenes, the formation of abstractions allows sophisticated forms of pattern recognition. For example, we have seen that deep networks trained on ImageNet learn neural codes that signal both objects and high-level categories. When we use multimodal input signals that mix language and visual information—as in giant foundation models—deep networks can even learn highly abstract semantic categories, such as *Christmas* and *African*. In this class of model, in which mappings are learnt among iconic representations (e.g. images) and symbolic representations (e.g. words), concepts act like keys that automatically unlock meaning. Thus, the concept of a cat automatically links together words and images referring to Cruikshanks, the Song of the Jellicles, and Halle Berry.[37] Similarly, an abstract representation coding for *small spheres in orbit around a large sphere* jointly refers to both atoms and solar systems, allowing a person equipped with such a representation (such as Bohr) to make the analogy. For this type of model, abstractions act like a

---

[37] Halle Berry is the actress that plays Catwoman. The Jellicle Song features in T. S. Elliot's poetry collection *Old Possum's Book of Practical Cats*.

multifaceted bunch of keys, allowing us to recognize the common ways in which the world is structured.

However, this class of computation alone is not sufficient for intelligence. Learning abstract patterns in data is undoubtedly an important part of what makes natural intelligence special. However, intelligent agents also need to act. Taking actions means engaging in a reciprocal cycle of interaction with the world, governed by a control policy. To date, RL is the most promising framework for describing how this happens, as demonstrated by the many recent successes in training agents to master complex tasks, such as MuZero. However, it seems unlikely—despite what some have argued—that 'RL is enough'. The RL framework is very well suited to problems (like board and video games) that have simple objectives, like winning or maximizing score. But life is not a game. Life is an open-ended problem with unclear objectives. Living long and well probably requires agents to optimize over homeostatic goals (keeping many things in balance, such as hunger and thirst) as much as heterostatic goals (obtaining as much of one thing as possible). Thus, it seems very likely that we will need to make significant advances in understanding intrinsic rewards—the way in which motivated behaviour is structured towards self-generated goals—before RL agents are viable across a wide range of naturalistic settings.

One of the most important innovations of recent years is the development of complex memory systems for RL agents. Memory systems untether RL agents from the present, and allow them to learn sophisticated, structured control policies that depend on past information. Memory is not just a temporary store for data. Memory systems allow agents to acquire highly structured control policies that can be reused in novel situations. For example, meta-RL can be used to train agents to rapidly adapt to new tasks. Thus, whereas large generative models allow us to transfer *abstract concepts*, sophisticated RL systems are beginning to allow us to generalize *structured programs*. This means that in addition to recognizing new patterns in data—to rapidly make sense of new sensory experiences—intelligent agents are beginning to be able to generalize control policy tasks, to grapple strategically with unseen tasks and achieve novel goals.

Both cognitive scientists and AI researchers have attempted to discover the primitive mental operations from which tasks in the real world tend to be composed. For example, neural networks or probabilistic programs have been equipped with operations like gating, recursion, or branching; or the computation of conjunction (AND) and disjunction (NOT) operations for program induction. This is a very fundamental project: to define the natural space of tasks, the atomic set of operations that an intelligent agent needs, given the way that sensory data, time, space, objects, relations, and rewards are organized in the natural world. This work is the modern-day descendent of the earliest approaches to AI that were based on symbolic computation and highly constrained logical inference. However, unlike the classic approaches, in which these operations were endowed by hand, in many modern systems, they are partly or wholly learnt from experience.

As always, researchers have to decide how to trade off the generality and data efficiency of their systems. Bayesian approaches to this problem usually involve a hand-engineered state space or specific assumptions about the prior, which can limit their generality. By contrast, connectionist approaches are more flexible, but often painfully hungry for data. The highly structured patterns of computation that are observed in the PFC and hippocampus of humans and other primates seem to imply that natural intelligence has settled on a good compromise, involving a minimal set of maximally general constraints on control processes. Meta-RL similarly offers a promising compromise, but via a different approach. It eschews handcrafting but instead uses curriculum learning—control over the set of tasks encountered during meta-training—to constrain the neural programs that can be learnt and generalized. As such, it evokes a principle observed in the natural world, whereby young members of a species are raised in highly stereotyped conditions that shepherd their learning in directions that are favourable for the adult environment. For humans, this prominently includes the fact that, where possible, we send our children to school.

By generalizing both programs and concepts, intelligent agents can use both thinking and knowing to solve new problems. Where one route fails, the other can take up the slack. It is interesting to observe that many of the oft-quoted feats of extraordinary human abstraction—from Eratosthenes devising his sieve for prime numbers to Bohr seeing the analogy between atoms and the solar system—seem to involve exceptional, once-in-a-generation geniuses whose flashes of creative insight dramatically reshaped the course of their field. Thus, whilst generalization of the most abstract concepts—spontaneously grasping the relational similarities across wildly different domains—is a characteristic of human thinking, it may be a vanishingly rare one. For the rest of us, intellectual mere mortals, our quotidian polymathy probably does not come from such grandiose feats of understanding. Rather, our mental models are more patchy and fragmentary than we would hope—the mind is flat. A more ragged conceptual universe makes it hard to apprehend complex problems with a single take or to spot deep relational patterns at a single glance, so we have to fall back on other means.

Fortunately, another route exists. We can generalize an ability to deploy mental operations—or transfer programs—to devise new solutions on the fly. Thus, where *knowing* falls short, *thinking* steps up. By generalizing programs for control, we can rapidly adapt to new settings. Thus, whilst most people's capacity for zero-shot far transfer is limited, we can solve complex tasks by rapidly composing new policies out of a handful of primitive building blocks, just as meta-RL agents redeploy the task solutions acquired during meta-training. When asked to tidy a room, items of different shapes and sizes might be strewn in random positions, but you apply a structure program for gathering, sorting, shelving, and discarding the various items. If you are finding your way through a new city, you can apply a program that involves following major thoroughfares, keeping track of landmarks, or asking for directions. Of course, language—the substrate we use both to communicate and to order our own thoughts—is fundamentally compositional in nature. Thus, whilst you have probably never imagined an elephant playing a trumpet whilst riding a bicycle before, you can do so effortlessly now you have read those words. The ability to think compositionally is at the heart of natural intelligence.

Composition promotes representational efficiency, by allowing infinite productivity from finite means. Thus, natural systems have evolved a bias to learn neural programs that facilitate the on-the-fly composition of ad hoc solutions to novel problems. This is presumably how we all become quotidian polymaths: we learn to think. The immense complexity of the natural world and the limits that physics and biology place on the time and capacity available for information processing mean that we all come to rely on a minimal set of useful mental operations. These include biases to explore the world in ways that facilitate this very process, by seeking out information, satisfying curiosity, exerting control, and meeting self-generated objectives. In other words, natural intelligence learns how to learn over multiple timescales, from the cradle to the grave. It seems likely that building systems that learn increasingly sophisticated forms of structured computation—that learn to generate and compose yet more versatile programs over longer timescales—is going to be an important way forward for AGI research.

This leaves one final question. What is the outlook for AGI? Is it plausible that we will ever actually build a general intelligence—an AI system whose intellectual versatility rivals our own?

8.6 Artificial intelligibility

The iconic image known as *The March of Progress* has inspired a thousand imitators (Figure 8.1A). First published in 1965, it shows a line of anthropoid figures. The forms at the rear are ape-like, but they gradually give way to the noble, upright, and hairless form of modern man. The image conveys a compelling idea: that evolution is synonymous with progress towards the well-groomed ideal represented by modern-day *Homo sapiens*.

However, that idea is wrong. Evolution does not march along a single axis, gradually perfecting organisms towards human likeness. Rather, it branches

(A)

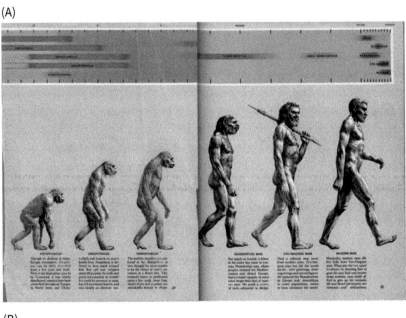

(B)

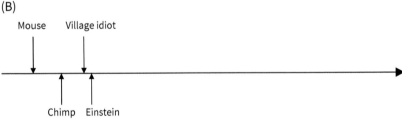

Fig. 8.1 (**A**) The abbreviated version of 'The Road to Homo Sapiens', also known as 'The March of Progress' from *Early Man* (1965).
(**B**) A one-dimensional view of intelligence.
Adapted from *Superintelligence*, 2014 (Figure 8).

and buckles as each organism adapts idiosyncratically to its environment—acquiring the physical and behavioural characteristics best suited to its niche. In his book *Wonderful Life*, the evolutionary biologist Stephen Jay Gould described the many pathways that evolution has followed and then abandoned (such as five-eyed fish discovered in the fossil-bearing deposit known as the Burgess Shale).[38] His conclusion is that:

> life is a copiously branching bush, continually pruned by the grim reaper of extinction, not a ladder of predictable progress.

Today, *orthogenic* theories of evolution—the idea that organisms evolve towards a single, well-defined goal—are discredited and largely obsolete.

However, our vision of intelligence still has this teleological ring to it. AI researchers, cognitive scientists, and assorted futurists conceive of mental ability as varying on a single axis that runs from subhuman to human to superhuman intelligence. The lowliest organisms are defined by their lack of human-like capacities, and we imagine future AI systems as those with human brains scaled to extraordinary heights. We administer tests of reasoning such as RPM to our primate cousins and note where they fail, and we imagine that AGI will use superlative reason to turbocharge science and technology beyond human limits. We question whether non-human species are capable of metacognition, whilst imagining that future AI systems will read our minds. In his book *Superintelligence*, Nick Bostrom depicts this march of intelligence, with *mouse* and *chimp* giving way to *village idiot* and then *Einstein*, but with the axis continuing on the way into the far reaches of intellectual omnipotence (Figure 8.1B).

However, this picture ignores the diversity in intelligence that is found in the natural world. In his book *Are We Smart Enough to Know How Smart Animals Are?*, the ethologist Frans de Waal charts the extraordinary variation in cognitive abilities across the animal kingdom.[39] Simultaneously, he decries our narrow view of the intellect:

> We love to compare and contrast animal and human intelligence, taking ourselves as the touchstone. [But] the comparison is not between humans and animals, but between one animal species—ours—and a vast array of others. I look at human cognition as a variety of animal cognition. It is not even clear how special ours is relative to a cognition distributed over eight independently moving arms, each

---

[38] See (Gould 1989).
[39] See (de Waal 2016). His answer is a resounding 'no'.

with its own neural supply, or one that enables a flying organism to catch mobile prey by picking up the echoes of its own shrieks.

The theme of de Waal's book is that every animal displays its own unique form of intelligence, adapted to its goals and environment. Humans are blind to the intelligence that other animals display. With typical human exceptionalism, we tend to recognize that animals are smart only when this claim fits with our own anthropocentric vision of what intelligence entails. We struggle to understand the politics that unfold in a community of orangutangs, we are perplexed by the games dolphins play whilst hunting, and we cannot fathom the principles of collective organization that allow a colony of termites to build megastructures a thousand times their height. Thus, psychologists are sceptical that animals can form abstract concepts, and whether they strategize, plan, or think creatively—because they assume that animals equipped with these skills will display them in exactly the same way that people do.

We fail to recognize the intelligence of other species because we do not share their *umwelt*. The concept of the umwelt was developed by the biologist Jakob von Uexküll in the early twentieth century. It refers to the internal model by which an animal understands the world. An animal's umwelt depends on its local environment, its embodied form, its desires and goals, and its interactions with conspecifics. Thus, agents with different bodies, habitats, and social structures struggle to understand one another. This is why your cat looks at you with such disdain, why you probably haven't yet persuaded your dog to play hide-and-seek, and why zoo animals occasionally eat their keeper. It is also the basis of the philosophical argument that we cannot understand what it is like to be a bat, or that if a lion could speak, we would not be able to understand it.[40] Even humans from different societies struggle to understand each other, which is, of course, why Western psychologists have historically demeaned or dismissed the intelligence of cultural groups living outside of their own WEIRD enclave.

If we ever build strong AI, it will have its own umwelt. This umwelt will be moulded by the information provided to its sensors, its action space, the structure of its world knowledge, the organization of its memory, the nature of its goals, and how it is motivated to act. For AI researchers, there are a vast number of ways in which these variables can be specified. One important consideration is that we are not attempting to build AGI just to satisfy our scientific curiosity. We are doing so for a purpose—to help humans in their

---

[40] Thomas Nagel and Ludwig Wittgenstein, respectively.

endeavours. In the words of optimistic start-ups and frontline tech companies, we are building AI to *make the world a better place*. But if we want AI to be useful to people, it will need to share our umwelt. If we build an AI that sees the world in a radically different way to us, its behaviour and mental states will be unintelligible. Such an agent will be at best unreliable and at worst unsafe.[41] Thus, the probability that we will succeed—building a system with which we can usefully interact—depends on whether the design principles we choose lend themselves to AI systems that share our umwelt. In other words, when building *Artificial Intelligence*, we need to consider *Artificial Intelligibility*.

During the heyday of classical AI, one of the field's most excoriating critics was the philosopher Hubert Dreyfus. Dreyfus is best known for a prescient endorsement of sub-symbolic AI systems at a time when the field was largely contemptuous of neural networks. But in his 1986 book *Mind Over Machine*, he makes a more subtle point that is levelled at connectionist models:

> If it is to learn from its own 'experiences' to make associations that are humanlike rather than be taught to make associations that have been specified by its trainer, a net must also share our sense of appropriateness of output, and this means it must share our needs, desires, and emotions and have a humanlike body with appropriate physical movements, abilities, and vulnerability to injury.

Dreyfus is arguing that if we want to build AI systems that exhibit human-like intelligence, with whom we can interact in pursuit of human-centred goals, these agents will need to think in ways that make sense to us. Presumably, we want systems with which we can converse, which will be able to use theory of mind to infer our beliefs and desires, and that perform tasks in ways that we think are reasonable, effective, and safe. For this to be realized, AI systems will need to at least partially form mental states that overlap with ours, via experiences that at least partly resemble our own, using a brain that is not radically different from those found in the natural world.

Dreyfus also notes the extent to which the ways that we understand the world are grounded in our physical nature (we have bodies) and our social and affective nature (we occupy a place in the community). Critically, it seems questionable whether AI systems will ever share these properties with us. If we were to build AGI, it would probably not have a body like ours. It would be unlikely to have feelings or desires that resemble those of people. We would

---

[41] The argument being made here is related to the idea that we need to build AI that is aligned to human values. But here, a stronger case is being made. I am arguing that if AI systems do not share our way of looking at the world, they will not be considered 'intelligent' by any reasonable definition of the term.

presumably not want it to occupy the same place in society as humans do. Thus, it seems quite unlikely that any system we build will ever share our umwelt. However, it is incumbent upon us, as we build stronger systems, to consider the extent to which their intelligence is intelligible to us. This project has already begun, with an upswing of interest in the ethics and safety of machine learning research and the foregrounding of human value alignment as a primary desideratum for AI.

Across this book, we discussed the question: should we try to build AI systems that emulate the structure and function of the human mind? In the AI community, some people advocate strongly against this view. The prevailing view among many researchers—those who accept the *bitter lesson*—is that attempts to mimic the way humans learn, or to copy the way biological brains have evolved, are a distraction that will lead us astray in our pursuit of general intelligence. Instead, they argue that we should allow structured computation to emerge by itself, fostered by the twin engines of powerful optimization and massive computation.

The use of self-play to solve board games—a method that allows for the development of novel strategies, beyond those that humans may have discovered—is emblematic of this approach. For example, AlphaZero played against instances of themselves to gradually learn from scratch, to becomes the strongest ever player of Chess, Shogi, and Go—even beating variants of itself that had been trained directly on human data.[42] The resulting policies were, in some cases, unrecognizable to other human players. For example, in Shogi, AlphaZero was prone to moving its King to the centre of the board, defying conventional wisdom. In chess, a whole book was written discussing the merits of its unconventional play.[43]

The fact that AlphaZero made discoveries that enlarged human knowledge of chess and Go is remarkable. But adversarial games are special in that they entail a crisply defined goal. As we move out of the sandbox and into the real world, the risk is that allowing AI systems to learn in ways that are untethered to human knowledge and thought will encourage agents to spiral off into modes of thinking and patterns of behaviour that are unintelligible to people. If future AI systems learn sophisticated policies that are divorced from human goals or concerns, or form mental states that we do not either agree with or understand, then their utility to us will be limited. We can already begin to see what happens when the data on which AI systems are trained are chosen indiscriminately. When supervised models learn from large-scale digital data

---

[42] See (Silver et al. 2018).
[43] See (Sadler & Regan 2019).

selected for their availability and convenience, they often make decisions which are unfair, opaque, or illogical. This is because these data are not curated to align their decisions with those that humans might make.

The argument made here thus is that AI systems without human-like intelligence risk being either useless or unsafe. This further motivates the argument that when building AI, we should study and learn from natural intelligence. David Marr—a pioneer of theoretical neuroscience who died tragically young—bequeathed to the field a tripartite structure for describing a computational system. The highest level defines its computational goals, the intermediate level describes the algorithms developed to meet those goals, and the lowest level specifies the substrate in which those algorithms are implemented.[44] When I say that we should emulate nature, I do not mean that we should slavishly try to mirror how neurons produce action potentials or mimic the varieties of transmitters and peptides it uses for signalling. The utility of studying natural intelligence is at the computational and algorithmic levels.

At the computational level, the natural world constrains the ways in which intelligence works. Time runs forwards, and so we need memory systems. The world is composed of features, objects, and scenes, so our sensory systems must be hierarchically organized. The world varies smoothly, so we need to learn generalizable functions; but it also contains exceptions, so we need to store instances and one-off events. Many courses of action are possible, so we need to reason, plan, and strategize. Our goals can be far off, and the trajectory towards them uncertain, so we need intrinsic and extrinsic motivational signals to keep us going. The world is noisy and uncertain, so our policies and inferences must be robust. The world contains other agents, so we need to impute and infer beliefs and desires and learn socially adaptive responses. As we have seen, natural intelligence is exquisitely honed to account for the way the world is structured.

It remains to be seen whether we will ever build systems with human-like general intelligence. But if we want any such systems to be safe, and if we wish to employ them to make the world a better place, then we should think carefully about the way in which evolution has given rise to natural general intelligence.

---

[44] Other terminology that has been used to make this distinction includes 'semantic, syntactic, and physical', or 'content, form, and medium'. See (Glass et al. 1979) and (Pylyshyn 1989).

References

Abramson J, Ahuja A, Barr I, et al. 2021. Imitating interactive intelligence. *arXiv:2012.05672 [cs]*

Aggleton JP, Vann SD, Denby C, et al. 2005. Sparing of the familiarity component of recognition memory in a patient with hippocampal pathology. *Neuropsychologia*. 43(12):1810–23

Ahmed Z, Roux NL, Norouzi M, Schuurmans D. 2019. Understanding the impact of entropy on policy optimization. *arXiv:1811.11214 [cs, stat]*

Aitchison L, Lengyel M. 2017. With or without you: predictive coding and Bayesian inference in the brain. *Curr Opin Neurobiol*. 46:219–27

Alcorn MA, Li Q, Gong Z, et al. 2019. Strike (with) a pose: neural networks are easily fooled by strange poses of familiar objects. *arXiv:1811.11553 [cs]*

Alderson-Day B, Fernyhough C. 2015. Inner speech: development, cognitive functions, phenomenology, and neurobiology. *Psychol Bull*. 141(5):931–65

Alexander WH, Brown JW. 2018. Frontal cortex function as derived from hierarchical predictive coding. *Sci Rep*. 8(1):3843

Androulidakis Z, Lulham A, Bogacz R, Brown MW. 2008. Computational models can replicate the capacity of human recognition memory. *Netw Comput Neural Syst*. 19(3):161–82

Aral S. 2020. *The Hype Machine*. London: Harper Collins

Arendt D, Tosches MA, Marlow H. 2016. From nerve net to nerve ring, nerve cord and brain—evolution of the nervous system. *Nat Rev Neurosci*. 17(1):61–72

Aronov D, Nevers R, Tank D. 2017. Mapping of a non-spatial dimension by the hippocampal-entorhinal circuit. *Nature*. 543:719–22

Baddeley AD, Hitch G. 1974. Working memory. *Psychol Learn Motiv*. 8:47–89

Badre D, D'Esposito M. 2009. Is the rostro-caudal axis of the frontal lobe hierarchical? *Nat Rev Neurosci*. 10(9):659–69

Banino A, Barry C, Uria B, et al. 2018. Vector-based navigation using grid-like representations in artificial agents. *Nature*. 557(7705):429–33

Bao X, Gjorgieva E, Shanahan LK, Howard JD, Kahnt T, Gottfried JA. 2019. Grid-like neural representations support olfactory navigation of a two-dimensional odor space. *Neuron*. 102(5):1066–75.e5

Bar M. 2004. Visual objects in context. *Nat Rev Neurosci*. 5(8):617–29

Bara BG, Bucciarelli M, Johnson-Laird PN. 1995. Development of syllogistic reasoning. *Am J Psychol*. 108(2):157–93

Barak O, Tsodyks M. 2014. Working models of working memory. *Curr Opin Neurobiol*. 25:20–4

Barto AG, Sutton RS. 1982. Simulation of anticipatory responses in classical conditioning by a neuron-like adaptive element. *Behav Brain Res*. 4(3):221–35

Bashivan P, Kar K, DiCarlo JJ. 2019. Neural population control via deep image synthesis. *Science*. 364(6439)

Bastos AM, Usrey WM, Adams RA, Mangun GR, Fries P, Friston KJ. 2012. Canonical microcircuits for predictive coding. *Neuron*. 76(4):695–711

Beattie C, Leibo JZ, Teplyashin D, et al. 2016. DeepMind Lab. *arXiv:1612.03801 [cs, AI]*

Beery S, van Horn G, Perona P. 2018. Recognition in terra incognita. *arXiv:1807.04975 [cs, q-bio]*

Behrens TE, Woolrich MW, Walton ME, Rushworth MF. 2007. Learning the value of information in an uncertain world. *Nat Neurosci*. 10(9):1214–21

Behrens TEJ, Muller TH, Whittington JCR, et al. 2018. What is a cognitive map? Organizing knowledge for flexible behavior. *Neuron*. 100(2):490–509

Bellemare MG, Naddaf Y, Veness J, Bowling M. 2013. The Arcade Learning Environment: an evaluation platform for general agents. *JAIR*. 47:253–79

Bellmund JLS, Gardenfors P, Moser EI, Doeller CF. 2018. Navigating cognition: spatial codes for human thinking. *Science*. 362(6415):eaat6766

Bender EM, Gebru T, McMillan-Major A, Shmitchell S. 2021. On the dangers of stochastic parrots: can language models be too big? *Proceedings of the 2021 ACM Conference on Fairness, Accountability, and Transparency*. pp. 610–23. Virtual Event Canada: ACM

Benjamin W. 1933. On the mimetic faculty. In *Selected Writings, 1926–1934*, pp. 720–2

Berkes P, Orban G, Lengyel M, Fiser J. 2011. Spontaneous cortical activity reveals hallmarks of an optimal internal model of the environment. *Science*. 331(6013):83–7

Bernhardt C. 2017. *Turing's Vision: The Birth of Computer Science*. Cambridge, MA: MIT Press

Bhattacharya A. 2022. *The Man from the Future: The Visionary Life of John von Neumann*. New York, NY: W.W. Norton & Company. First American edition

Bicanski A, Burgess N. 2020. Neuronal vector coding in spatial cognition. *Nat Rev Neurosci*. 21(9):453–70

Biederman I. 1987. Recognition-by-components: a theory of human image understanding. *Psychol Rev*. 94(2):115–47

Bisley JW, Goldberg ME. 2010. Attention, intention, and priority in the parietal lobe. *Annu Rev Neurosci*. 33:1–21

Blair, C. 1957. Passing of a great mind. *Life*, pp. 89–108. Feb. 25

Bommasani R, Hudson DA, Adeli E, et al. 2021. On the opportunities and risks of Foundation Models. *arXiv:2108.07258 [cs]*

Bonnen T, Yamins DLK, Wagner AD. 2021. When the ventral visual stream is not enough: a deep learning account of medial temporal lobe involvement in perception. *Neuron*. 109(17):2755–66.e6

Bornstein AM, Khaw MW, Shohamy D, Daw ND. 2017. Reminders of past choices bias decisions for reward in humans. *Nat Commun*. 8(1):15958

Bornstein B, Sroka H, Munitz H. 1969. Prosopagnosia with animal face agnosia. *Cortex*. 5(2):164–9

Botvinick M, Barrett DG, Battaglia P, et al. 2017. Building machines that learn and think for themselves. *Behav Brain Sci*. 40: E255

Botvinick M, Ritter S, Wang JX, Kurth-Nelson Z, Blundell C, Hassabis D. 2019. Reinforcement learning, fast and slow. *Trends Cogn Sci*. 23(5):408–22

Botvinick M, Wang JX, Dabney W, Miller KJ, Kurth-Nelson Z. 2020. Deep reinforcement learning and its neuroscientific implications. *Neuron*. 107(4):603–16

Botvinick MM, Niv Y, Barto AC. 2009. Hierarchically organized behavior and its neural foundations: a reinforcement learning perspective. *Cognition*. 113(3):262–80

Bowers JS, Davis CJ. 2012. Bayesian just-so stories in psychology and neuroscience. *Psychol Bull*. 138(3):389–414

Boyd R, Richerson PJ, Henrich J. 2011. The cultural niche: why social learning is essential for human adaptation. *Proc Natl Acad Sci U S A*. 108(Suppl 2):10918–25

Brady TF, Konkle T, Alvarez GA, Oliva A. 2008. Visual long-term memory has a massive storage capacity for object details. *Proc Natl Acad Sci U S A*. 105(38):14325–9

Bright P, Hale E, Gooch VJ, Myhill T, van der Linde I. 2018. The National Adult Reading Test: restandardisation against the Wechsler Adult Intelligence Scale—fourth edition. *Neuropsychol Rehabil*. 28(6):1019–27

Bromberg-Martin ES, Matsumoto M, Hong S, Hikosaka O. 2010. A pallidus-habenula-dopamine pathway signals inferred stimulus values. *J Neurophysiol.* 104(2):1068–76

Brown RE. 2016. Hebb and Cattell: the genesis of the theory of fluid and crystallized intelligence. *Front Hum Neurosci.* 10:606

Brown TB, Mann B, Ryder N, et al. 2020. Language models are few-shot learners. *arXiv:2005.14165 [cs, CL]*

Burda Y, Edwards H, Storkey A, Klimov O. 2018. Exploration by random network distillation. *arXiv:1810.12894 [cs, stat]*

Cai J, Shin R, Song D. 2017. Making neural programming architectures generalize via recursion. *arXiv:1704.06611 [cs]*

Calhoun AJ, Chalasani SH, Sharpee TO. 2014. Maximally informative foraging by *Caenorhabditis elegans. eLife.* 3:e04220

Carey S. 2011. Precis of 'The Origin of Concepts'. *Behav Brain Sci.* 34(3):113–24; discussion 124–62

Carr MF, Jadhav SP, Frank LM. 2011. Hippocampal replay in the awake state: a potential substrate for memory consolidation and retrieval. *Nat Neurosci.* 14(2):147–53

Casasanto D, Bottini R. 2014. Mirror reading can reverse the flow of time. *J Exp Psychol Gen.* 143(2):473–9

Chaisangmongkon W, Swaminathan SK, Freedman DJ, Wang XJ. 2017. Computing by robust transience: how the fronto-parietal network performs sequential, category-based decisions. *Neuron.* 93(6):1504–17.e4

Chance P. 1999. Thorndike's puzzle boxes and the origins of the experimental analysis of behavior. *J Exp Anal Behav* 72(3):433–40

Chase WG, Simon HA. 1973. Perception in chess. *Cogn Psychol.* 4(1):55–81

Chaudhuri R, Knoblauch K, Gariel M-A, Kennedy H, Wang X-J. 2015. A large-scale circuit mechanism for hierarchical dynamical processing in the primate cortex. *Neuron.* 88(2):419–31

Chmiel A, Schubert E. 2017. Back to the inverted-U for music preference: a review of the literature. *Psychology of Music.* 45(6):886–909

Chowdhery A, Narang S, Devlin J, et al. 2022. PaLM: scaling language modeling with pathways. *arXiv:2204.02311 [cs, CL]*

Christian B. 2020. *The Alignment Problem: Machine Learning and Human Values.* New York, NY: W.W. Norton & Company. First edition

Clerkin EM, Hart E, Rehg JM, Yu C, Smith LB. 2017. Real-world visual statistics and infants' first-learned object names. *Phil Trans R Soc B.* 372(1711):20160055

Cobbe K, Hesse C, Hilton J, Schulman J. 2020. Leveraging procedural generation to benchmark reinforcement learning. *arXiv:1912.01588 [cs, stat]*

Cobbe K, Kosaraju V, Bavarian M, et al. 2021. Training verifiers to solve math word problems. *arXiv:2110.14168 [cs]*

Cohen JD, Perlstein WM, Braver TS, et al. 1997. Temporal dynamics of brain activation during a working memory task. *Nature.* 386(6625):604–8

Constantinescu AO, O'Reilly JX, Behrens TEJ. 2016. Organizing conceptual knowledge in humans with a gridlike code. *Science.* 352(6292):1464–8

Corkin S. 2014. *Permanent Present Tense: The Man with No Memory, and What He Taught the World.* New York, NY: Basic Books

Cortese JM, Dyre BP. 1996. Perceptual similarity of shapes generated from fourier descriptors. *Journal of Experimental Psychology: Human Perception and Performance.* 22(1):133–43

Cosmides L, Barrett HC, Tooby J. 2010. Adaptive specializations, social exchange, and the evolution of human intelligence. *Proc Natl Acad Sci U S A.* 107(Suppl 2):9007–14

Cox D, Meyers E, Sinha P. 2004. Contextually evoked object-specific responses in human visual cortex. *Science*. 304(5667):115–17

Cox JR, Griggs RA. 1982. The effects of experience on performance in Wason's selection task. *Mem Cognit*. 10(5):496–502

Cremer C. 2021. Deep limitations? Examining expert disagreement over deep learning. *Progress in Artificial Intelligence*. 10:449–64

Cueva CJ, Wei XX. 2018. Emergence of grid-like representations by training recurrent neural networks to perform spatial localization. *arXiv:1803.07770 [cs, q-bio]*

Cushman F. 2020. Rationalization is rational. *Behav Brain Sci*. 43:e28

Davies A, Veličković P, Buesing L, et al. 2021. Advancing mathematics by guiding human intuition with AI. *Nature*. 600(7887):70–4

Daw ND, Gershman SJ, Seymour B, Dayan P, Dolan RJ. 2011. Model-based influences on humans' choices and striatal prediction errors. *Neuron*. 69(6):1204–15

Daw ND, Niv Y, Dayan P. 2005. Uncertainty-based competition between prefrontal and dorsolateral striatal systems for behavioral control. *Nat Neurosci*. 8(12):1704–11

Dayan P. 1991. Reinforcing connectionism: learning the statistical way. Doctoral thesis, http://hdl.handle.net/1842/14754

Decker JH, Otto AR, Daw ND, Hartley CA. 2016. From creatures of habit to goal-directed learners: tracking the developmental emergence of model-based reinforcement learning. *Psychol Sci*. 27(6):848–58

Dehaene S, Bossini S, Giraux P. 1993. The mental representation of parity and number magnitude. *J Exp Psychol Gen*. 122(3):371–96

DeLong AJ. 1981. Phenomenological space-time: toward an experiential relativity. *Science*. 213(4508):681–3

Dember WN, Earl RW. 1957. Analysis of exploratory, manipulatory, and curiosity behaviors. *Psychol Rev*. 64(2):91–6

Detterman DK. 1993. The case for the prosecution: Transfer as an epiphenomenon. In: DK Detterman & RJ Sternberg, editors. *Transfer on trial: Intelligence, cognition, and instruction*, pp. 1–24. Ablex Publishing

de Waal F. 2016. *Are We Smart Enough to Know How Smart Animals Are?* New York, NY: W. W. Norton & Company

Diamond JM. 2012. *The World until Yesterday: What Can We Learn from Traditional Societies?* New York, NY: Viking

Doeller CF, Barry C, Burgess N. 2010. Evidence for grid cells in a human memory network. *Nature*. 463(7281):657–61

Dolan RJ, Dayan P. 2013. Goals and habits in the brain. *Neuron*. 80(2):312–25

Dolscheid S, Shayan S, Majid A, Casasanto D. 2013. The thickness of musical pitch: psychophysical evidence for linguistic relativity. *Psychol Sci*. 24(5):613–21

Domingos P. 2015. *The Master Algorithm: How the Quest for the Ultimate Learning Machine Will Remake Our World*. Basic Books: New York, NY

Dordek Y, Soudry D, Meir R, Derdikman D. 2016. Extracting grid cell characteristics from place cell inputs using non-negative principal component analysis. *eLife*. 5:e10094

Dosovitskiy A, Beyer L, Kolesnikov A, et al. 2021. An image is worth 16x16 words: transformers for image recognition at scale. *arXiv:2010.11929 [cs]*

Duan Y, Schulman J, Chen X, Bartlett PL, Sutskever I, Abbeel P. 2016. RL^2: Fast reinforcement learning via slow reinforcement learning. *arXiv:1611.02779 [cs, AI]*

Duncan J, Burgess P, Emslie H. 1995. Fluid intelligence after frontal lobe lesions. *Neuropsychologia*. 33(3):261–8

Durstewitz D, Seamans JK, Sejnowski TJ. 2000. Neurocomputational models of working memory. *Nat Neurosci*. 3(S11):1184–91

Egner T, Hirsch J. 2005. Cognitive control mechanisms resolve conflict through cortical amplification of task-relevant information. *Nat Neurosci.* 8(12):1784–90

Eichenbaum H. 2016. Still searching for the engram. *Learn Behav.* 44(3):209–22

Elias P. 1955. Predictive coding—I. *IEEE Trans Inform Theory.* 1(1):16–24

Elman JL. 1990. Finding structure in time. *Cogn Sci.* 14(2):179–211

Faisal AA, Selen LPJ, Wolpert DM. 2008. Noise in the nervous system. *Nat Rev Neurosci.* 9(4):292–303

Farmelo G. 2010. *The Strangest Man: The Hidden Life of Paul Dirac; Quantum Genius.* London: Faber and Faber

Feher da Silva C, Hare TA. 2020. Humans primarily use model-based inference in the two-stage task. *Nat Hum Behav.* 4(10):1053–66

Feigenbaum EA, McCorduck P. 1983. *The Fifth Generation: Artificial Intelligence and Japan's Computer Challenge to the World.* Boston, MA: Addison-Wesley

Feldman J. 2000. Minimization of Boolean complexity in human concept learning. *Nature.* 407(6804):630–3

Fikes RE, Nilsson NJ. 1971. Strips: a new approach to the application of theorem proving to problem solving. *Artificial Intelligence.* 2(3–4):189–208

Findling C, Skvortsova V, Dromnelle R, Palminteri S, Wyart V. 2019. Computational noise in reward-guided learning drives behavioral variability in volatile environments. *Nat Neurosci.* 22(12):2066–77

Findling C, Wyart V. 2020. Computation noise promotes cognitive resilience to adverse conditions during decision-making. *bioRxiv.* https://doi.org/10.1101/2020.06.10.145300

Fine JM, Hayden BY. 2022. The whole prefrontal cortex is premotor cortex. *Phil Trans R Soc B.* 377(1844):20200524

Finn C, Abbeel P, Levine S. 2017. Model-agnostic meta-learning for fast adaptation of deep networks. *arXiv:1703.03400 [cs]*

Fitzgerald JK, Freedman DJ, Fanini A, Bennur S, Gold JI, Assad JA. 2013. Biased associative representations in parietal cortex. *Neuron.* 77(1):180–91

Fleuret F, Li T, Dubout C, Wampler EK, Yantis S, Geman D. 2011. Comparing machines and humans on a visual categorization test. *Proc Natl Acad Sci U S A.* 108(43):17621–5

Fodor JA. 1980. Methodological solipsism considered as a research strategy in cognitive psychology. *Behav Brain Sci.* 3(1):63–73

Fortunato M, Azar MG, Piot B, et al. 2019. Noisy networks for exploration. *arXiv:1706.10295 [cs, stat]*

Foster DJ. 2017. Replay comes of age. *Annu Rev Neurosci.* 40(1):581–602

Frank MJ, Loughry B, O'Reilly RC. 2001. Interactions between frontal cortex and basal ganglia in working memory: a computational model. *Cogn Affect Behav Neurosci.* 1(2):137–60

Freedman DJ, Miller EK. 2008. Neural mechanisms of visual categorization: insights from neurophysiology. *Neurosci Biobehav Rev.* 32(2):311–29

Frey U, Morris RGM. 1997. Synaptic tagging and long-term potentiation. *Nature.* 385(6616):533–6

Friedman-Hill SR, Robertson LC, Treisman A. 1995. Parietal contributions to visual feature binding: evidence from a patient with bilateral lesions. *Science.* 269(5225):853–5

Friston K. 2009. The free-energy principle: a rough guide to the brain? *Trends Cogn Sci.* 13(7):293–301

Friston K. 2010. The free-energy principle: a unified brain theory? *Nat Rev Neurosci.* 11(2):127–38

Friston K. 2013. Life as we know it. *J R Soc Interface.* 10(86):20130475

Friston K, Adams R, Montague R. 2012. What is value—accumulated reward or evidence? *Front Neurorobot.* 6:11

Fuster JM. 2001. The prefrontal cortex—an update. *Neuron*. 30(2):319–33

Fuster JM, Alexander GE. 1971. Neuron activity related to short-term memory. *Science*. 173(3997):652–4

Garnelo M, Schwarz J, Rosenbaum D, et al. 2018. Neural processes. *arXiv:1807.01622 [cs, stat]*

Garnelo M, Shanahan M. 2019. Reconciling deep learning with symbolic artificial intelligence: representing objects and relations. *Curr Opin Behav Sci*. 29:17–23

Garvert MM, Dolan RJ, Behrens TE. 2017. A map of abstract relational knowledge in the human hippocampal-entorhinal cortex. *Elife*. 6:e17086

Geirhos R, Medina Temme CRM, Rauber J, Schutt HH, Bethge M, Wichmann FA. 2018. Generalisation in humans and deep neural networks. Available from: https://papers.nips.cc/paper/7982-generalisation-in-humans-and-deep-neural-networks.pdf

Gentner D, Holyoak KJ, Kokinov BN, eds. 2001. *The Analogical Mind: Perspectives from Cognitive Science*. Cambridge, MA: MIT Press

Gershman SJ. 2019. What does the free energy principle tell us about the brain? *arXiv:1901.07945 [q-bio]*

Gershman SJ. 2021. *What Makes Us Smart: The Computational Logic of Human Cognition*. Princeton, NJ: Princeton University Press

Gershman SJ, Daw ND. 2017. Reinforcement learning and episodic memory in humans and animals: an integrative framework. *Annu Rev Psychol*. 68(1):101–28

Gerstner W, Lehmann M, Liakoni V, Corneil D, Brea J. 2018. Eligibility traces and plasticity on behavioral time scales: experimental support of neoHebbian three-factor learning rules. *Front Neural Circuits*. 12:53

Gick ML, Holyoak KJ. 1980. Analogical problem solving. *Cogn Psychol*. 12:306–55

Gittins JC. 1979. Bandit processes and dynamic allocation indices. *Journal of the Royal Statistical Society: Series B (Methodological)*. 41(2):148–64

Giurfa M, Zhang S, Jenett A, Menzel R, Srinivasan MV. 2001. The concepts of 'sameness' and 'difference' in an insect. *Nature*. 410(6831):930–3

Glass AL, Holyoak KJ, Santa JL. 1979. *Cognition*. Boston, MA: Addison-Wesley

Glimcher PW. 2004. *Decision, Uncertainty and the Brain: The Science of Neuroeconomics*. Cambridge, MA: MIT Press

Goh G, Cammarata N, Voss C, et al. 2021. Multimodal neurons in artificial neural networks. *Distill*. 6(3):10.23915/distill.00030

Gold JI, Shadlen MN. 2007. The neural basis of decision making. *Annu Rev Neurosci*. 30:535–74

Goldman-Rakic PS. 1995. Cellular basis of working memory. *Neuron*. 14(3):477–85

Goodfellow IJ, Pouget-Abadie J, Mirza M, et al. 2014. Generative adversarial networks. *arXiv:1406.2661 [cs, stat]*

Goodman N, Mansinghka V, Roy DM, Bonawitz K, Tenenbaum JB. 2014. Church: a language for generative models. *arXiv:1206.3255 [cs]*

Goodman ND, Tenenbaum JB, Feldman J, Griffiths TL. 2008. A rational analysis of rule-based concept learning. *Cognitive Science*. 32(1):108–54

Gopnik A. 2012. Scientific thinking in young children: theoretical advances, empirical research, and policy implications. *Science*. 337(6102):1623–7

Gopnik A, Sobel DM, Schulz LE, Glymour C. 2001. Causal learning mechanisms in very young children: two-, three-, and four-year-olds infer causal relations from patterns of variation and covariation. *Dev Psychol*. 37(5):620–9

Gopnik A, Wellman HM. 2012. Reconstructing constructivism: causal models, Bayesian learning mechanisms, and the theory theory. *Psychol Bull*. 138(6):1085–108

Gould SJ. 1989. *Wonderful Life: The Burgess Shale and the Nature of History*. New York, NY: W.W. Norton. First edition

Grace K, Salvatier J, Dafoe A, Zhang B, Evans O. 2018. When will AI exceed human performance? Evidence from AI experts. *arXiv:1705.08807 [cs, AI]*

Graesser AC, Long DL, Mio JS. 1989. What are the cognitive and conceptual components of humorous text? *Poetics.* 18(1–2):143–63

Graves A, Wayne G, Reynolds M, et al. 2016. Hybrid computing using a neural network with dynamic external memory. *Nature.* 538(7626):471–6

Gregor K, Rezende DJ, Wierstra D. 2016. Variational intrinsic control. *arXiv:1611.07507 [cs]*

Griffiths TL, Tenenbaum JB. 2006. Optimal predictions in everyday cognition. *Psychol Sci.* 17(9):767–73

Grigorenko EL, Meier E, Lipka J, Mohatt G, Yanez E, Sternberg RJ. 2004. Academic and practical intelligence: a case study of the Yup'ik in Alaska. *Learning and Individual Differences.* 14(4):183–207

Grigorenko EL, Sternberg RJ. 2001. Analytical, creative, and practical intelligence as predictors of self-reported adaptive functioning: a case study in Russia. *Intelligence.* 29(1):57–73

Gross CG. 2002. Genealogy of the 'grandmother cell'. *Neuroscientist.* 8(5):512–18

Gupta AS, van der Meer MAA, Touretzky DS, Redish AD. 2010. Hippocampal replay is not a simple function of experience. *Neuron.* 65(5):695–705

Ha D, Schmidhuber J. 2018. World models. *arXiv:1803.10122 [cs, stat]*

Haber, S. 2016. Corticostriatal circuitry. *Dialogues Clin Neurosci.* 18(1):7–21

Hadsell R, Rao D, Rusu AA, Pascanu R. 2020. Embracing change: continual learning in deep neural networks. *Trends Cogn Sci.* 24(12):1028–40

Haenlein M, Kaplan A. 2019. A brief history of artificial intelligence: on the past, present, and future of artificial intelligence. *California Management Review.* 61(4):5–14

Hall L, Johansson P, Tärning B, Sikström S, Deutgen T. 2010. Magic at the marketplace: choice blindness for the taste of jam and the smell of tea. *Cognition.* 117(1):54–61

Hammer M. 1993. An identified neuron mediates the unconditioned stimulus in associative olfactory learning in honeybees. *Nature.* 366(6450):59–63

Hanks TD, Summerfield C. 2017. Perceptual decision making in rodents, monkeys, and humans. *Neuron.* 93(1):15–31

Harlow H. 1949. The formation of learning sets. *Psychol Rev.* 56:51–65

Harlow HF, Harlow MK, Meyer DR. 1950. Learning motivated by a manipulation drive. *J Exp Psychol.* 40(2):228–34

Harnad S. 1990. The symbol grounding problem. *Physica D: Nonlinear Phenomena.* 42(1–3):335–46

Haskell RE. 2001. *Transfer of Learning: Cognition, Instruction, and Reasoning.* San Diego, CA: Academic Press

Hassabis D, Kumaran D, Summerfield C, Botvinick M. 2017. Neuroscience-inspired artificial intelligence. *Neuron.* 95(2):245–58

Hasson U, Nastase SA, Goldstein A. 2020. Direct fit to nature: an evolutionary perspective on biological and artificial neural networks. *Neuron.* 105(3):416–34

Hawkins J. 2004. *On Intelligence.* Times Books: New York, NY

Hazy TE, Frank MJ, O'Reilly RC. 2006. Banishing the homunculus: making working memory work. *Neuroscience.* 139(1):105–18

Henderson JM, Hollingworth A. 1999. High-level scene perception. *Annu Rev Psychol.* 50(1):243–71

Hernández-Orallo J, Martínez-Plumed F, Schmid U, Siebers M, Dowe DL. 2016. Computer models solving intelligence test problems: progress and implications. *Artificial Intelligence.* 230:74–107

Higgins I, Chang L, Langston V, et al. 2021. Unsupervised deep learning identifies semantic disentanglement in single inferotemporal face patch neurons. *Nat Commun.* 12(1):6456

Higgins I, Matthey L, Glorot X, et al. 2016. Early visual concept learning with unsupervised deep learning. *arXiv:1606.05579*

Higgins I, Sonnerat N, Matthey L, et al. 2017. SCAN: learning hierarchical compositional visual concepts. *arXiv:1707.03389*

Hochreiter S, Younger AS, Conwell PR. 2001. Learning to learn using gradient descent. In: G Dorffner, H Bischof, K Hornik, editors. *Artificial Neural Networks—ICANN 2001*, Vol. 2130, pp. 87–94. Berlin, Heidelberg: Springer

Hoffmann J, Borgeaud S, Mensch A, et al. 2022. Training compute-optimal large language models. *arXiv:2203.15556*

Holding DH. 1992. Theories of chess skill. *Psychol Res.* 54(1):10–16

Hopfield JJ. 1982. Neural networks and physical systems with emergent collective computational abilities. *Proc Natl Acad Sci U S A.* 79(8):2554–8

Hunt GR. 1996. Manufacture and use of hook-tools by New Caledonian crows. *Nature.* 379(6562):249–51

Ison MJ, Quian Quiroga R, Fried I. 2015. Rapid encoding of new memories by individual neurons in the human brain. *Neuron.* 87(1):220–30

Itti L, Baldi P. 2009. Bayesian surprise attracts human attention. *Vision Res.* 49(10):1295–306

Jacobsen CF. 1935. Functions of frontal association area in primates. *Arch NeurPsych.* 33(3):558

Jazayeri M, Shadlen MN. 2015. A neural mechanism for sensing and reproducing a time interval. *Curr Biol.* 25(20):2599–609

Jerde TA, Merriam EP, Riggall AC, Hedges JH, Curtis CE. 2012. Prioritized maps of space in human frontoparietal cortex. *J Neurosci.* 32(48):17382–90

Jiang L, Hwang JD, Bhagavatula C, et al. 2021. Delphi: towards machine ethics and norms. *arXiv:2110.07574 [cs]*

Johansson P, Hall L, Sikström S, Olsson A. 2005. Failure to detect mismatches between intention and outcome in a simple decision task. *Science.* 310(5745):116–19

Johnson J, Hariharan B, van der Maaten L, Fei-Fei L, Zitnick CL, Girshick R. 2016. CLEVR: a diagnostic dataset for compositional language and elementary visual reasoning. *arXiv:1612.06890 [cs]*

Johnson-Laird PN. 2010. Mental models and human reasoning. *Proc Natl Acad Sci U S A.* 107(43):18243–50

Jonas E, Kording KP. 2017. Could a neuroscientist understand a microprocessor? *PLoS Comput Biol.* 13(1):e1005268

Jumper J, Evans R, Pritzel A, et al. 2021. Highly accurate protein structure prediction with AlphaFold. *Nature.* 596(7873):583–9

Kahneman D, Slovic P, Tversky A. 1982. *Judgment Under Uncertainty: Heuristics and Biases.* New York, NY: Cambridge University Press

Kakade S, Dayan P. 2002. Dopamine: generalization and bonuses. *Neural Netw.* 15(4–6):549–59

Kang MJ, Hsu M, Krajbich IM, et al. 2009. The wick in the candle of learning: epistemic curiosity activates reward circuitry and enhances memory. *Psychol Sci.* 20(8):963–73

Kaplan J, McCandlish S, Henighan T, et al. 2020. Scaling laws for neural language models. *arXiv:2001.08361 [cs, stat]*

Kapturowski, Ostrovski,G., Quan, J., Munos R., Dabney, W. 2018. Recurrent experience replay in distributed reinforcement learning. https://openreview.net/pdf?id=r1lyTjAqYX

Kar K, Kubilius J, Schmidt K, Issa EB, DiCarlo JJ. 2019. Evidence that recurrent circuits are critical to the ventral stream's execution of core object recognition behavior. *Nat Neurosci.* 22(6):974–83

Karpathy A. 2015. The unreasonable effectiveness of recurrent neural networks. https://karpathy.github.io/2015/05/21/rnn-effectiveness/

Keil FC. 1979. *Semantic and Conceptual Development: An Ontological Perspective*. Cambridge, MA: Harvard University Press

Kemp C, Tenenbaum JB. 2008. The discovery of structural form. *Proc Natl Acad Sci U S A*. 105(31):10687–92

Kidd C, Piantadosi ST, Aslin RN. 2012. The Goldilocks effect: human infants allocate attention to visual sequences that are neither too simple nor too complex. *PLoS One*. 7(5):e36399

Kim J, Ricci M, Serre T. 2018. Not-so-CLEVR: learning same–different relations strains feed-forward neural networks. *Interface Focus*. 8(4):20180011

Kirk R, Zhang A, Grefenstette E, Rocktäschel T. 2022. A survey of generalisation in deep reinforcement learning. *arXiv:2111.09794 [cs]*

Kirkpatrick J, Pascanu R, Rabinowitz N, et al. 2017. Overcoming catastrophic forgetting in neural networks. *Proc Natl Acad Sci U S A*. 114(13):3521–6

Koechlin E, Ody C, Kouneiher F. 2003. The architecture of cognitive control in the human prefrontal cortex. *Science*. 302(5648):1181–5

Koechlin E, Summerfield C. 2007. An information theoretical approach to prefrontal executive function. *Trends Cogn Sci*. 11(6):229–35

Kosinski M, Stillwell D, Graepel T. 2013. Private traits and attributes are predictable from digital records of human behavior. *Proc Natl Acad Sci U S A*. 110(15):5802–5

Kubota K, Niki H. 1971. Prefrontal cortical unit activity and delayed alternation performance in monkeys. *J Neurophysiol*. 34(3):337–47

Kurby CA, Zacks JM. 2008. Segmentation in the perception and memory of events. *Trends Cogn Sci*. 12(2):72–9

Kurth-Nelson Z, Economides M, Dolan RJ, Dayan P. 2016. Fast sequences of non-spatial state representations in humans. *Neuron*. 91(1):194–204

Laird J. 2012. *The Soar Cognitive Architecture*. Cambridge, MA: MIT Press

Lake BM, Baroni M. 2018. Generalization without systematicity: on the compositional skills of sequence-to-sequence recurrent networks. *arXiv:1711.00350 [cs]*

Lake BM, Salakhutdinov R, Tenenbaum JB. 2015. Human-level concept learning through probabilistic program induction. *Science*. 350(6266):1332–8

Lake BM, Ullman TD, Tenenbaum JB, Gershman SJ. 2017. Building machines that learn and think like people. *Behav Brain Sci*. 40:e253

Lakoff G. 1987. *Women, Fire, and Dangerous Things: What Categories Reveal about the Mind*. Chicago, IL: University of Chicago Press

Larriva-Sahd JA. 2014. Some predictions of Rafael Lorente de NÃ3 80 years later. *Front Neuroanat*. 8:147

Lave J. 1988. *Cognition in Practice: Mind, Mathematics and Culture in Everyday Life*. New York, NY: Cambridge University Press. First edition

Law CT, Gold JI. 2009. Reinforcement learning can account for associative and perceptual learning on a visual-decision task. *Nat Neurosci*. 12(5):655–63

LeCun Y, Bengio Y, Hinton G. 2015. Deep learning. *Nature*. 521(7553):436–44

Legg S, Hutter M. 2007. A collection of definitions of intelligence. *arXiv:0706.3639*

Lehmann MP, Xu HA, Liakoni V, Herzog MH, Gerstner W, Preuschoff K. 2019. One-shot learning and behavioral eligibility traces in sequential decision making. *eLife*. 8:e47463

Leibo JZ, Hughes E, Lanctot M, Graepel T. 2019. Autocurricula and the emergence of innovation from social interaction: a manifesto for multi-agent intelligence research. *arXiv:1903.00742 [cs, AI]*

Lenat DB, Guha RV, Pittman K, Pratt D, Shepherd M. 1990. Cyc: toward programs with common sense. *Commun ACM*. 33(8):30–49

Lengyel M, Dayan P. 2007. Hippocampal contributions to control: the third way. https://papers.nips.cc/paper/2007/file/1f4477bad7af3616c1f933a02bfabe4e-Paper.pdf

Levitt GM. 2006. *The Turk, Chess Automaton*. Jefferson, NC: McFarland & Co

Levitt JB, Lewis DA, Yoshioka T, Lund JS. 1993. Topography of pyramidal neuron intrinsic connections in macaque monkey prefrontal cortex (areas 9 and 46). *J Comp Neurol.* 338(3):360–76

Li Y, Gimeno F, Kohli P, Vinyals O. 2020. Strong generalization and efficiency in neural programs. *arXiv:2007.03629 [cs, stat]*

Lloyd K, Becker N, Jones MW, Bogacz R. 2012. Learning to use working memory: a reinforcement learning gating model of rule acquisition in rats. *Front Comput. Neurosci.* 6:87

Loetscher T, Schwarz U, Schubiger M, Brugger P. 2008. Head turns bias the brain's internal random generator. *Curr Biol.* 18(2):R60–2

Lubow RE, Moore AU. 1959. Latent inhibition: the effect of nonreinforced pre-exposure to the conditional stimulus. *J Comp Physiol Psychol.* 52(4):415–19

Luyckx F, Nili H, Spitzer B, Summerfield C. 2019. Neural structure mapping in human probabilistic reward learning. *Elife.* 8:e42816

Lynch G. 2009. *Big Brain: The Origins and Future of Human Intelligence*. Palgrave Macmillan: London, UK

Mandler G. 1980. Recognizing: the judgment of previous occurrence. *Psychol Rev.* 87(3):252–71

Mante V, Sussillo D, Shenoy KV, Newsome WT. 2013. Context-dependent computation by recurrent dynamics in prefrontal cortex. *Nature.* 503(7474):78–84

Marcus G. 2020. The next decade in AI: four steps towards robust artificial intelligence. *arXiv:2002.06177 [cs]*

Marcus G, Davis E. 2019. *Rebooting AI: Building Artificial Intelligence We Can Trust*. New York, NY: Pantheon Books. First edition

Martinho A, Kacelnik A. 2016. Ducklings imprint on the relational concept of 'same or different'. *Science.* 353(6296):286–8

Mattar MG, Daw ND. 2018. Prioritized memory access explains planning and hippocampal replay. *Nat Neurosci.* 21(11):1609–17

McClelland JL, Botvinick MM, Noelle DC, et al. 2010. Letting structure emerge: connectionist and dynamical systems approaches to cognition. *Trends Cogn Sci.* 14(8):348–56

McCloskey M, Cohen NJ. 1989. Catastrophic Interference in Connectionist Networks: The Sequential Learning Problem. In: G Bower, editor. *Psychology of Learning and Motivation* 24:109–65. Academic Press

McCorduck P. 2004. *Machines Who Think: A Personal Inquiry into the History and Prospects of Artificial Intelligence*. Natick, MA: A. K. Peters. 25th anniversary update edition

McCulloch WS, Pitts W. 1943. A logical calculus of the ideas immanent in nervous activity. *Bull Math Biol.* 5(4):115–33

Medin DL, Schaffer MM. 1978. Context theory of classification learning. *Psychol Rev.* 85:207–38

Menon V. 2016. Memory and cognitive control circuits in mathematical cognition and learning. *Prog Brain Res.* 227:159–86

Mercado E, Killebrew DA, Pack AA, Mácha IVB, Herman LM. 2000. Generalization of 'same–different' classification abilities in bottlenosed dolphins. *Behav Processes.* 50(2–3):79–94

Messer WS, Griggs RA. 1989. Student belief and involvement in the paranormal and performance in introductory psychology. *Teaching of Psychology.* 16(4):187–91

Mikulik V, Delétang G, McGrath T, et al. 2020. Meta-trained agents implement Bayes-optimal agents. *arXiv:2010.11223 [cs]*

Miller EK, Cohen JD. 2001. An integrative theory of prefrontal cortex function. *Annu Rev Neurosci.* 24:167–202

Mineault PJ, Bakhtiari S, Richards BA, Pack CC. 2021. Your head is there to move you around: goal-driven models of the primate dorsal pathway. *Neuroscience*

Minsky M. 1979. A framework for representing knowledge. In: D Metzing, editor. *Frame Conceptions and Text Understanding*, pp. 1–25. Berlin: de Gruyter

Mischel W, Shoda Y, Rodriguez ML. 1989. Delay of gratification in children. *Science*. 244(4907):933–8

Mitchell CT, Davis R. 1987. The perception of time in scale model environments. *Perception*. 16(1):5–16

Mnih V, Kavukcuoglu K, Silver D, et al. 2015. Human-level control through deep reinforcement learning. *Nature*. 518(7540):529–33

Mongillo G, Barak O, Tsodyks M. 2008. Synaptic theory of working memory. *Science*. 319(5869):1543–6

Montague PR, Dayan P, Person C, Sejnowski TJ. 1995. Bee foraging in uncertain environments using predictive hebbian learning. *Nature*. 377(6551):725–8

Moore BR, Stuttard S. 1979. Dr. Guthrie and *Felis domesticus* or: tripping over the cat. *Science*. 205(4410):1031–3

Moravcik M, Schmid M, Burch N, et al. 2017. DeepStack: expert-level artificial intelligence in heads-up no-limit poker. *Science*. 356(6337):508–13

Morrens J, Aydin Ç, Janse van Rensburg A, Esquivelzeta Rabell J, Haesler S. 2020. Cue-evoked dopamine promotes conditioned responding during learning. *Neuron*. 106(1):142–53.e7

Morris RGM, Garrud P, Rawlins JNP, O'Keefe J. 1982. Place navigation impaired in rats with hippocampal lesions. *Nature*. 297(5868):681–3

Mugny G, Carugati F. 2009. *Social Representations of Intelligence*. Cambridge: Cambridge University Press

Mumford D. 2020. The convergence of AI code and cortical functioning—a commentary. *arXiv:2010.09101 [cs]*

Murray E, Wise S, Baldwin M, Graham KS. 2019. *The Evolutionary Road to Human Memory*. Oxford: Oxford University Press

Murray EA, Bussey TJ, Saksida LM. 2007. Visual perception and memory: a new view of medial temporal lobe function in primates and rodents. *Annu Rev Neurosci*. 30(1):99–122

Murray JD, Bernacchia A, Freedman DJ, et al. 2014. A hierarchy of intrinsic timescales across primate cortex. *Nat Neurosci*. 17(12):1661–3

Murray JD, Bernacchia A, Roy NA, Constantinidis C, Romo R, Wang X-J. 2017. Stable population coding for working memory coexists with heterogeneous neural dynamics in prefrontal cortex. *Proc Natl Acad Sci U S A*. 114(2):394–9

Nakazawa K, Sun LD, Quirk MC, Rondi-Reig L, Wilson MA, Tonegawa S. 2003. Hippocampal CA3 NMDA receptors are crucial for memory acquisition of one-time experience. *Neuron*. 38(2):305–15

Nicolas S. 1996. Experiments on implicit memory in a Korsakoff patient by Claparede (1907). *Cogn Neuropsychol*. 13(8):1193–9

Nieder A, Dehaene S. 2009. Representation of number in the brain. *Annu Rev Neurosci*. 32(1):185–208

Nieder A. 2012. Supramodal numerosity selectivity of neurons in primate prefrontal and posterior parietal cortices. *Proc Natl Acad Sci U S A*. 109(29):11860–5

Nisbett RE, Wilson TD. 1977. Telling more than we can know: verbal reports on mental processes. *Psychol Rev*. 84(3):231–59

Norman DA, Shallice T. 1986. Attention to action: willed and automatic control of behaviour. In: GE Schwartz, D Shapiro, editors. *Consciousness and Self-Regulation*, pp. 1–18. New York, NY: Plenum Press

Nosofsky RM, Palmeri TJ, McKinley SC. 1994. Rule-plus-exception model of classification learning. *Psychol Rev*. 101(1):53–79

Nunes T, Schliemann AD, Carraher DW. 1993. *Street Mathematics and School Mathematics.* New York, NY: Cambridge University Press

O'Doherty J, Dayan P, Schultz J, Deichmann R, Friston K, Dolan RJ. 2004. Dissociable roles of ventral and dorsal striatum in instrumental conditioning. *Science.* 304(5669):452–4

Ólafsdóttir HF, Bush D, Barry C. 2018. The role of hippocampal replay in memory and planning. *Curr Biol.* 28(1):R37–50

Oliva A, Torralba A. 2007. The role of context in object recognition. *Trends Cogn Sci.* 11(12):520–7

Op de Beeck H, Wagemans J, Vogels R. 2001. Inferotemporal neurons represent low-dimensional configurations of parameterized shapes. *Nat Neurosci.* 4(12):1244–52

Ord T. 2020. *The Precipice: Existential Risk and the Future of Humanity.* New York, NY: Hachette Books. First edition

O'Reilly RC, Frank MJ. 2006. Making working memory work: a computational model of learning in the prefrontal cortex and basal ganglia. *Neural Comput.* 18(2):283–328

Orhan AE, Ma WJ. 2017. Efficient probabilistic inference in generic neural networks trained with non-probabilistic feedback. *Nat Commun.* 8(1):138

Orhan AE, Ma WJ. 2019. A diverse range of factors affect the nature of neural representations underlying short-term memory. *Nat Neurosci.* 22(2):275–83

Otto A, Gershman S. 2013. The curse of planning: dissecting multiple reinforcement learning systems by taxing the central executive. *Psychological Science.* 24(5):751–61

Oudeyer P, Kaplan F. 2007. What is intrinsic motivation? A typology of computational approaches. *Front Neurorobotics.* 1:6

Park IM, Meister ML, Huk AC, Pillow JW. 2014. Encoding and decoding in parietal cortex during sensorimotor decision-making. *Nature Neurosci.* 17(10):1395–403

Parker ES, Cahill L, McGaugh JL. 2006. A case of unusual autobiographical remembering. *Neurocase.* 12(1):35–49

Parkinson C, Liu S, Wheatley T. 2014. A common cortical metric for spatial, temporal, and social distance. *J Neurosci.* 34(5):1979–87

Passingham R, Wise S. 2012. *The Neurobiology of the Prefrontal Cortex: Anatomy, Evolution, and the Origin of Insight.* Oxford: Oxford University Press

Pavlides C, Winson J. 1989. Influences of hippocampal place cell firing in the awake state on the activity of these cells during subsequent sleep episodes. *J. Neurosci.* 9(8):2907–18

Pearl J. 1984. *Heuristics: Intelligent Search Strategies for Computer Problem Solving.* Boston, MA: Addison-Wesley

Penn DC, Holyoak KJ, Povinelli DJ. 2008. Darwin's mistake: explaining the discontinuity between human and nonhuman minds. *Behav Brain Sci.* 31(2):109–30; discussion 130–78

Pepperberg IM. 1987. Acquisition of the same/different concept by an African grey parrot (*Psittacus erithacus*): learning with respect to categories of color, shape, and material. *Animal Learning & Behavior.* 15(4):423–32

Pérez J, Marinković J, Barceló P. 2019. On the Turing completeness of modern neural network architectures. *arXiv:1901.03429 [cs, stat]*

Pezzulo G, Baldassarre G, Butz MV, Castelfranchi C, Hoffmann J. 2007. From Actions to Goals and Vice-Versa: Theoretical Analysis and Models of the Ideomotor Principle and TOTE. In: MV Butz, O Sigaud, G Pezzulo, G Baldassarre, editors. *Anticipatory Behavior in Adaptive Learning Systems. ABiALS 2006. Lecture Notes in Computer Science*, Vol. 4520. Springer: Berlin, Heidelberg. https://doi.org/10.1007/978-3-540-74262-3_5

Piantadosi ST, Tenenbaum JB, Goodman ND. 2016. The logical primitives of thought: empirical foundations for compositional cognitive models. *Psychol Rev.* 123(4):392–424

Piketty T, Goldhammer A. 2014. *Capital in the Twenty-First Century.* Cambridge, MA: The Belknap Press of Harvard University Press

Pinker S. 2010. Colloquium paper: the cognitive niche: coevolution of intelligence, sociality, and language. *Proc Natl Acad Sci U S A.* 107(Suppl 2):8993–9

Plappert M, Houthooft R, Dhariwal P, et al. 2018. Parameter space noise for exploration. *arXiv:1706.01905 [cs, stat]*

Platt ML, Glimcher PW. 1999. Neural correlates of decision variables in parietal cortex. *Nature.* 400(6741):233–8

Plunkett K, Sinha C. 1992. Connectionism and developmental theory. *Br J Dev Psychol.* 10(3):209–54

Poe EA. 1836. Maelzel's chess-player. Available from: https://www.eapoe.org/works/essays/maelzel.htm

Popham SF, Huth AG, Bilenko NY, et al. 2021. Visual and linguistic semantic representations are aligned at the border of human visual cortex. *Nat Neurosci.* 24(11):1628–36

Prakash C, Stephens KD, Hoffman DD, Singh M, Fields C. 2021. Fitness beats truth in the evolution of perception. *Acta Biotheor.* 69(3):319–41

Premack D. 2010. Why humans are unique: three theories. *Perspect Psychol Sci.* 5(1):22–32

Pylyshyn ZW. 1973. What the mind's eye tells the mind's brain: a critique of mental imagery. *Psychol Bull.* 80(1):1–24

Pylyshyn ZW. 1989. *Computation and Cognition: Toward a Foundation for Cognitive Science.* Cambridge, MA: MIT Press

Quiroga RQ, Reddy L, Kreiman G, Koch C, Fried I. 2005. Invariant visual representation by single neurons in the human brain. *Nature.* 435(7045):1102–7

Rae JW, Borgeaud S, Cai T, et al. 2022. Scaling language models: methods, analysis and insights from training gopher. *arXiv:2112.11446 [cs]*

Ralph MAL, Jefferies E, Patterson K, Rogers TT. 2017. The neural and computational bases of semantic cognition. *Nat Rev Neurosci.* 18(1):42–55

Ramesh A, Dhariwal P, Nichol A, Chu C, Chen M. 2022. Hierarchical text-conditional image generation with CLIP latents. *arXiv:2204.06125 [cs]*

Ramesh A, Pavlov M, Goh G, et al. 2021. Zero-shot text-to-image generation. *arXiv:2102.12092 [cs]*

Rao RP, Ballard DH. 1999. Predictive coding in the visual cortex: a functional interpretation of some extra-classical receptive-field effects. *Nature Neurosci.* 2(1):79–87

Rao SC, Rainer G, Miller EK. 1997. Integration of what and where in the primate prefrontal cortex. *Science.* 276(5313):821–4

Raven J. 2000. The Raven's progressive matrices: change and stability over culture and time. *Cogn Psychol.* 41(1):1–48

Redgrave P, Gurney K. 2006. The short-latency dopamine signal: a role in discovering novel actions? *Nat Rev Neurosci.* 7(12):967–75

Redgrave P, Rodriguez M, Smith Y, et al. 2010. Goal-directed and habitual control in the basal ganglia: implications for Parkinson's disease. *Nat Rev Neurosci.* 11:760–72

Regier T, Kay P, Cook RS. 2005. Focal colors are universal after all. *Proc Natl Acad Sci U S A.* 102(23):8386–91

Rey HG, Gori B, Chaure FJ, et al. 2020. Single neuron coding of identity in the human hippocampal formation. *Curr Biol.* 30(6):1152–9.e3

Reynolds JN, Hyland BI, Wickens JR. 2001. A cellular mechanism of reward-related learning. *Nature.* 413(6851):67–70

Rhinehart N, Wang J, Berseth G, et al. 2021. Information is power: intrinsic control via information capture. *arXiv:2112.03899 [cs]*

Richards BA, Lillicrap TP, Beaudoin P, et al. 2019. A deep learning framework for neuroscience. *Nat Neurosci.* 22(11):1761–70

Rips LJ. 1983. Cognitive processes in propositional reasoning. *Psychol Rev.* 90(1):38–71

Robertson L, Treisman A, Friedman-Hill S, Grabowecky M. 1997. The interaction of spatial and object pathways: evidence from Balint's syndrome. *J Cogn Neurosci.* 9(3):295–317

Robertson L. 2003. Binding, spatial attention and perceptual awareness. *Nat Rev Neurosci.* 4:93–102

Rocke AJ. 2010. *Image and Reality: Kekulé, Kopp, and the Scientific Imagination.* Chicago, IL: University of Chicago Press

Roitman JD, Brannon EM, Platt ML. 2007. Monotonic coding of numerosity in macaque lateral intraparietal area. *PLoS Biol.* 5(8):e208

Rose NS, LaRocque JJ, Riggall AC, et al. 2016. Reactivation of latent working memories with transcranial magnetic stimulation. *Science.* 354(6316):1136–9

Roth G, Dicke U. 2005. Evolution of the brain and intelligence. *Trends Cogn Sci.* 9(5):250–7

Russakovsky O, Deng J, Su H, et al. 2015. ImageNet large scale visual recognition challenge. *arXiv:1409.0575*

Russell S. 2019a. *Human Compatible: AI and the Problem of Control.* Penguin Random House: New York, NY

Russell S. 2019b. Defining AI wireheading. https://www.lesswrong.com/posts/vXzM5L6njDZSf4Ftk/defining-ai-wireheading

Russell S, Norvig P. 1995. *Artificial Intelligence: A Modern Approach.* Upper Saddle River, NJ: Prentice Hall

Sadler M, Regan N. 2019. *Game Changer: AlphaZero's Groundbreaking Chess Strategies and the Promise of AI.* Alkmaar: New in Chess

Saez E, Zucman G. 2019. *The Triumph of Injustice: How the Rich Dodge Taxes and How to Make Them Pay.* New York, NY: W. W. Norton & Company. First edition

Saharia C, Chan W, Saxena S, et al. 2022. Photorealistic text-to-image diffusion models with deep language understanding. *arXiv:2205.11487 [cs, CV]*

Salge C, Glackin C, Polani D. 2013. Empowerment—an introduction. *arXiv:1310.1863 [nlin]*

Samborska V, Butler J, Walton M, Behrens TEJ, Akam T. 2021. Complementary task representations in hippocampus and prefrontal cortex for generalising the structure of problems. *bioRxiv,* https://doi.org/10.1101/2021.03.05.433967

Samuelson W, Zeckhauser R. 1988. Status quo bias in decision making. *J Risk Uncertainty.* 1(1):7–59

Santoro A, Bartunov S, Botvinick M, Wierstra D, Lillicrap T. 2016. One-shot learning with memory-augmented neural networks. *arXiv:1605.06065 [cs]*

Sawamura H, Shima K, Tanji J. 2002. Numerical representation for action in the parietal cortex of the monkey. *Nature.* 415(6874):918–22

Saxe A, Nelli S, Summerfield C. 2021. If deep learning is the answer, what is the question? *Nat Rev Neurosci.* 22(1):55–67

Saxe AM, McClelland JL, Ganguli S. 2019. A mathematical theory of semantic development in deep neural networks. *Proc Natl Acad Sci U S A.* 116(23):11537–46

Saxena S, Cunningham JP. 2019. Towards the neural population doctrine. *Curr Opin Neurobiol.* 55:103–11

Saxton D, Grefenstette E, Hill F, Kohli P. 2019. Analysing mathematical reasoning abilities of neural models. *arXiv:1904.01557 [cs, stat]*

Schapiro AC, Kustner LV, Turk-Browne NB. 2012. Shaping of object representations in the human medial temporal lobe based on temporal regularities. *Curr Biol.* 22(17):1622–7

Schapiro AC, Turk-Browne NB, Botvinick MM, Norman KA. 2017. Complementary learning systems within the hippocampus: a neural network modelling approach to reconciling episodic memory with statistical learning. *Philos Trans R Soc Lond B Biol Sci.* 372(1711):20160049

Schaul T, Quan J, Antonoglou I, Silver D. 2016. Prioritized experience replay. *arXiv:1511.05952 [cs]*

Schrittwieser J, Antonoglou I, Hubert T, et al. 2020. Mastering Atari, Go, chess and shogi by planning with a learned model. *Nature*. 588(7839):604–9

Schultz W, Apicella P, Ljungberg T. 1993. Responses of monkey dopamine neurons to reward and conditioned stimuli during successive steps of learning a delayed response task. *J. Neurosci*. 13(3):900–13

Schultz W, Dayan P, Montague PR. 1997. A neural substrate of prediction and reward. *Science*. 275(5306):1593–9

Schulz LE, Gopnik A, Glymour C. 2007. Preschool children learn about causal structure from conditional interventions. *Dev Sci*. 10(3):322–32

Sejnowski TJ. 2018. *The Deep Learning Revolution*. Cambridge, MA: MIT Press

Shadlen MN, Newsome WT. 2001. Neural basis of a perceptual decision in the parietal cortex (area LIP) of the Rhesus monkey. *J Neurophysiol*. 86(4):1916–36

Shafir E. 1993. Choosing versus rejecting: why some options are both better and worse than others. *Mem Cognit*. 21(4):546–56

Shallice T. 1982. Specific impairments of planning. *Philos Trans R Soc Lond B Biol Sci*. 298(1089):199–209

Shallice T, Burgess PW. 1991. Deficits in strategy application following frontal lobe damage in man. *Brain*. 114(Pt 2):727–41

Shanahan M. 2015. *The Technological Singularity*. Cambridge, MA: MIT Press

Sharma A, Gu S, Levine S, Kumar V, Hausman K. 2020. Dynamics-aware unsupervised discovery of skills. *arXiv:1907.01657 [cs, stat]*

Sharot T. 2011. The optimism bias. *Curr Biol*. 21(23):R941–5

Shepard RN, Hovland CI, Jenkins HM. 1961. Learning and memorization of classifications. *Psychological Monographs: General and Applied*. 75(13):1–42

Shiffrin RM, Schneider W. 1977. Controlled and automatic human information processing: II. Perceptual learning, automatic attending and a general theory. *Psychol Rev*. 84(2):127–90

Shima K, Isoda M, Mushiake H, Tanji J. 2007. Categorization of behavioural sequences in the prefrontal cortex. *Nature*. 445(7125):315–18

Silver D, Hubert T, Schrittwieser J, et al. 2018. A general reinforcement learning algorithm that masters chess, shogi, and Go through self-play. *Science*. 362(6419):1140–4

Silver D, Singh S, Precup D, Sutton RS. 2021. Reward is enough. *Artificial Intelligence*. 299:103535

Simoncelli EP. 2003. Vision and the statistics of the visual environment. *Curr Opin Neurobiol*. 13(2):144–9

Slonim N, Bilu Y, Alzate C, et al. 2021. An autonomous debating system. *Nature*. 591(7850):379–84

Smith FW, Muckli L. 2010. Nonstimulated early visual areas carry information about surrounding context. *Proc Natl Acad Sci U S A*. 107(46):20099–103

Song HF, Yang GR, Wang X-J. 2017. Reward-based training of recurrent neural networks for cognitive and value-based tasks. *eLife*. 6:e21492

Spelke ES, Breinlinger K, Macomber J, Jacobson K. 1992. Origins of knowledge. *Psychol Rev*. 99(4):605–32

Spelke ES, Kinzler KD. 2007. Core knowledge. *Developmental Science*. 10(1):89–96

Sperling G. 1960. The information available in brief visual presentations. *Psychological Monographs: General and Applied*. 74(11):1–29

Stachenfeld KL, Botvinick MM, Gershman SJ. 2017. The hippocampus as a predictive map. *Nat Neurosci*. 20(11):1643–53

Stahl AE, Feigenson L. 2015. Observing the unexpected enhances infants' learning and exploration. *Science*. 348(6230):91–4

Standing L. 1973. Learning 10,000 pictures. *Q J Exp Psychol*. 25(2):207–22

Stewart N, Chater N, Brown GDA. 2006. Decision by sampling. *Cogn Psychol*. 53(1):1–26

Stokes MG. 2015. 'Activity-silent' working memory in prefrontal cortex: a dynamic coding framework. *Trends Cogn Sci*. 19(7):394–405

Strandberg T, Olson JA, Hall L, Woods A, Johansson P. 2020. Depolarizing American voters: democrats and republicans are equally susceptible to false attitude feedback. *PLoS One*. 15(2):e0226799

Strange BA, Henson RNA, Friston KJ, Dolan RJ. 2000. Brain mechanisms for detecting perceptual, semantic, and emotional deviance. *NeuroImage*. 12(4):425–33

Sullivan J, Mei M, Perfors A, Wojcik EH, Frank MC. 2020. SAYCam: a large, longitudinal audio-visual dataset recorded from the infant's perspective. PsyArXiv, https://psyarxiv.com/fy8zx/

Summerfield C, Luyckx F, Sheahan H. 2019. Structure learning and the posterior parietal cortex. *Prog Neurobiol*. 184:101717

Sun W, Advani M, Spruston N, Saxe A, Fitzgerald JE. 2021. Organizing memories for generalization in complementary learning systems. *bioRxiv*, https://doi.org/10.1101/2021.10.13.463791

Sun Z, Firestone C. 2020. The dark room problem. *Trends Cogn Sci*. 24(5):346–8

Sutton R. 2019. The bitter lesson. http://www.incompleteideas.net/IncIdeas/BitterLesson.html

Szczepanski SM, Knight RT. 2014. Insights into human behavior from lesions to the prefrontal cortex. *Neuron*. 83(5):1002–18

Szegedy C, Zaremba W, Sutskever I, et al. 2014. Intriguing properties of neural networks. *arXiv:1312.6199 [cs]*

Tanji J, Shima K, Mushiake H. 2007. Concept-based behavioral planning and the lateral prefrontal cortex. *Trends Cogn Sci*. 11(12):528–34

Teeuwen RRM, Wacongne C, Schnabel UH, Self MW, Roelfsema PR. 2021. A neuronal basis of iconic memory in macaque primary visual cortex. *Curr Biol*. 31(24):5401–14.e4

Tegmark M. 2017. *Life 3.0: Being Human in the Age of Artificial Intelligence*. Allen Lane:, London, UK

Tenenbaum JB, Kemp C, Griffiths TL, Goodman ND. 2011. How to grow a mind: statistics, structure, and abstraction. *Science*. 331(6022):1279–85

Thom R. 1970. Topologie et linguistique. In: *Essays on Topology and Related Topics*, pp. 226–47. Berlin, Heidelberg: Springer

Tolman EC. 1933. Gestalt and sign-gestalt. *Psychol Rev*. 40(5):391–411

Tolman EC. 1948. Cognitive maps in rats and men. *Psychol Rev*. 55(4):189–208

Tolman EC, Ritchie BF, Kalish D. 1946. Studies in spatial learning. I. Orientation and the short-cut. *J Exp Psychol*. 36(1):13–24

Tolman H. 1930. Introduction and removal of reward, and maze performance in rats. *University of California Publications in Psychology*. 4:257–75

Treisman A, Schmidt H. 1982. Illusory conjunctions in the perception of objects. *Cogn Psychol*. 14(1):107–41

Tsitsiklis JN, Van Roy B. 1997. An analysis of temporal-difference learning with function approximation. *IEEE Trans Automat Contr*. 42(5):674–90

Tsividis PA, Loula J, Burga J, et al. 2021. Human-level reinforcement learning through theory-based modeling, exploration, and planning. *arXiv:2107.12544 [cs]*

Tsividis PA, Pouncy T, Xu JL, Tenenbaum JB, Gershman SJ. 2017. Human learning in Atari. Available from: https://cbmm.mit.edu/sites/default/files/publications/Tsividis%20et%20al%20-%20Human%20Learning%20in%20Atari.pdf

Tsutsui K-I, Grabenhorst F, Kobayashi S, Schultz W. 2016. A dynamic code for economic object valuation in prefrontal cortex neurons. *Nat Commun.* 7(1):12554

Turing AM. 1950. I.—Computing machinery and intelligence. *Mind.* 59:433–60

van den Herik HJ, Uiterwijk JWHM, van Rijswijck J. 2002. Games solved: now and in the future. *Artificial Intelligence.* 134(1–2):277–311

van den Oord A, Dieleman S, Zen H, et al. 2016. WaveNet: a generative model for raw audio. *arXiv:1609.03499 [cs]*

van den Oord A, Li Y, Vinyals O. 2019. Representation learning with contrastive predictive coding. *arXiv:1807.03748 [cs, stat]*

van Opheusden B, Galbiati G, Kuperwajs I, Bnaya Z, li Y, Ji W. 2021. Revealing the impact of expertise on human planning with a two-player board game. *PsyArXiv.* https://psyarxiv.com/rhq5j/

Vaswani A, Shazeer N, Parmar N, et al. 2017. Attention is all you need. *arXiv:1706.03762 [cs]*

Veit L, Nieder A. 2013. Abstract rule neurons in the endbrain support intelligent behaviour in corvid songbirds. *Nat Commun.* 4(1):2878

Vinyals O, Blundell C, Lillicrap T, Kavukcuoglu K, Wierstra D. 2017. Matching networks for one shot learning. *arXiv:1606.04080 [cs, stat]*

von Restorff H. 1933. Über die Wirkung von Bereichsbildungen im Spurenfeld. *Psychol Forsch.* 18(1):299–342

Wagner DA. 1978. Memories of Morocco: the influence of age, schooling, and environment on memory. *Cogn Psychol.* 10(1):1–28

Wais PE. 2008. fMRI signals associated with memory strength in the medial temporal lobes: a meta-analysis. *Neuropsychologia.* 46(14):3185–96

Wais PE, Mickes L, Wixted JT. 2008. Remember/know judgments probe degrees of recollection. *J Cogn Neurosci.* 20(3):400–5

Wallis JD, Anderson KC, Miller EK. 2001. Single neurons in prefrontal cortex encode abstract rules. *Nature.* 411(6840):953–6

Walsh V. 2003. A theory of magnitude: common cortical metrics of time, space and quantity. *Trends Cogn Sci.* 7(11):483–8

Wang JX, Kurth-Nelson Z, Kumaran D, et al. 2018a. Prefrontal cortex as a meta-reinforcement learning system. *Nat Neurosci.* 21(6):860–8

Wang JX, Kurth-Nelson Z, Tirumala D, et al. 2017. Learning to reinforcement learn. *arXiv:1611.05763 [cs, stat]*

Wang X, Ma T, Ainooson J, et al. 2018b. The Toybox dataset of egocentric visual object transformations. *arXiv:1806.06034 [cs]*

Wang XJ. 2002. Probabilistic decision making by slow reverberation in cortical circuits. *Neuron.* 36(5):955–68

Wang X-J. 2021. 50 years of mnemonic persistent activity: quo vadis? *Trends Neurosci.* 44(11):888–902

Wason PC. 1960. On the failure to eliminate hypotheses in a conceptual task. *Quarterly Journal of Experimental Psychology.* 12:129–40

Watanabe K, Funahashi S. 2014. Neural mechanisms of dual-task interference and cognitive capacity limitation in the prefrontal cortex. *Nat Neurosci.* 17(4):601–11

Wayne G, Hung C, Amos D, et al. 2018. Unsupervised predictive memory in a goal-directed agent. *arXiv:1803.10760 [cs, LG]*

Wei J, Wang X, Schuurmans D, et al. 2022. Chain of thought prompting elicits reasoning in large language models. *arXiv:2201.11903 [cs, CL]*

Weston J, Chopra S, Bordes A. 2015. Memory networks. *arXiv:1410.3916 [cs, stat]*

White L. 1961. Eilmer of Malmesbury, an eleventh century aviator: a case study of technological innovation, its context and tradition. *Technology and Culture.* 2(2):97

Whittington JCR, Muller TH, Mark S, et al. 2020. The Tolman-Eichenbaum machine: unifying space and relational memory through generalization in the hippocampal formation. *Cell.* 183(5):1249–63.e23

Whittington JCR, Warren J, Behrens TEJ. 2021. Relating transformers to models and neural representations of the hippocampal formation. *arXiv:2112.04035 [cs, q-bio]*

Whorf BL, Carroll JB. 2007. *Language, Thought, and Reality: Selected Writings.* Cambridge, MA: MIT Press

Wilson MA, McNaughton BL. 1994. Reactivation of hippocampal ensemble memories during sleep. *Science.* 265(5172):676–9

Winter E. 1998. Napoleon Bonaparte and chess. Available from: https://www.chesshistory.com/winter/extra/napoleon.html

Wolff MJ, Jochim J, Akyurek EG, Stokes MG. 2017. Dynamic hidden states underlying working-memory-guided behavior. *Nat Neurosci.* 20(6):864–71

Woodworth RS, Thorndike EL. 1901. The influence of improvement in one mental function upon the efficiency of other functions. (I). *Psychol Rev.* 8(3):247–61

Wunderlich K, Smittenaar P, Dolan RJ. 2012. Dopamine enhances model-based over model-free choice behavior. *Neuron.* 75(3):418–24

Yamins DL, Hong H, Cadieu CF, Solomon EA, Seibert D, DiCarlo JJ. 2014. Performance-optimized hierarchical models predict neural responses in higher visual cortex. *Proc Natl Acad Sci U S A.* 111(23):8619–24

Yates JF, Lee J-W, Bush JGG. 1997. General knowledge overconfidence: cross-national variations, response style, and 'reality'. *Organizational Behavior and Human Decision Processes.* 70(2):87–94

Yonelinas AP. 2002. The nature of recollection and familiarity: a review of 30 years of research. *Journal of Memory and Language.* 46:441–517

Yonelinas AP, Aly M, Wang W-C, Koen JD. 2010. Recollection and familiarity: examining controversial assumptions and new directions. *Hippocampus.* 20(11):1178–94

Yonelinas AP, Kroll NEA, Dobbins I, Lazzara M, Knight RT. 1998. Recollection and familiarity deficits in amnesia: convergence of remember-know, process dissociation, and receiver operating characteristic data. *Neuropsychology.* 12(3):323–39

Yosinski J, Clune J, Nguyen A, Fuchs T, Lipson H. 2015. Understanding neural networks through deep visualization. *arXiv:1506.06579 [cs]*

Yuste R. 2015. From the neuron doctrine to neural networks. *Nat Rev Neurosci.* 16(8):487–97

Zaremba W, Sutskever I. 2014. Learning to execute. *arXiv preprint.* arXiv:1410.4615

Zenke F, Poole B, Ganguli S. 2017. Continual learning through synaptic intelligence. *arXiv:1703.04200*

Zhang C, Bengio S, Hardt M, Recht B, Vinyals O. 2017. Understanding deep learning requires rethinking generalization. *arXiv:1611.03530 [cs]*

Zhou J, Jia C, Montesinos-Cartagena M, Gardner MPH, Zong W, Schoenbaum G. 2021. Evolving schema representations in orbitofrontal ensembles during learning. *Nature.* 590(7847):606–11 *Guardian Newspaper.* https://www.theguardian.com/commentisfree/2020/sep/08/robot-wrote-this-article-gpt-3

Index